PSYCHIATRYLAND

How to Protect Yourself from Pill-Pushing Psychiatrists and Develop a Personal Plan for Optimal Mental Health

Phillip Sinaikin, M.D.

iUniverse, Inc.
New York Bloomington

Psychiatryland
How to Protect Yourself from Pill-Pushing Psychiatrists and Develop a Personal Plan for Optimal Mental Health

iUniverse books may be ordered through booksellers or by contacting:

iUniverse
1663 Liberty Drive
Bloomington, IN 47403
www.iuniverse.com
1-800-Authors (1-800-288-4677)

ISBN: 978-1-4502-5290-4 (pbk)
ISBN: 978-1-4502-5289-8 (cloth)
ISBN: 978-1-4502-5288-1 (ebk)

Library of Congress Control Number: 2010912267

Printed in the United States of America

iUniverse rev. date: 8/30/2010

To my wife Jenni

To the other special ladies in my life:

Alice, Ariela, Benay, Christy,
Jamie, Karlye, Mia, Shara,
and Tatiana

And to some special guys:

Charlie, Jeff, Michael, Ron
and Tinus

Contents

Introduction ix

Chapter One: 1
BE AFRAID...BE VERY AFRAID

Chapter Two: 25
OIL FOR THE TINMAN

Chapter Three: 42
DIAGNOSTIC PRACTICES IN PSYCHIATRY:
Good Intentions...Bad Outcome

Chapter Four: 67
IF YOU ARE GOING TO LIE, MAKE SURE IT'S A GOOD ONE!
Diagnosis goes crazy

Chapter Five: 87
CASES IN POINT
Bipolar Spectrum & Adult Attention Deficit Disorder

Chapter Six: 108
SEROTONIN: The "X" Factor

Chapter Seven: 144
PSYCHOPHARMACOLGY
It Aint Rocket Science

Chapter Eight: 175
"PSYCHIATRY, MEET BIG BUSINESS"
"I'm sure this is going to be the beginning of a beautiful relationship!"

Chapter Nine: 206
SO, WHAT'S THE STORY?

Chapter Ten: 227
TO PILL OR NOT TO PILL?
Towards a Rational Psychiatry Part One

Chapter Eleven: 248
TOWARDS A RATIONAL PSYCHIATRY Part Two
Mood Disorders, Anxiety Disorders & Why Can't I Sleep?

Chapter Twelve: 276
SO...WHAT'S YOUR STORY?
The "Consumer" Narrative

Chapter Thirteen: 301
IS FREE CHEAP ENOUGH??
Emotions Anonymous and the Salvation of Mental Healthcare

Author Biography 335

Biblography 337

Appendix 343

Introduction

> Disneyland is a paradise: the United States is a paradise. Paradise is just paradise. Mournful, monotonous, and superficial though it may be, it is paradise. There is no other.
>
> Philosopher Jean Baudrillard

> From the standpoint of almost every culture and time except this era in the United States, the psychiatric approach to despair would be seen as naïve or nutty. The idea that only cheeriness is normal has a distinctly Brave New World feel. It's no wonder that despair, the darkest of the dark emotions, is virtually taboo in our society. Feeling this bad in a feel-good culture is transgressive; it goes against the grain in a culture of denial.
>
> Psychologist Miriam Greenspan
> *healing through the dark emotions*

We all know that Disneyland is the happiest place on earth, where magic happens and dreams come true. Every year millions of us spend billions of dollars at the Disney theme parks. We visit Frontierland, Adventureland and Tomorrowland. We go to Epcot and get to experience all the wonders of France, Switzerland, Germany, Spain and Mexico in just half a day. Baudrillard (quoted above) is reported to have remarked that the Swiss pavilion at Epcot is "more Swiss than Switzerland." What a place; the vacation of a lifetime!

Uh…

It is hot and very crowded and your legs ache from all the walking. You've spent much more money than you planned to and the kids are kind of cranky and tired. You begin to notice that a lot of kids look cranky and tired, even a little miserable. Of course there are the "attractions." But, come to think of it, they really aren't all that great. "Dumbo" was an absolute rip, waiting in line with a bunch of impatient kids and their families for forty five minutes for what felt like a thirty second ride. And "It's a Small World" looked like a slightly snazzier version of the haunted house rides at the local carnival. "Space Mountain", now that was a blast. Then again, it was just a roller coaster in the dark. The biggest disappointment for the kids, however, was the "character breakfast" (that cost you a bundle). Really, what did they expect, actual live cartoon characters? They expected to meet the "real" Mickey Mouse? Kids! But you have to admit…even you were a little disappointed at how fake and weird those costumed characters were. They didn't talk at all. Not a sound. Spooky.

But hey…what memories. You got tons of pictures and the kids said they had a great time, even though it didn't always look like it. You are driving out of the parking lot ("I can't believe they charge for parking") and your four-year-old exclaims "I love Mickey, when can we come back?" When we can get another home equity loan to pay for it, you silently think to yourself.

I am a psychiatrist. I've been in practice for twenty-five years, the last seventeen in Central Florida. So yes, I've been to Disneyworld (the Orlando version of Disneyland) a number of times. It is a nice amusement park with some unique attractions and rides. It is clean and well kept but it gets really crowded and it can be unbearably hot and humid in Orlando. And it is very expensive. There is a kind of informal wisdom passed around from the Central Florida veterans to the newcomers moving into the area. The newcomers are advised that when the inevitable visits from the relatives up north begin, send them off to Disneyworld by themselves. If you accompany all your relatives there you will get sick of the place and spend a fortune.

Here is the relevant point. After experiencing an *actual* trip to Disneyland it feels like there is some sort of a disconnect between the mental *image* of a trip to Disneyland and the *reality* of a trip to Disneyland. Why do so many of us share in and believe this image of Disneyland? What has led us to believe that this place really is a magic kingdom, the vacation of a lifetime? That, my readers, is the billion dollar question. The answer is that, in fact, billions of dollars have been spent carefully *crafting* the image of Disneyland that we have in our minds. From years of exposure to well designed marketing and advertising campaigns we have simply come to accept and believe the image of Disney that ***Disney wants us to have***. It has gone so far that I believe that in some fundamental way, the *reality* of Disneyland is the shared *image* we have of Disneyland.

THE IMAGE IS THE REALITY!

I hope this point is clear because now I want to take you to another magical kingdom, an "amusement" park of sorts, the place I call PSYCHIATRYLAND. I want to show you how the carefully crafted *image* of psychiatry as a **progressive medical science** has come to supplant the *reality* of an **unscientific, pseudo-medical specialty with imprecise and arbitrary diagnoses and questionably effective medications fraught with toxicities and side effects.** Yet millions of people rush to visit PSYCHIATRYLAND every day in pursuit of its promised journey to the magic kingdom of emotional stability and a happier life. To understand how this came to be, we can turn back to Disneyland and ask how they did it. We'll start by looking more closely at what Baudrillard was *really* saying when he observed that the Swiss pavilion is "more Swiss than Switzerland" because it was not a compliment.

Think about the country Switzerland. A lot of people live there. There is traffic, crime, a cold climate, roads under construction, feuding political parties, friendly people, unfriendly people, safe neighborhoods and dangerous ones...i.e. all of the complexities of a modern, industrialized Western nation. Of course there are also tourist attractions and vacation destinations. As in most countries, the tourist attractions are user-friendly, warm, welcoming and designed to maximize the separation of you from your money. The problem with seeing the tourist attractions of Switzerland *in* Switzerland are all of the hassles involved. First you need to get to Switzerland and then you need to travel between the tourist attractions, find places to sleep and eat, all while not understanding a word of the language. So what if we just skip all the hassles of actually traveling to Switzerland and create scaled down versions of the Swiss tourist attractions and then just put them all together in one convenient, tourist-friendly vacation destination? We can't build the Matterhorn, of course, but we could build a scale model of the Matterhorn and maybe even throw in a roller coaster. Sound familiar?

So what is Baudrillard really trying to say about Disney and its home, the "mournful, monotonous and superficial" paradise, the United States? I believe that he is asserting that many things here are simply duplicated, scaled down, user-friendly versions of the originals. He calls them simulations. Simulations are reproducible, sanitized, and grossly simplified versions of things in the real world that, through the intense marketing and image-making efforts of the brightest minds with the most money in this country, become their own reality, distinct and separate from the dirty and complicated nature of actual world in which we live. This manufactured reality is sometimes called "hypereality", the "more real than real." (Think of New York-New York or the Venetian in Las Vegas as other Disney-like examples).

This explains how, despite having a less than "magical" experience, maybe even having a lousy time, we can still feel and believe that our visit to Disneyland was the promised vacation of a lifetime. *The image has trumped the reality.* Do you buy this? If you don't, just give some thought to the role of image versus reality in our recent presidential elections in this country. Think about the advertising campaigns for everything from automobiles to beer to medications on TV. Think of how slogans and spin are used to shape our visions of life and truth. (Is there or isn't there a global warming crisis?) Or think about something more medical...placebos, those inert sugar pills used in scientific studies of medication. Do you know how often people in medical studies get "better" on placebos? ; a lot more than you think. In studies of psychiatric drugs so many people on placebos improve that it has led many medical scientists to question whether psychiatric "medications" such as antidepressants have any effect at all or are themselves simply acting as placebos (Greenberg and Fisher 1997). To me the "placebo" effect is the ultimate case of image trumping reality. The mental *idea* that a "pill" will make you feel better *actually making* you feel "better" is an inarguable triumph of "idea" over physical reality.

So now let's turn to that magical kingdom where pills make wishes and dreams *(appear to)* come true...PSYCHIATRYLAND.

In the quote opening this chapter psychologist Miriam Greenspan critiques the United States and its psychiatrists for trivializing despair while promoting "cheeriness" as the expected and desired "normal" mood state in our society. But how does something like that happen; how does being "cheerful" become defined as a culture's emotional norm? And how does psychiatry become assigned the task of medicating anyone who isn't? The answers to these questions are long and complicated and will be addressed in detail throughout this book. For the purpose of this introduction, however, let me briefly state that psychiatry has become defined as the overseer and guardian of "cheeriness" and "normality" in this country much in the same way that Disneyland has come to be defined as the greatest vacation destination and happiest place on earth, i.e. through relentless promotion. Medical model psychiatry has taken the "dirty", mysterious and *extremely complex* issues of human emotional pain and behavioral problems and sanitized, simplified and packaged them into a relentlessly promoted *user-friendly, checklist based diagnostic and medication managed subset of medical illnesses.* You no longer are seen as depressed, anxious or disturbed *about* something like society, the economy, injustice, trauma, racism, sexism, unremitting stress, your personal life experiences or even existential issues like the meaning of life. No...way too complicated (and not marketable). Now you are simply suffering from a depressive "illness" or anxiety "disorder", perhaps related to or stimulated by social or existential issues, but *in reality* rooted in an imbalance in brain chemistry, easily corrected by chemicals produced by the pharmaceutical industry. So understanding human emotional distress or behavioral problems is not complicated…its simple! Just go online and fill in the answers to a six question quiz and discover that the reason your life is going down the tubes (divorce, job loss, legal problems) is in reality a brain chemical imbalance causing you to have Adult Attention Deficit Disorder. Just go to your doctor and request some Adderall XR; that will do the trick. Not sleeping and eating, bothered by a lack of enthusiasm for life, and having feelings of low self-esteem and hopelessness about the future ever since you lost your job and your "adjustable" mortgage adjusted? Simple, you are suffering from an episode of depression (a "serious medical condition"); an SSRI antidepressant will fix you right up. It didn't work? No problem, we've got a lot more medications (and diagnoses) to try.

So am I being overly cynical? Do I really think PSYCHIATRYLAND "exists" like Disneyland exists? And am I saying that the promotion and marketing of this grossly oversimplified conceptualization of the nature of human emotional pain and behavioral problems has become its own reality, separate from the complexities and details of our personally unique lives?

YES, THAT IS EXACTLY WHAT I AM SAYING.

Only in the case of PSYCHIATRYLAND a lot more is at stake than simply a disappointing and costly visit to an amusement park. A lot more…

In May 2003 I was in San Francisco to give a paper at the annual meeting of the Association for the Advancement of Philosophy and Psychiatry (AAPP). To encourage attendance the AAPP would hold their meetings the weekend before the annual meeting of the American Psychiatric Association (APA), a massive get together attended by five to ten thousand psychiatrists. I remember how odd it felt to look out my hotel window and see a huge billboard advertisement for Abilify, a new medication that was at that time approved only for the treatment of schizophrenia. A billboard advertising a medication for schizophrenia; only in America I thought to myself. Just then something else caught my eye. It was one of those traveling billboards mounted on the back of a pickup truck, only it wasn't an advertisement aimed at the thousands of newly arriving psychiatrists. It was a warning. It read:

"THE PSYCHIATRISTS ARE IN TOWN:
HIDE YOUR CHILDREN."

I have to say, in the immortal words of Larry the Cable Guy, "That's funny. I don't care who you are, that's funny." It is also very good advice.

NEW YORK TIMES: February 15, 2007

> Early on the morning of Dec 13, police officers responding to a 911 call arrived at a house in Hull, Mass., a seaside town near Boston, and found a 4-year-old girl on the floor of her parents bedroom, dead.
>
> She was lying on her side, in a pink diaper, the police said, sprawled across some discarded magazines and a stuffedbrown bear.
>
> Last week, prosecutors in Plymouth County charged the parents, Michael and Carolyn Riley, with deliberately poisoning their daughter Rebecca by giving her overdoses of prescription drugs to sedate her.

Are you with me so far? What a horrible tragedy; parents poisoning their daughter with prescription medications. I wonder whose pills they used, the mother's or the father's? Let's read on.

> The police said the girl had been taking a potent cocktail of psychiatric drugs since age 2, when she was given a diagnosisof attention deficit disorder and bipolar disorder, which is characterized by mood swings.

WAIT A SECOND...REBECCA WAS
OVERDOSED ON HER OWN DRUGS?
FOR <u>BOTH</u> ATTENTION DEFICIT AND BIPOLAR DISORDER?
DIAGNOSED AT AGE TWO?

WHAT IS GOING ON HERE?

The terrifying truth is that what is going on here is nothing out of the ordinary (except for the poor child dying). The astounding fact that this child was diagnosed at age two as suffering from two incurable mental disorders and was being treated with three adult psychiatric medications should not surprise you; nor should you be shocked that her six-year-old and eleven-year-old siblings were *also* diagnosed with attention deficit disorder (ADD) and bipolar disorder and on the same medications. These children were not carelessly diagnosed by an inexperienced doctor at a walk-in clinic. They got psychiatric care at Tuft's New England Medical Center (which, by the way, quickly released a statement that their doctor's psychiatric care was "appropriate and within responsible professional standards"). The fact is that the practice of diagnosing and aggressively treating mental disorders in children is fully sanctioned by mainstream psychiatry and has been going on for years. Over seven years ago the cover story of Time Magazine's August 19, 2002 edition was titled:

"Inside the Volatile World of the YOUNG AND BIPOLAR".

Diagnosing bipolar disorder in pre-school children was presented there as non-controversial and both scientifically and medically justified along with the multi-drug cocktails being promoted as the treatment of choice. (Don't worry if you missed this article; I am going to pick it apart *in detail* for you in chapter one).

Have you ever heard of a presidential initiative called the New Freedom Commission on Mental Health? No? The commission was formed in 2002. Though apparently tabled for now, the plan they proposed was to perform massive mental health "screenings" on all pre-school and school-age children in the United States (MichNews 2004). That's over fifty million children!! You may or may not know this yet, but the outcome of such a screening program would be, without doubt, the finding that millions of children suffer from previously unrecognized and undiagnosed mental illnesses and need to be treated. (Trust me, this *would be* the outcome!) And in the vast majority of cases the primary modality of treatment would be psychiatric medications, most not even tested on nor approved for use in children. The "drugging of America" would take a giant leap forward if or when this program is in full swing, insuring customers for life for the psychiatric and pharmaceutical industries. But hold on a second, wouldn't the parents have a say here? Couldn't they object to their children being put on psychiatric medications? I'm sure that many would initially object but it won't be easy to hold out against the flood of dire warnings on the potential consequences of not treating childhood mood and anxiety disorders issued by the authoritative "thought leaders" in child psychiatry (more on this in chapter one). Ultimately, legal force could be used to require mandatory medication before a psychiatrically diagnosed child can return to school. (It's been done already in kids diagnosed with ADD!)

THIS SOUNDS LIKE SOME SORT OF ORWELLIAN NIGHTMARE! CAN ANYTHING BE DONE TO STOP THIS?

I think so (or at least I hope so). That is why I've decided to write this book. Understand, however, that this book is not simply about the over-diagnosis or misdiagnosis of psychiatric disorders in children. That problem is just the proverbial tip of a very large iceberg. As you will see (and probably already have seen) the over-diagnosis and overmedicating of adults is an even more worrisome and widespread problem. Tens of millions of American adults are now being medicated on a daily basis for psychiatric "illnesses", with the numbers climbing every year.

Is this because there has been a major breakthrough in psychiatry with the finding of identifiable chemical imbalances in the brain responsible for mental and emotional problems?

No.

Is it because new treatments have been developed that have a much higher success rate than older treatments?

No.

Is this because psychiatric medications are big money makers for the pharmaceutical industry?

Getting warmer.

Is this because there is an alliance between a group of psychiatrists and the pharmaceutical industry that has so much money and power that they own the market and effectively silence all other points of view?

Bingo.

So what exactly is going on…and how did it happen? In this book we will examine what underlies and supports the total dominance of mental healthcare by the so-called "medical model" of psychiatry. (A "medical-model" means that human emotional and mental problems are classified diagnosed and treated the same as physical problems in the other branches of medicine. We will be examining the fundamental flaws in this model throughout the book). By virtue of a close alliance with the pharmaceutical industry, medical-model psychiatry (also called biological psychiatry or just biopsychiatry) has managed to cast such a powerful spell over America that most of us unquestioningly and passively accept and submit to recommendations for psychiatric medication, even when the diagnosis and treatment plan is made by non-psychiatrists. In fact, most psychiatric medication is prescribed by family doctors, and other primary care physicians (PCP's) such as pediatricians and gynecologists.

True story: I was invited to give a lecture at an annual meeting of family physicians held at Walt Disney World. My topic was "Recognition and Management of Depression and Anxiety Disorders in Primary Care Medicine." The time allotted for the presentation: 30 minutes. I could give 30 hours on the topic of depression and anxiety and still have material left over. But that is not what the family physicians wanted. They wanted a simple plan to follow, one that was time and cost efficient and fit into the pressures and demands of their jobs. That need clearly trumped any concerns they might have that human emotional problems such as anxiety and depression should not be dealt with so simplistically. Or maybe they don't harbor any doubts or concerns. Maybe they are simply displaying their unwitting participation in the biopsychiatry belief system that so successfully dominates our culture.

This pervasive attitude of uncritical acceptance of biopsychiatry is the *fundamental problem* we will need to directly deal with in this book. As New York Times columnist Judith Warner puts it in her February 22, 2007 post on Rebecca Riley:

> Rebecca Riley was not killed by biological psychiatry or Astra Zeneca or the Massachusetts Department of Social Services or parents like you or me who may or may not be medicating our children but are, indisputably, part of a culture *in which doing so is now the norm.* (Italics mine)

Thus, the answer to what we must do about psychiatry spinning out of control lies in an in-depth examination and deep understanding of *how we have become* a culture in which psychiatrically medicating emotional, behavioral and cognitive problems in both children and adults has become the unquestioned norm. It wasn't always this way, not by a long shot. In fact, as you will see, I can pinpoint exactly when this cultural transformation began. It was in 1980, the year the Diagnostic and Statistical Manual of the American Psychiatric Association, Third Edition (DSM III) was published. Because that book, promoting a pseudo-scientific medical-model for psychiatry, would literally change the world and the lives of everyone in it. ("Bibles" tend to have that effect. Stay tuned...you'll see).

SO, WHO AM I?

As it says on the book cover my name is Phillip Sinaikin and I am an M.D., Board Certified in psychiatry. (I'd love to be called Dr. Phil but I think that name is already taken. How about Dr. Phill, think I can get away with it?) I graduated medical school in 1981 and entered my four year psychiatric residency at just about the time the DSM III was really starting to catch on. So I was there from the beginning. I have been in clinical psychiatry (directly treating patients) my entire career. I have experienced first-hand the impact of the medical model in clinical psychiatry and have witnessed its rise to total dominance in mental healthcare by virtue of what some critics have called its "unholy" alliance with the incredibly powerful and influential pharmaceutical industry. The thing is, I haven't been on board with this way of thinking from the beginning. When I saw the 2002 article in Time magazine I decided it was time to do something. But do what? It wasn't like I was the only psychiatrist, psychologist, therapist, philosopher or patient who knew that something had gone terribly wrong in mental healthcare. Dozens of books had been written about the problem (I'll have a list in the appendix), but none of them seemed to me to be designed to specifically address the right target audience.

I believe that the people most in need of this information are the American *consumers.* Perhaps this is merely semantics, but I don't think so. I think that the label "consumer" speaks to an aspect of daily American life that not only forms the economic foundation for a world economy, but also describes how the American people are viewed by the powerful corporate entities that really run the show. So I've written this book specifically for you, the reader, *in your role as a consumer* because, as you will see, that is a much more appropriate label for the way you are *targeted* by medical model psychiatry and the drug companies. Americans are viewed by all corporations as consumers of or potential customers for the products they sell. It doesn't matter if the product is a new movie, a car, a political candidate or, as you will see, a pill for a mental disorder. Marketing is marketing. (Except in the case of pills for mental disorders, there are two things being marketed, the medication *and* the illness). I believe that the day is coming when an *overwhelming majority* of the population in this country will be taking psychiatric medications for a wide range of "conditions", many of which used to be thought of as problems in living (such as grief, the emotional turmoil of divorce, or economic stress). And that will suit the pharmaceutical industry just fine. Looking at the situation in psychiatry from this perspective keeps the issue of ***marketing*** (to both doctors and their patients) ***front and center***, where it deserves to be. Because, as you will see, the explosive growth of medical model psychiatry is not grounded in its progress (there isn't much) or its growth as a legitimate medical science (it isn't one), but in its capacity for persuasion and influence by virtue of its carefully crafted *image* as a legitimate and growing medical science. Billions of dollars in marketing of this model by the pharmaceutical industry and we arrive at where we are today, labeling tens of millions of Americans, from two years old to one hundred and two, mentally ill, and just passively accepting this or feeling powerless to do anything about it.

So my approach in this book is most like Ralph Nader's was when he wrote the book *Unsafe at Any Speed* and exposed the manipulative marketing tactics and dangerous practices of the automotive industry. I see this as a ***consumer empowerment*** book because I believe that medical model psychiatry itself is unassailable; it will only keep growing in power and influence. The only hope for any sanity to be restored is through the educated and discerning consumer to take control by making intelligent and informed decisions when dealing with mental and emotional problems in themselves and their loved ones. That is exactly what I will teach you to do!

WHY ME?

What qualifies me to be the one to write this book? I do have twenty-six years of clinical experience but that alone is not enough. I said above that I was "not on board" with the medical model from the beginning. In part that's because I was not your typical student when I entered medical school. Before I enrolled in medical school I had already earned a Master's degree in humanistic psychology from West Georgia College, the only program of its kind in the United States. Grounded in the work of Abraham Maslow and his concepts of human potential and self actualization (Maslow 1962), humanistic psychology focuses more on human emotional growth and less on psychopathology. In general terms humanistic psychology is *holistic* which means that spiritual, social, familial, ethnic, sexual, historical, cultural and biological factors are *all* incorporated into a comprehensive understanding of the individual. Medical science is *reductionistic* which means that medical science (and by extension medical model psychiatry) tries to understand the functioning of the whole by breaking it down into the function of its parts. Thus, in a reductionistic model, the psychological functioning (or dysfunction) of the human *mind* is determined by the function of the neurons (nerve cells) that make up the physical *brain*. Since neurons communicate chemically you end up with concepts like "chemical imbalance" explaining alleged brain dysfunctions manifesting as depression or anxiety. I came into medical school with a commitment to holistic thinking, especially as it relates to psychology. I was then and remain today what you would call a "radical critic" of reductionistic biologic explanations for emotional and mental problems, especially since *no direct evidence of neuronal dysfunction in emotional disorders has ever been discovered. NO CHEMICAL IMBALANCES HAVE EVER BEEN DEMONSTRATED IN A HUMAN BRAIN!*

An important foundation for holistic thinking in humanistic psychology derives from the discipline of philosophy. Many people I meet seem turned off by philosophy because it seems too obscure and abstract. And it can be, no doubt. But I like to define philosophy as simply "thinking about thinking." In philosophy questions are asked about the nature of reality and how we come to know things about ourselves and the world we live in. There are many schools of thought in philosophy, and some are admittedly diametrically opposed to each other. Through my work in humanistic psychology I was exposed to a school of thought called continental philosophy, the forerunner of what is now called postmodern philosophy. The point here is that through my study of postmodern philosophy I was able to more clearly state and define my critique of medical model psychiatry and understand and communicate with other like-minded critics. (As you will see, there are plenty of them). Now here is how this is relevant to this book: I am going to ***teach you*** how to think like a postmodern philosopher because that is how you are going to gain the power and confidence you will need to resist the onslaught of marketing and (let's just call it what it is) propaganda by biopsychiatry and the drug companies. And don't kid yourself…it is an onslaught. I have the May 14, 2007 issue of Newsweek sitting in front of me. In the front section of this issue there are not one, but two multi-page full color ads for drugs that "treat" bipolar disorder. One is a two page ad for Abilify. You may be familiar with this ad because it has been running in national publications for a long time. The other is for a new player in the bipolar treatment game, Seroquel. It is a full five pages long. It must have cost a small fortune (but don't worry too much, the drugs they are advertising cost a small fortune themselves; I've heard anywhere from $8.00 to $14.00 PER PILL!).

HOW WE ARE GOING TO DO THIS?

You may be wondering to yourself (and rightfully so) what goes on in my office. What do I do with patients (consumers) who come to me expecting to receive a definitive diagnosis and psychiatric medication for their emotional problems? The answer to that question is complicated. I will be addressing it throughout this book. But I want you to know that I often do prescribe medication. I am not anti-medication. I do believe that there are biologically based mental disorders that require medication but that they are grossly over-diagnosed. I also believe that psychiatric medications can be and sometimes are helpful *as a part of* a comprehensive treatment program that prioritizes specific therapies for the presenting problem. I am also keenly aware that there are a multitude of other causes of mental and emotional distress that doctors can't do anything about. It is complicated! I can't ignore that fact despite what the "marketplace" demands.

What I try to do in my office is remain true to my belief in a holistic, individual approach to each patient. What that translates into in real life is what can best be described as a sort of ongoing conversation between me and my patients where we explore together the many ways to potentially understand and deal with their problems. I use the word conversation to describe this because that word denotes a sense of equality; I do not see myself as an authority figure making pronouncements about what is wrong with the patient and what needs to be done to fix it (a practice that is far too common in psychiatry). Some patients like this approach, others do not. Either way, I insist that my patients get actively involved in the decision-making about their treatment, including medication issues. To accomplish this requires my educating them about the lack of certainty in psychiatry and the gross distortions and inadequacies of the medical model. I have to then acquaint them with other ways to understand and approach their problems so that they can make informed choices about their lives and sometimes about the lives of their loved ones. It is serious business and needs to be taken seriously. I've written this book as an extended and more detailed version of the conversation I have with my patients. Here is how it is organized:

In chapters one and two you will be introduced to postmodern philosophical concepts that will assist you in understanding precisely what is going on in psychiatry and how and why a pseudo-scientific checklist model of mental disorders has come to dominate the field. I will use many examples and stories to help you understand the philosophical principles I will be teaching you. As a concrete illustration of the importance of critical thinking skills you learn in postmodern philosophy I will (as I said above) "pick apart" the article on bipolar disorder in children from Time magazine. (Except you will now understand this process of evaluation by the philosophical term "deconstruction"). You will be shocked and amazed to see the flagrant manipulation and gross distortion of reality that goes into a seemingly "informative" article like this. You will learn how dominant points of view attain and maintain their dominance through "discourse control", i.e. by muffling or silencing alternate points of view. In chapter two I will use an old story we are all familiar with, the story of the Tinman in the Wizard of Oz, to illustrate important philosophical points about the role that our unbridled faith in technology and other social beliefs play in shaping our day to day lives and the choices we make. You will now be prepared to take on psychiatry, which we will do in chapters three through eight.

Something that is a little different about my book is the amount of space I devote to a critique of the **diagnostic** practices in psychiatry (chapters three, four and five). That is because I think this topic is overlooked, even in articles and books critical of the overuse of psychiatric medications. You will learn, to your horror I think, that the business of psychiatric diagnosis is often sloppy, imprecise and completely unscientific; and yet so very much is at stake when these diagnostic labels are attached to you or someone you love. Then in chapters six and seven we will go on to take a hard look at psychiatric medications. The information in these chapters will startle, amaze and sometimes even terrify you. Then in chapter eight we will explore in detail the exact nature of the alliance between psychiatry and the pharmaceutical industry including all of the tricks of the trade they have used and still are using to maintain the dominance of the biopsychiatry perspective. It too is downright scary.

But do not despair…there is hope. There is ***always hope.*** And here is the good news. The help we need to fix mental healthcare in America is ***already in place***. Alternate and complimentary theories and practices abound. The problem for the "consumer" is that the dominance of the biopsychiatry model is so singular and powerful that there is little exposure to (or even awareness of the existence of) other paths to mental wellbeing and peace of mind. In chapter nine I will teach you about narratives and social constructionism. These philosophical concepts will help you understand that, at the core, our reality is based on the "stories" we tell ourselves about our lives. In grasping this concept you, as the "consumer" of mental healthcare, will be fully empowered and able to see that you have ***choices*** in deciding which storyline works best for you. Once you understand this we will explore alternative storylines together in chapters ten to thirteen. In chapters ten and eleven I will give full and fair voice to the DSM "storyline" so that you can decide when this might be the most appropriate, when it could be a complimentary choice, and when it would be just plain destructive for you and your family and loved ones. In chapter twelve I will introduce you to cognitive therapy, positive psychology, existential psychotherapy, new age spirituality and other approaches and techniques you might choose to better your emotional state. The final chapter, chapter thirteen, will be devoted to exploring the widely available and *cost free* twelve step programs, including Emotions Anonymous.

Then we will be done.

I hope this book works for you.
Writing it is certainly helping me.

Chapter One:
BE AFRAID...BE VERY AFRAID

Pete (not his real name, but a real patient) was thirty-six years old when I was still in private practice and wrote this case history. Five years prior his wife left him for another man. The other man was his cousin. Pete went into a major funk and couldn't pull himself out. His mother took him to a psychiatrist and then another one…

Three years later…

Pete came to see me because the current psychiatrist treating him was over an hour away and every time he needed a refill or medication adjustment he had to drive to the psychiatrist's office to see the nurse, or, occasionally the doctor. He also didn't like being on so many pills. He was on a very complex treatment regimen. These were his medications:

1. *Tofranil (an antidepressant) 50 mg. three times a day.*
2. *Keppra (an anticonvulsant being used as a mood stabilizer) 500 mg twice a day*
3. *Inderal (a blood pressure pill being used to treat anxiety) 10 mg three times a day*
4. *Wellbutrin (an antidepressant) 150 mg once a day*
5. *Abilify (an antipsychotic also approved for Bipolar I disorder) 15 mg once a day*
6. *Eskalith (a form of lithium, a mood stabilizer) 450 mg twice a day*
7. *Klonopin (a tranquilizer) 0.5 mg twice a day*

8. *Adderall (an amphetamine used for "ADD") 20 mg. twice a day*

Totaling this up, my new patient Pete was on sixteen pills a day prescribed by his psychiatrist. Was this shocking to me? Yes! But not surprising because I have been watching the trend of "polypharmacy" (prescribing more than one medication at a time) growing in psychiatry for a number of years and Pete was far from being my first new patient presenting on so many medications at once. What stands out more about this case was that after interviewing Pete and carefully reviewing his medical records from the treating psychiatrist I came to the conclusion that ***psychiatrically*** *there was:*

NOTHING WRONG WITH HIM!
ABSOLUTELY NOTHING!

So why did he end up on more pills than a cancer patient with heart disease? Because as I said…Pete went to a psychiatrist…which I believe is becoming an increasingly dangerous decision. Let's look at Pete's history and see how he ended up on all those pills.

As mentioned above Pete cites the onset of his problems to his wife leaving him. He didn't handle this too well. He admittedly "went into a deep funk" for eight months after she left. There were other "pre-existing" problems as well. Pete had found himself on the wrong side of the law more than once and did enjoy his pot, even though it got him into trouble. When he finally (at the urging of his mother with whom he was living at the time) sought help for his post-divorce "depression" he found himself on trials of medication that didn't seem to make much difference. Various diagnoses were kicked around, including bipolar disorder. That diagnosis (and the medications used to treat it) bothered him enough that he decided to do a little research on his own. When he read about bipolar disorder on the internet he decided that one thing was certain…he was NOT bipolar. Nevertheless, his first psychiatrist had him on a "trial" of a bipolar medication (Abilify) when he switched to a second psychiatrist three years before seeing me. The new psychiatrist opined that Pete "does not believe that he is bipolar; however, according to his mother and her description of her son, he does appear to have some mild bipolar spectrum."

Another statement from the doctor, however, reports that Pete disagreed with even the concept of mild bipolar spectrum. Pete tried to explain his view of the problem: "He indicates that his wife cheated on him with his cousin and left him to marry the cousin, which is the reason why he became depressed and he believes that this was situational and not part of his bipolar spectrum."

That seems reasonable. Infidelity with a relative and then an unwanted divorce, ouch! But, for some reason (which happens to be my reason for writing this book) the psychiatrist ***persisted*** *in promoting his belief that Pete was seriously mentally ill and needed medication treatment. In fact, on that first visit the doctor added yet another "diagnosis", adult attention deficit disorder. He recommended that Pete stay on the Abilify and added the amphetamine Adderall to his treatment.*

Okay doc, you are starting to scare me. But how did Pete go from being on two medications to eight? He MUST have gotten worse, had more symptoms; you just don't add medications willy-nilly for no reason. Are you sure we don't? We'll peek over the doctor's shoulder and see as soon as we set the scene in greater detail.

At thirty-three years old, Pete had been back living at home with his parents. Devastated by his divorce, it was taking him time to come back to life. Although this is perfectly understandable, (especially to anyone who has been divorced), viewed through the lens of modern psychiatry Pete was displaying "symptoms" of a mental illness and tracking and treating those symptoms was the task at hand. On every visit to the doctor Pete was accompanied by his mother. She was in the office with Pete and the doctor and was often noted to be the source of information upon which treatment decisions would be made. For his part Pete would usually endorse the fact that he remained unmotivated and often had a hard time just getting out of bed to go to work. He wasn't dating and rarely pursued his previously enjoyed social outlets. Neither the mother nor the doctor could just sit back and watch this previously gregarious and cheerful young man vegetate. So on nearly every visit early in treatment, a change or adjustment was made in Pete's medication regimen. Two months into treatment Pete's psychiatrist notes: "We talked at length about the 'alphabet soup' of medications that are necessary when there is bipolar spectrum disorder." On that visit two new medications were added, an antidepressant and an antipsychotic. He was now two months into "treatment" and up to six medications a day. The doctor wrote: "Once we get him stabilized on the medications we will try to eliminate those medications that have not been of benefit."

Obviously the promised simplification of the medication regimen never occurred. How could it when it was so complex to maintain Pete in what the doctor described as a "delicately balanced" emotional state? And there were other complications as well. Pete needed to comply with a medication regimen which required him to take multiple pills three times a day. Try as she would, mom could not insure that Pete did this. On top of that there were problems getting the medication. Some of them were so expensive that Pete had to apply to the drug companies' patient assistance programs to be able to afford the pills. Some of the drug companies ship the pills directly to the patient's home; others will only ship them to the doctor's office where they need to get picked up. But these nuisances were small potatoes compared to the mother's task of maintaining a vigilant watch over Pete's emotional symptoms. The fact that Pete was diagnosed ***bi****-polar created* *a whole new set of concerns. Because now she not only had to alert the doctor when Pete started getting depressed, she also had to watch out for that much more subtle and insidious expression of bipolar disease…getting too happy. As reflected in the doctor's progress notes, she did the best she could:*

"His mother set up this appointment, because she has been concerned for a couple of weeks now, about some of Pete's behavior. He has been acting more erratic than he had for the past several months. We had him delicately stable on the medication. She reports that he is more easily distracted, going out at night, drinking more, and has also learned that he has been smoking marijuana more frequently, and that he has been smoking pot the entire time of treatment. The patient's mother's concerns are valid."

And it wasn't helping that Pete was being stubborn and had to be continually re-convinced that he was bipolar. In a progress note ten months after the above:

"His mother reports that…he continues to become more manic every day. He was not attending to the business in the family store. He has become involved in skiing and outlandish business opportunities. He has been going out late at night to bars. His mother reports in the morning, if she were to go to his room, it would smell like cigarettes and alcohol. He is most likely smoking marijuana again. He appears agitated and irritated. He reports that it is only because he is busy and ***he should not have to come in for appointments so often.*** *He is angry. His words are, 'I'm pissed off.' We talk about it and soon he begins to* ***surrender*** *to the fact that he is manic. His concern is that he prefers being manic to being depressed. He is coming out of a very long period of depression, and he* ***does not want to get medicated back into a depression.*** *He would much rather be in a manic state but* ***neither phase is appropriate****. He is impulsive when he is in a manic state, and he is unmotivated off-putting when he is in a depressed phase. I am hoping to find* ***a nice balance****." (Emphases mine)*

GEE, I DON'T KNOW; IS IT JUST ME OR DOES THIS SOUND A LITTLE ***"BRAVE NEW WORLDISH"*** *TO YOU TOO?*

From the beginning Pete's mother was obviously overly-involved in her thirty-three year old son's psychiatric care. It sometimes seemed as if the doctor was treating the mother, not Pete. (Watch out, good insight. You could hypothesize the same with the parents of Rebecca Riley and her misbehaving siblings). In fact, eerily similar to the reports I've read about Rebecca Riley, Pete's psychiatrist would, in fact, make medication adjustments on the phone as a response to concerns expressed by the mother. One time mom called the office with a concern that Pete was getting manic because "he did not come home last night." She called his work and he was there "but he is playing on his computer rather than doing his job." The mother "points out that this is typical of the behavior he displayed last year, just before going into a manic phase." She expresses worry "that the medications may be hyping him up, and wants to know if anything can be done to hold him over the weekend, when we can see him on Monday." The doctor recommended ***an increase in the dose of one of his antipsychotic medications.***

Okay, let's pause here a second. We are talking about a human being, right? Because this is sounding a lot more like someone going to a mechanic to get an engine fine-tuned than it sounds like talking about the emotional status of living, breathing human being. Guess what? That is the point. This "mechanistic" view of people is a central feature of medical psychiatry. We'll get to exploring that in detail shortly. For now though, let's get back to Pete's saga because, believe it or not, the worst is yet to come.

From what I can gather from the notes Pete eventually started to get a little tired of his mother micromanaging his life. Did I mention that due to the side effects of his many psychiatric drugs that Pete began to have sexual potency problems? Would you like to hazard a guess what his doctor did?

Viva, Viva Viagra!

Here is a strange notation from the doctor: "Patient became annoyed with his mother, and told her that his continued treatment would be contingent on her helping him pick up or pay for the Viagra." Whoa.

The schism between mother and son widened and that did not work out too well (for Pete). He moved out to his own place and moved his new girlfriend in. Soon after, a frantic phone call by the mother to the doctor resulted (THIS IS TOTALLY TRUE) in the ***police going to Pete's apartment to see if he needed to be taken by force and committed to the psychiatric hospital****. The police did go to the apartment and spoke to Pete and his girlfriend but reported to the doctor that "he seemed okay." However, there is another way to get people committed to a psychiatric hospital in Florida. It's called an ex-partie Baker act. Concerned families make an appointment with a judge to whom they report their "observations." If the judge is convinced that involuntary hospitalization is indicated (that the patient is a "danger to self or others") an order is issued for the police to pick the patient up. Of course the judge only hears one side of the story but in Pete's case the fact that there was a pre-existing diagnosis of a serious mental illness carried a lot of weight…so…Pete got committed. At the psychiatric hospital they changed a lot of his medications and took him off his amphetamines. That, at least, made some sense. However, soon after, the mother (herself fully under the magical spell of the medical model) called the doctor expressing concern that her son was "having trouble with concentration because the ADD is not being addressed. She has inquired with Social Security whether he might be eligible for benefits."*

(Hey taxpayers...he got them)

Okay; time to stop. I'm sure you are wondering if I am making this whole thing up or at least exaggerating. A man that I am saying has no mental illness is treated with obscene amounts of medication, gets committed to a psychiatric hospital and now has a mother getting him social security disability. **But I am not making this up**...not one word of it! I told you psychiatry is spinning totally out of control and these kinds of cases are the proof. Now let me tell you about my time as Pete's doctor.

On my first visit with Pete (about a year before I am writing this) I changed his "official" diagnosis to major depression, single episode, resolved. I needed his medical records to see why he had been diagnosed bipolar before I got too aggressive in decreasing his medication. I simplified his medication regimen and told him that after I got his records we would re-evaluate his whole case. I scheduled him to see me in a month. The records arrived but Pete didn't come back until nearly two months later. The first thing he did was hand me a newspaper article. I had a little trouble understanding it but apparently he and his new wife (the previously mentioned girlfriend) were involved in an auto accident on a local interstate. In the car was "an 11 year old girl." The girl complained that she had hurt her back but Pete and his wife refused to let the police examine her, saying that she was faking. The police arrested them both. The reason Pete had not come to his scheduled appointment was because he was in jail, for a total of 35 days. In jail, THEY STOPPED ALL OF HIS PSYCHIATRIC MEDICATIONS...ALL OF THEM. So when I saw him, he had been off all of his medications for six weeks. Since I had already received and reviewed his medical records I was pleased because I saw no evidence of him having what I consider bipolar disorder (a lot more about how I make diagnoses later). The real hassle was going to be getting him off all of his medications. It's not easy to get off of medicines that work in the central nervous system; there are a lot of withdrawal symptoms. But jail had taken care of that. Since Pete never thought he was bipolar anyhow we agreed to just do some watchful waiting. He would see me again in two weeks but under no circumstances could he tell his mother that he was no longer on psychiatric drugs. I wanted her to think that he was doing just what the (previous) doctor ordered. I sat back and waited for the "frantic mother" phone call. It never came. It never has. And Pete has never gone manic, or manic spectrum, or depressed or anything else. He's happily married, his business has picked up and he no longer has much contact with his mother. I did prescribe some Adderall for a while because he truly seemed to me to be unable to focus at times but now he is off that as well.

So is it possible that this young man, who submitted to insane drug combinations for years, who was committed to a psychiatric hospital under a judge's order, who has been arrested twice in the past year (the above mentioned arrest and one for domestic disturbance) is normal?? YES! A normal, complex, at times psychologically unstable, pot smoking, surfing, artistically talented, one time divorced all-American dude; a far from perfect, mistake making, traumatized and troubled human being...just like the rest of us. But seriously mentally ill needing lifetime medication?

There is no doubt that many psychiatrists out there would agree that the doctor in this case went overboard in both diagnosis and treatment. But, the basic approach here is *completely mainstream* and consistent with accepted psychiatric practice. It is the MEDICAL MODEL of mental healthcare and it is spinning terrifyingly out of control.

The single most powerful incentive to write this book came from an unlikely source, Time magazine. It was the August 19, 2002 issue. On the cover of that issue was the face of a cute nine year old boy identified as Ian Palmer. Certainly nothing looked to be wrong with him. The picture caption tells us, however, that nine year old Ian is "being treated for bipolar disorder". The large caption on the cover tells us that the story inside is titled:

> *"Inside the Volatile World of the YOUNG AND BIPOLAR. Why are so many kids being diagnosed with the disorder once known as MANIC DEPRESSION?"*

I have always liked and basically trusted Time magazine and figured that this story was probably an expose on *over*-diagnosing and *over*-medicating children. But I was dead wrong. Among the many astonishing and alarming aspects of this Time magazine article is that in its total of eleven pages the idea that very young children can have diagnosable bipolar disorder, a serious lifelong mental illness, is presented as scientific fact; not speculation or hypothesis...*fact*. They go so far as to include a forty-item checklist so parents can assess their children and get them to the doctor ASAP. In the entire eleven pages there is only one use of the word "controversial" which is barely even noticeable among the dire warnings about the horrendous outcome of untreated childhood bipolar disorder issued by expert after expert in the field. Only here is what you need to know. Every statement, every warning, every prediction and treatment recommendation in this article is, in fact, pure speculation. It is not fact! And it is not science!

So how did a speculative and terribly one-sided article like this, one that could directly impact so many lives, end up published in Time magazine looking for all the world like a scientific and factual account? That is the question we will be exploring in the first two chapters of this book. It is not an easy question to answer because it requires an understanding of some fundamental and foundational issues that are most directly addressed in the field of study called philosophy. But we will take it slowly, one concept at a time. This is a necessary first step because to *empower yourself* to deal with emotional and behavioral problems in yourself or loved ones without automatically falling into the trap of being "diagnosed" and "medicated" will require this deeper understanding about what is going on in mental healthcare. So take a deep breath, because here we go!

The Time magazine article is merely one example of an extremely widespread phenomenon. It is simply one of the thousands of stories "planted" in magazines, journals, newspapers and on TV by two very powerful groups: mainstream psychiatry and the pharmaceutical industry. And I don't mean planted by payola or bribes; I mean planted by a much more powerful, insidious and invisible process called *discourse control* (your first philosophical term). When I teach you what this means you will see why you should be very afraid of what is going on here and how and why Time magazine, Oprah, Web MD, The CBS Evening News, and *even your own doctor* cannot and will not protect you from being flagrantly manipulated by the psychiatrists and drug companies who control mental healthcare in this country. So we need to ask; what exactly is a "discourse" and how does one "control" it?

The dictionary defines discourse as "a set of connected utterances" but that doesn't tell us very much. For our purposes in this book, I will turn to philosopher Ludwig Wittgenstein's compact definition of discourses as "language games." As many contemporary philosophers have come to realize, language is far from simply a neutral way to describe an "objective" reality. Instead, they say, language is the way we constitute reality. The words we choose as well as the finite number of words available to choose from delimit our possible conceptions of reality. Just think, for example, of the difference between naming Pete's behavior towards his mother as "rebellious" versus naming it "manicky" and you can see what I'm getting at. Within every language there are self-contained and self-defining discourses which *presuppose* a certain truth about the nature of reality for the discourse to make any sense. A famous teaching example is the act of moving pieces on a chessboard. For our purposes we will consider a chess piece move to be a "word" in the chess discourse. The meaning and significance of each "move" (word) is totally dependant on the rules of the game of chess which each player *presupposes* that the other player is following. Without both players working within the discourse of chess (understanding the game and following the rules) then moving a piece from one square to another would make no sense, it would be a meaningless, random action. I like this example; it's easy to understand yet really gives you the sense of what discourse means. Understanding this, you will be able to begin to see discourses all around you. For example, astrology is a discourse. Similar to how "pawn to queen four" makes sense in the chess discourse, the "moon is in the seventh house" makes sense and has significance to those who accept the presuppositions and assumptions (the rules of the "language game") of the astrology discourse. To those who don't, it either sounds like a vaguely familiar song lyric or just plain bunk.

Turning back to the mental health field, let's look at a familiar but dated example of a psychiatry discourse. Here are some words from it: id, ego and super-ego. Recognize them? These are terms from the discourse of psychoanalysis. These words make sense within the view of reality espoused by Sigmund Freud, the most important component of which is the acceptance of the existence of the unconscious mind. You simply have to accept as true that our mind is at work at a level we are not aware of or Freud's famous so-called "topography" makes no sense. If you are speaking within the Freudian discourse then you can talk and argue endlessly about specifics, e.g. why this particular person is acting or feeling this way or that based on an analysis of the operations of their id, ego and super ego. Freudian psychoanalysts have filled libraries with their books and papers that dialog within this particular "language game." But, what if you step outside the Freudian discourse; can you still use the words ego, id and superego? Of course you can, but when you say them they will have a different meaning and significance. For example I might say that in writing this book I am "putting my ego on the line" but not mean what Freud meant by ego. I would be talking about the idea of ego as my self esteem or feelings of self worth. This is the essence of the concept of "language games." The words we use and the context we use them in will always reflect what "reality" we are assuming underlies the meaning of those words. But don't think that the stakes in language games are just matters of interest to philosophers and intellectuals. For example, think about religions, if you will pardon the sacrilegious expression, as "language games." Think about all that is presupposed and assumed before words like salvation, sin, atonement or even jihad make any sense. Here we can begin to see that there can be a lot at stake in our choice of and allegiances to particular discourses. We may call them language games but they are often very serious games where ways of life and even life itself are at stake because our discourses are about more than just words or views of reality, they are about *power*.

Michel Foucault is the philosopher who is famous for drawing attention to the often unseen relationship between power and knowledge. Foucault was an historian and by "knowledge" he was referring to the dominant discourses in human history, not to the notion of knowledge as factual truth (Caputo 1993). Basically he came to believe that there is no knowledge that is not supported by and/or supportive of a particular power. And he is not just talking about obvious examples such as the "language games" of Soviet dictatorships or Nazi regimes (which we often think of as propaganda), he is talking about the relationship of power to knowledge in everyone's life, everyday. There was a time when the Freudian discourse *dominated* thinking in psychiatry. When that was the case many doctors chose to learn Freudian psychoanalysis in special training programs after they finished medical school. They learned how to use techniques such as free association, dream analysis and interpretation to assist the troubled souls seeking help for their problems with depression, anxiety, obsessions and the like. These are the *very same problems* that now have untold millions of people taking tranquilizers, mood stabilizers and antidepressants. (Are you starting to see how discourses work?) When you presented to a psychoanalyst with emotional problems the analyst would *not* give you a diagnosis and write a prescription. You would be asked to lie down on a couch and start free associating and recounting your dreams. The Freudians had their books and journals and they had their experts with authoritarian positions of power and influence in medical schools, in courts, in all walks of life. And as long as one stayed within the domain of the Freudian discourse it all made perfect sense. But what about those outside of the Freudian discourse? What about people who opposed this perspective and its widespread influence? Here is where the *power* comes in. As hard as this might be to believe today, not so long ago in America there wasn't much heard, spoken of or promoted outside the Freudian discourse that exercised any significant power or influence in society. Foucault calls this dominating type of discourse, one that silences or muffles other points of view a "regime of truth."

Patrick Bracken MD and Phillip Thomas MD, founders of the "postpsychiatry" movement summarize Foucault's concept this way: "According to Foucault, in modern societies, power is exercised most often through 'regimes of truth': expert discourses through which we understand ourselves and our motives, our desires and our behaviors. Furthermore, such discourses have their expert commentators, advisors and judges. We come to live our lives through these discourses and think about our priorities and values in terms they have given us. Because they are 'regimes of truth' they provide the backdrop to our ethical debates and through them it becomes possible to utter the 'truth'. In fact, what is regarded as true or false is set by these discourses" (Bracken and Thomas 2005, p.93).

I know this is pretty abstract but I'm sure you are beginning to see what I'm getting at and where this is going. (Meditate for a minute on how you perceive reality, the role played by "experts" and the guidelines and principles of living outlined by them and then followed by us. "Should I spank Johnny when he disobeys me and runs into traffic?") ***Regimes of truth run the show***! If you were a depressed person sixty years ago, or if the court wanted expert psychiatric testimony or if you wanted to understand why your child was misbehaving in school, you turned to the Freudian discourse for the answer, the then current "regime of truth." And you would have had *no reason* to question the validity of what you heard because an army of highly trained experts would be standing by to back up this language of id, ego, and superego. Doesn't it sound strange now? Isn't it hard to believe that less than a lifetime ago these were the dominant ideas in psychiatry and psychology? It sounds strange because, like they have in every culture throughout history, the discarded ideas of the previous generation sound so dated and wrong. "How could they have believed this stuff?" every generation asks about previous generations. And we are no different today.

However I think most people today believe that the age of strange and esoteric language games in psychology is finally behind us. We wonder how humans have survived so long with one group of expert psychologists and psychiatrists after another expressing such bizarre ideas about the nature of human behavior and emotion. Thank goodness there is now one accurate, reliable and rational source of truth to turn to that isn't based on superstition, faith or somebody like Freud's zany ideas about Oedipus complexes and childhood sexuality. Thank goodness for the real source of truth:

SCIENCE!

But wait a second… Science has been around for hundreds of years. When Freud was alive so was the scientific method we still rely on today. In fact, Freud, trained as a neurologist, considered his work to be science. And the critical philosophers I've mentioned like Foucault and Wittgenstein lived and wrote in the twentieth century, the age of science and scientific achievements! What gives?

Well, hold onto your hats because what I am going to contend (as have many others) is that science is itself *merely a discourse*, a "regime of truth", as intimately tied to power as any other belief system and not the be all and end all road to "real" reality we have come to believe! OK, this is a lot to digest so let's slow down and (as philosophers like to say) "unpack" what I've just said.

Perhaps we need to first ask, what exactly do we mean by science? (Debates on this can fill many volumes so understand that this is going to be a very simplified discussion). Think back to high school and you'll probably recall when you were first exposed to the definition of science. It seemed mostly to do with method, how to ask and answer questions. The questions were framed as hypotheses or "educated guesses" and the answers were sought empirically, through rigidly defined rules of experimentation. "Variables" needed to be controlled so that whatever hypothesis was being tested in an experiment would not be contaminated by the influence of too many uncontrolled variables. Mathematics also played a big role, allowing scientists to determine whether the outcome of an experiment was the result of chance alone or whether a true effect was being observed. Enough experiments repeated by enough people in enough labs yielding the same outcome could result in the identification of timeless truths called "laws of nature." The overall concept is that slowly but surely, (inexorably really), science progresses, gaining more and more truths about reality until what? I suppose until we humans have it all figured out, the nature and workings of true reality finally fully revealed. And, most importantly, science is "objective", free of the contamination of false beliefs, superstitions, or the self-interests of any particular group of people. Isn't that true? Sometimes it is; it all depends on what you are talking about. Here is a case in point:

I had polio. It was 1954 and I was three years old living in Pittsburgh, Pennsylvania. You know who else lived and worked in Pittsburgh in 1954? Jonas Salk, the man who developed the polio vaccine. My brother, who is two years older and was already in school, got the vaccine; I didn't. Fortunately my polio only affected my left arm and hand and, as an adult, I fully realize that I am indeed most fortunate. As a child who had a deformed and weak left hand (my friends called me "the claw") I was deeply affected even by my mild case of this horrible illness. Was the man who discovered the polio vaccine and spared countless millions this crippling disease a scientist working within the scientific method? Yes! Using the best scientific techniques he was able to isolate and weaken the polio virus so that it could be safely injected into humans and create immunity to the real virus. What an incredible achievement! And this is just one among the tens of thousands of scientific discoveries, inventions and theories that have improved the lives of all human beings. So I am not anti-science, not by a long shot. But I do contend that science is a discourse, a powerful one, often fruitful, but still just *one* way, not *the only* way to understand all aspects of existence.

This is where a lot of authors might go on to remind the readers that there is a dark side to science as well, mentioning that science has also invented ways to cruelly and efficiently kill as well as cure. While this is true it would deflect us from the concern I have about science in the context of mainstream psychiatry. And that is to question whether science and the scientific method is the best, or as some would argue, the only legitimate way to investigate the most complex puzzle in the universe, ourselves. Human existence, human consciousness, human emotion, human beliefs, human morality, the quality of human life, are these appropriate topics for scientific investigation?

While the scientific method often yields important positive results in areas of inquiry that fit well with science, it is not so clear that the methods and techniques of science are as well suited for inquiry in all disciplines, especially those considered the humanities. We can probably all agree that the creative arts such as music, literature and painting are not areas of human culture where science holds some privileged position as a source of final truth or knowledge. The trickier subjects are disciplines that study and try to make sense of human existence such as sociology, theology, anthropology and our main topic of interest, psychology. The scientific method has, in a way, come in and out of prominence in psychology over the years. For example, behaviorism, as articulated by B. F. Skinner, heavily involved experimentation grounded in the scientific method while something like Rogerian client-centered therapy did not. To be honest we have gained valuable insights and knowledge from many theories in psychology, both science based and not. But that is not really the issue here. The concern here is that the theories of modern biological psychiatry are not meant to complement and enrich other theories of human nature, *they are meant to supplant them*! Let's get back to the relationship of knowledge to power.

Because science and the scientific method have yielded such visible and impressive results in many areas of life it is only natural that this method of inquiry has earned a privileged position in modern society. We now live in the era of the unquestioned triumph of science although some rather interesting conflicts between fundamentalist religion and scientific theories are surprisingly re-emerging. Analyzing this phenomenon is beyond the scope of this book (although the spiritual hunger this reflects will be discussed in later chapters); suffice it to say that the recent battles about issues such as creationism versus evolution clearly highlight the relationship of power to knowledge Foucault was talking about. It also reminds us that these battles are not distant or inconsequential; they affect everyone. They are extremely complex battles too, not yielding to simplistic explanations or solutions. Because when it comes to understanding human behavior and emotion there are no simple answers yet so very, very much is at stake. It shouldn't be surprising then that the burning desire to gain a greater understanding of human behavior and emotion would eventually yield to the method of inquiry that has enjoyed the most visible and influential success, science. But is science up to the task? Can science and the scientific method really bring about an understanding of the human mind and heart? Obviously to do so would require that somehow the incalculable complexity of human behavior, emotion and cognition would need to be simplified or reduced in some way to make it amenable to study by the scientific method of hypothesis generation and experimental investigation. Why? We previously discussed the concept of variables in scientific experiments. Let's look into that a little deeper.

The ideal biology experiment is one that is done on genetically identical organisms raised in precisely the same environment. Give organism A compound X while organism B gets a "placebo." Then you can measure the effect of compound X (the controlled variable) on this organism. Repeat and repeat and repeat the experiment in different labs and voila…you find out something useful. But what if they used non-genetically identical organisms? What if they used organisms from different species? What if they used identical organisms raised in different environments? All of these changes would weaken the findings on the effect of compound X because now there would be more variables to consider that might contaminate or alter the observed effect of compound X and result in inaccurate findings. These are the uncontrolled variables. In ANY scientific experiment you try to keep the number of uncontrolled variables to a minimum. I'm sure you can see why. So, let's get back to the human organism.

Do you have a neighbor? How alike are you? How different are you? If I asked you to write a list of the ways you are different from your neighbor genetically and biologically and then asked you to list all of the ways that you are sociologically and psychologically different and then asked you to list all of the environmental and experiential differences between you and your neighbor from birth ……you get the picture. Human beings "differ" from one another in an apparently infinite number of ways. So even if both you and your neighbor complained about "feeling depressed" how would I know that you were both talking about the same thing? Maybe by depression you mean feeling less motivated and energetic than usual while to your neighbor depression means "I miss my dog that died last month." Obviously, these two would not be very good subjects for a scientific experiment on the effectiveness of antidepressants. In fact, how could you ever find humans suitable for such an experiment when the word "depression" can mean so many things? You can't. You have to do something first. You have to simplify and organize things by *pre-defining* what depression means. In medical model terms, that would mean identifying the *symptoms* of the "illness" of depression. Then you need to identify the frequency, severity and duration of those symptoms. This is called developing a set of operational criteria. By choosing the specific criteria that you do, you automatically eliminate a vast number of variables by simply ***not including them*** in the diagnostic evaluation. To study the human being scientifically, you must *reduce* the complexity of being human. Psychiatry has done just such a reduction. As mentioned in the introduction, it happened in 1980, the year of the publication of the Diagnostic and Statistical Manual of the American Psychiatric Association, third edition, the DSM III.

We will be talking about DSM III in great detail in this book. Among the many things that made the publication of DSM III a monumental event was that its way of classifying and diagnosing mental problems by clusters of *allegedly* observable, objectifiable and countable "symptoms" could be utilized in scientific experiments, something that the lack of precision and quantification in previous diagnostic systems (such as Freudian) did not allow. (In the Freudian discourse "neurosis" was a very important diagnostic term. Even though it was not precisely defined, we all knew what it meant and it was powerfully descriptive of the core problem in most of our patients. But because it was not precisely defined and did not involve assessing or counting visible symptoms it was dropped from the DSM nomenclature. I and many of my colleagues still use the term among ourselves to describe our patients to each other). With DSM III, psychiatrists could join their medical colleagues and evaluate the treatment of mental illnesses the same way other researchers evaluated the treatment of physical illnesses. I am sure you are aware that, for example, antidepressants, have garnered an impressive track record of triumphs over placebo in countless scientific studies. So, how can you argue with success? You can if the experiments are fatally and fundamentally flawed from the beginning because not all science experiments, including medical science's "gold standard", double blind placebo controlled medication trials, are created equal. And when it comes to comparing medication trials in other branches of medicine to studies in psychiatry, we are truly not even in the same ballpark! But I am getting way ahead of myself. This issue is very complex and will be dealt with throughout the book. Suffice it to say for now that there are very real and very serious concerns about the application of the scientific method to study questions about normal and abnormal human behavior, emotions and cognition. What this chapter is about is why that should frighten you. To explain that I want to begin to turn back towards analyzing the previously mentioned Time magazine article about bipolar disorder in children by first doing some teaching on the philosophical concept of "deconstruction."

Deconstruction is a term used in postmodern philosophy. Stated simply, the difference between modern (or analytic) philosophy and postmodern (or continental) philosophy is that postmodernists believe that there is no absolute truth and that all knowing is incomplete, contingent and historically situated. In plain terms, there are a lot of ways to look at things and no one perspective or point of view is THE truth. That doesn't mean, however, that postmodernists believe that every point of view is equally compelling, useful and valid. That would simply be "relativism", a weakness often ascribed to postmodernism by its critics. I'd like to offer a response to that criticism right now. Once in a while I will refer in this book to Rick Roderick, a *postmodern* philosopher who I never met but got to know by watching a series of his lectures videotaped by The Teaching Company. His lecture series was recorded in 1992 and was entitled *The Self Under Siege.* I love Rick's irreverence (think of Jon Stewart doing philosophical instead of political satire) and will sometimes refer to quotes from his lectures. I like to call them **"Roderickisms".** Here is one that Rick said in response to the critique that postmodern philosophy is just relativism:

> **"There is no one who ever lived, lives now, or will ever live in the future who believes that any point of view is just as good as any other point of view".**

In other words, that criticism leveled at postmodernism is just plain weak and silly. What postmodernism is really about is recognizing that the human mind can understand phenomena in many different ways and that any system of inquiry investigating and exploring the nature of human existence must take that into account. One way is to struggle with multiple perspectives and somehow "negotiate" between them (more on this later). But let me give you a brief example of what I'm talking about because I hate reading anything philosophical that doesn't give some illustrative concrete examples.

Let's imagine there is a very nervous person who wants your help with some life problems. His wife died suddenly two and a half years ago and he still misses her terribly and is having trouble maintaining his faith in God, a real comfort to him for most of his life. His company downsized six months ago and his contract was bought out. He isn't hurting for money but is having a difficult time filling his days and wonders what exactly the purpose of his life is now. You feel for this man and want to help him. Where do you start? That will depend a lot on what *perspective* you take in understanding the nature of his problem. If you approach his problem spiritually (his changing relationship with God), that would lead to one form of help. Approach it existentially (coming to grips with mortality and the seeming meaninglessness of life), it would lead to another. You could focus on socioeconomic issues and deal with his job loss and difficulty feeling he has worth without being a productive worker. You could inquire about his relationships and see what is going on with friends, his family and whether he has someone special in his life or feels like even a date would be somehow "cheating" on his dead wife. You could evaluate what "stage of grief" he is in and perhaps try to assist him in that process. And yes, you could ask about "symptoms" and diagnose and treat his problem with medication. Do you see how each one of these approaches is reasonable and how it would be impossible to decide with certainty which is "right" or "wrong"? That is a muti-perspectival evaluation. You'll notice there are not any bizarre or crazy perspectives in the bunch. They are all perfectly reasonable, complementary but incomplete areas of inquiry. What would be totally unreasonable is to decide *a priori* (that means ahead of time) which evaluative perspective is *best* because that would mean you wouldn't even bother with considering the other perspectives or the therapeutic interventions they entail. But guess what? That is exactly what modern psychiatry does! If you are reading this book there is a good chance your interest has been sparked by a personal experience of you or a loved one having "problems in living" and seeking help from a doctor, therapist or psychiatrist and being told you are suffering from a chemical imbalance which can be corrected by medication. End of story. No further discussion required; fifteen minutes and we've got the problem both named and treatment initiated. This type of limiting and what I will call "reductionistic" and "dehumanizing" evaluation is going on RIGHT NOW in thousands of doctor's offices around this country. This should scare you, a lot! If it doesn't I'm going to teach you how and why it should by using the most powerfully persuasive topic in America today: the health and safety of our children. Let's get back to defining deconstruction and then move onto the article in Time magazine.

You can more fully understand the idea of deconstruction by imagining that there is this building and you decide to find out how it was built by carefully taking it apart, brick by brick, doing a kind of backwards construction…a "deconstruction" for the purpose of understanding the original construction. In this deconstruction you would get a chance to see what building techniques or ideas were used to construct the building and, by extension, what techniques *were not used.* Applied to something like a book, deconstruction means a careful reading to try to reconstruct the intended meaning of a text by looking at how it was written, what words and ideas and perspectives were chosen, and, by extension, *not chosen* in the writing. It's that "not chosen" part that is the crux of deconstruction (or at least my understanding of it). So a deconstructive reading looks at not only what is said, but what is not said, *but could have been.* This type of reading helps you to see the biases, prejudices and manipulations in a text that might otherwise not be noticed (Caputo 1997). You can see how nicely this fits into Foucault's concern about the influence of power on what we call knowledge. Now I will show you how nicely it can help us gain a very different understanding of a Time magazine article ostensibly written to educate you about a very serious mental illness that might be affecting your children and possibly damaging them beyond repair.

If you can, get a copy of the August 19, 2002 issue of Time magazine so you can read the article along with me. If not, don't worry, my point will still be crystal clear. The article was co written by Jeffrey Kluger and Sora Song. Without ever having met or spoken to them, I guarantee that they did not get paid off by medical psychiatrists or pharmaceutical companies to write a hyperbolic and terrifying one-sided article on mental illness in our children or to push us to drug them. It just turned out that way. All they did was consult the experts. (Remember that a community of "experts" is crucial to maintaining "regimes of truth"). Like most magazine and newspaper articles this one starts out with a dramatic anecdote.

The subject of the anecdote is Nicole and she is 16 years old. She began to withdraw and isolate at 14 years old. At age 16 she started to go manic. She went without sleep but didn't feel tired. Her mind and thoughts raced. Finally she became frankly delusional, calling herself the "chosen one", becoming a clear-cut risk of danger to herself and others. She had no insight into her condition and had to be forcibly hospitalized and medicated. Does Nicole have bipolar disorder? Sure sounds like it to me. I want you to understand I am not one of the radical critics who refute the existence of mental illnesses. Unless Nicole is secretly abusing some heavy-duty drugs or has a brain tumor then an early onset Bipolar Type One disorder is the right diagnosis. (As I will explain in later chapters, the distinction of a Bipolar Type One disorder from other hypothesized types of bipolar disorder is a crucial one) Like all good writers then, the authors start their story with a dramatic attention-getting, "potential tragedy averted by the miracles of modern science" real life drama, the story of Nicole. But then the hype, distortion, misrepresentation and manipulation begin. As expected (do you learn this in writing 101?) the authors leap from the specific to the general. They say that this "ferocious" (how's that for a fear word?) illness "seems to be showing up in children at an increasing rate, and that has taken a lot of mental health professionals by surprise." Now that is just out and out distortion. The mental health professionals the authors interviewed could not possibly be "surprised" by the growing prevalence of bipolar disorder in children because they are *the cause* of it. Let me explain. Children have generally not been diagnosed as bipolar because, except in rare cases like the almost-adult teenager, *16 year old* Nicole, children (especially pre-teens) have *never* displayed the characteristic diagnostic signs and symptoms of bipolar disorder. The increased prevalence of bipolar disorder in children occurred only *after* some mental health professionals actually ***changed the criteria*** for diagnosis and then, by applying these new criteria, fit more and more troubled and troubling kids into this diagnostic category. So the more accurate statement is that this "ferocious" illness is *being diagnosed* in children at an increasing rate. The only psychiatrists that this genuinely "surprised" perhaps are ones, like me, who were already alarmed by the massive, often careless over-diagnosis of bipolar disorder in adults and simply can't believe that the so-called "thought leaders" in psychiatry are endorsing this same practice in children as young as two years old. But what is really "surprising" is that no one is trying to stop them!

As mentioned above, children do not display classic bipolar symptomatology with circumscribed and lasting periods of depression or mania. So here is what the psychiatrists did. One of the diagnostic rules for bipolar disorder (Type 1) is that the manic episode, the high energy, no sleep, grandiose and delusional phase "must last at least one week" (DSM IV p.328). Even the less severe (and more controversial) Bipolar Type II disorder requires four consecutive days of unremitting hypomania, a less severe type of manic pathology. The child psychiatrists behind the increasing rates of diagnosis of bipolar disorder in children know that no young child goes into an observable stage of unremitting mania for a week or even four days. Rather than acknowledging that and therefore, by the rules of logic, NOT labeling young children bipolar, they just decided to change the rules. (Why psychiatrists would even think of doing this will be dealt with later in the book when we look deeper into the benefits of discourse control). In contrasting the presentation of bipolar disorder in children and adults the article says: "Most children with the condition are ultra-rapid cyclers, flitting back and forth among mood states several times a day." Well that solves the problem. Finding kids with sustained periods of high or low mood states lasting days or weeks at a time might be a little tough. But kids with mood changes up and down throughout the day, no problem! Wait, isn't that every kid? Well, the authors didn't question this so why should I? After all they did get that quote from a world "expert" on bipolar disorder in children, Dr. Demetri Papolos "research director of the Juvenile Bipolar Research Foundation and co-author of *The Bipolar Child*", published by Broadway Books in 1999. (Thank goodness Dr. Papolos is a "scientist" because otherwise someone cynical might suspect some hidden self-serving agenda here). I would like to hear from some other doctors who are concerned with how Dr. Papolos seems to be playing it loose and easy with the diagnostic criteria. But I can't find any in this article. ***This is a classic case of discourse control!*** It is not unreasonable to suggest that opposing points of view should be included in this article since it is in a widely read and highly influential news magazine. Instead, Dr. Papolos is given free reign, unchallenged even when he makes easily disputed, illogical statements. For example, Dr. Papolos is credited with "discovering" a characteristic pattern of mood swings in bipolar children. The authors write: [Dr. Papolos] "studied 300 bipolar kids, ages 4 through 18, and he believes he spotted a characteristic pattern. In the morning, bipolar children are more difficult to rouse than the average child. They resist getting up, getting dressed, heading to school. They are either irritable, with a tendency to snap and gripe, or sullen and withdrawn". Aside from making rather obvious all-inclusive covering statements (they can be irritable and snappy or sullen and withdrawn) there is a core violation of logic in this statement. Papolos contends that he identified this characteristic pattern of mood instability by observing a cohort (study group) of 300 children with bipolar disorder. But, if the central diagnostic criterion for bipolar disorder is mood instability, how were they diagnosed in the first place? Wouldn't, in fact, the pattern of mood instability be the basis for the diagnosis? This might not sound terribly illogical because it so closely mimics legitimate findings in other areas of medicine, for example, studying the clinical course of a hepatitis C infection. Could you not identify a "cohort" of 300 people infected with hepatitis C and follow them over a period of time to see if any characteristic pattern of symptoms is observed? Yes, definitely. However, in the hepatitis case the diagnosis is not made (and the study group identified) by the characteristic pattern of symptoms you discover in the study. The study subjects would be diagnosed by the physically demonstrable presence of hepatitis C viruses in their livers. Dr. Papolos could not use a lab study or X-ray or any other test to pre-identify his study group and then look for patterns of symptoms because in psychiatry there is no lab test or X-ray or biopsy that identifies illness; psychiatric disorders are diagnosed *on the basis of* characteristic patterns of symptoms. Do you see the circularity of reasoning here? Perhaps this is confusing because you think that there is an identifiable physical abnormality in psychiatric illness, a "chemical imbalance" or faulty circuit in the brain. After all, you've been hearing that on TV commercials for years and there is a very scientific looking multicolored cross section picture of the brain in the article with a complicated array of labels, charts, and arrows attached to it. That's just got to be scientific!

Yes there is a color-coded cross-section of a human brain in the article. The fact is that most popular magazine articles promoting the progress in psychiatry manage to fit in a picture of a cross-section of the brain. It looks very convincing. But as will be documented throughout this book (by direct quotes from medical psychiatrists and mainstream textbooks) there is NO DIRECT EVIDENCE of any specific lesion or defect in any part of the brain that is the demonstrable cause of any psychiatric illness. The inclusion of brain cross section pictures in popular magazine articles and psychiatric drug advertisements is for speculation, hype and show, period.

The idea that young children can have bipolar disorder remains a hot topic of debate in mainstream psychiatry. I have seen articles discussing the battle between two groups, one who insists that some symptoms resembling adult bipolar disorder (like grandiosity or pressured speech) must be present to make the diagnosis, the other group asserting that "mania" in children presents as irritability and that kids with dramatic "temper tantrums" need to be evaluated. (Be afraid…). One debate I read was so ridiculous that I would have thought it was a satire…but it wasn't. Two well respected "thought leaders" in psychiatry were debating the underlying "pathology" of a three year old girl who carelessly ran out into traffic. The first doctor believed that her dangerous behavior was indicative of an Oppositional-Defiant disorder, a condition diagnosed in children who defy rules and authority. The other doctor argued that her impulsive act represented grandiose delusions where this little girl believed that she was "special" and cars could not hurt her. She was, therefore bipolar. This was a serious debate, I kid you not! (…be very afraid!)

In the Time magazine article the section on psychiatric drugs reflects the incredible power of the pharmaceutical industry to influence journalists and the media. It says "Pharmacologists are *perfecting* combinations of new drugs that are increasingly capable of leveling the manic peaks and lifting the disabling lows" (my italics). I swear I must be living on a different planet. What I have witnessed happening in psychiatry is a parade of "promising" new mood stabilizers being embraced by psychiatry only to later be found to be ineffective in clinical trials. Two that come to mind are Neurontin and Topomax. I cannot tell you how many patients were put on these agents when they first came out by enthusiastic psychiatrists. I can clearly remember attending a conference where research psychiatrists from a university hospital were presenting data about their successful treatment of bipolar disorder using obscenely high dosages of Neurontin, 5000 to 6000 mg., a drug usually used in dosages of around 900 to 1200 mg (for epilepsy or pain control). What I have observed in actuality is not some clear-cut progress in stabilizing moods but a massive increase in the willingness of psychiatrists to use more and more drugs at the same time, the previously mentioned phenomenon called polypharmacy. (Even some mainstream psychiatrists have noticed and criticized this trend). I'll have a lot more to say about this in the chapters on psychiatric medicines but now that we have identified what voices and opinions were silenced in this part of the article, let's move on with our deconstruction by addressing another terrifying and flagrantly obvious weakness that is totally glossed over in the article, which has to do with the response to treatment by these children diagnosed as bipolar.

OK, you've diagnosed a bunch of children as suffering from bipolar disorder and warned us that if they don't get treatment they are going to end up being burnt out suicidal drug addicts…seriously! Here is a quote directly from the article: "bipolar disorder is not an illness that can be allowed to go untreated. Victims have an alcoholism and drug-abuse rate triple that of the rest of the population and a suicide rate that may approach 20%." To add an exclamation point to this fear mongering, Time quotes our friend Dr. Papolos who tells us that in bipolar disorder: "If you don't catch it early on, it gets worse, like a tumor." OK, I don't know about you but I've had it with this Papolos guy, invoking the terrifying images we all have of cancerous tumors to get us to do what? Accept his dire warnings and drug our kids?

This is a mainstream biopsychiatry inspired article, so there is no way that the central and irreplaceable foundation of treatment will be anything other than psychiatric medications. After all, we've already had our world class legion of "experts", our brain picture and a symptom checklist to "prove" that this is a medical illness. So, let's start our discussion of treatment with the butt-covering statement; again, quoting directly from the article: "For any bipolar, the sheer number of drug options is a real boon, as what works for one patient will not necessarily work for another." End of explanation. No scientific sounding speculation on why that would be or whether it has any implications of weakness or imprecision in our diagnostic or treatment practices, just say it, don't explain it, and move on to case histories. (This maneuver is very common in psychiatric research). Next we are told about Brandon Kent, a 9 year old Texas boy diagnosed bipolar. When Brandon "started taking Depakote and Risperdal, his body began to swell (Whoa, that's a little scary, his body swelled?). Then he switched to Topomax, (remember my mentioning Topomax as an example of how psychiatrists keep using drugs even after they are proven ineffective), which made him lethargic. Eventually he was put on a mix of Tegretol and Risperdal, which have stabilized him with few side effects". Kyle Broman, another youngster the article profiles "is having a harder time but has grown calmer on a combination of Risperdal and Celexa, an antidepressant *that for now at least doesn't appear to be flipping him into mania*." For some reason Lewis Black the comedian just popped into my head. I was picturing the diatribe he would come up with after reading that little kids being treated for a serious mood disorder are being put on drugs (antidepressants) that can *cause* the mania you are trying to prevent. I guess I thought of Lewis Black because he loves to satirize obvious examples of insane irrationality. Well here it is Lewis, right in Time magazine. But of course it might be a little scary to satirize an article talking about doctors treating mentally ill children. But not NEARLY AS SCARY as dosing our children with wild combinations of medications that act by unknown mechanisms in their ***still developing*** central nervous systems which also have serious side effects and potentially fatal complications. I am not making this up! I will address these medications one by one in the chapters on psychiatric meds and, just by reading off the package inserts, scare the heck out of every parent who has agreed to let their children be treated with these compounds!

THE PSYCHIATRISTS ARE IN TOWN:
HIDE YOUR CHILDREN.
Do you get it?

Of course, for our children to be protected from dangerous psychiatric speculation, we need parents to resist being seduced by the biopsychiatrist's point of view. That is not easy to do. Here is a very scary quote from the Time magazine article: "Preverbal toddlers and infants cannot manifest the disorder so clearly, and there is no agreement about whether they exhibit any symptoms at all. However, many parents of a bipolar say they noticed something off about their baby almost from birth, reporting that he or she was fidgety or difficult to soothe. Broman insists she knew her son Kyle (he is the one stabilized on Risperdal and Celexa) was bipolar *even when he was in the womb*. 'This child never slept inside,' she says. 'He was active 24 hours a day.'" C'mon, are you kidding me? What's ironic is that these types of understandably desperate parents are the same ones who have been convinced over the last few decades by mental health professionals that their misbehaving children's mental disorder was ADD. Thank goodness these professionals have come to recognize the consequences of their overly enthusiastic support of that diagnosis. Time reports that up to 15% of the children diagnosed as having ADD may actually be bipolar and that mistakenly treating them with stimulants like Ritalin "can deepen an existing cycle or trigger one anew", causing what Time describes as "plenty of kids suffering needlessly." Alarmingly, "At least half the people who have this disorder don't get treated", bemoans Dr. Terrence Ketter, director of the bipolar disorder clinic at Stanford.

Wow, Stanford! That's almost as prestigious a source as Harvard...or Yale, alma mater of our former president. What those people say must be true. They are the best of the best, the cream of the crop. Real experts! But Dr. Papolos and Dr. Ketter are just two people. Who is going to be out there uncovering the subtle signs and symptoms of bipolar disorder in children, signs and symptoms less expert observers might mistakenly identify as ADD, or Oppositional Defiant Disorder, or worse yet, not even recognize as childhood mental illness at all? The authors state in their conclusion to the article: "Doctors who recognize bipolar disorder and know how to handle it are in *critically short supply*. Growing up is hard enough for children who are bipolar. The last thing they need is a misdiagnosis and treatment for something they don't have." How about that; from curious reporters to biopsychiatry zealots in only eleven pages?

Okay, I know that I have regressed from a philosophical deconstruction to plain old sarcasm. But really, can you believe this? I could write an entire book poking holes in this one article! In fact, I can't help myself. I have to share one last item with you. It's about bipolar kids needing their sleep (and how to make sure they get it). The warning is that bipolar kids are especially susceptible to destabilizing in response to an irregular sleep schedule. Here are the article's recommendations: "For this reason, parents of bipolar kids are urged to enforce sleep schedules firmly and consistently. Bedtime must mean bedtime and morning must mean morning. While that can be hard when an actively manic child is still throwing a tantrum two hours after lights-out, a combination of mood- stabilizing drugs and an enforced routine may even bring some of the most symptomatic kids into line." To me this sounds like something out of a training manual for animal handlers at a circus. These "mood stabilizing drugs", (like the Risperdal and Tegretol Brandon Kent takes), are often *extremely sedating*, even in adults. So I see another side to this recommendation, a license for the exasperated parents of temper tantrum throwing kids to knock them out with powerful tranquilizers and feel justified in doing it. End of problem. In my mind it is this message from biopsychiatry that lead to the death of Rebecca Riley. If this doesn't scare you, if this doesn't anger you, then you can stop reading right now; you've picked up the wrong book. Because I think my profession of psychiatry has gone nuts, over the deep end, off its rocker. I don't think that the biopsychiatrists and pharmaceutical industry are going to stop until every living American is taking psychotropic drugs...or worse. Brain implants are right around the corner...oops, spoke too soon—they are here already!! (See discussion of non-medication "treatments" for depression in chapter seven).

That is the tone and philosophy of this book. But I am not going to even attempt to "scientifically" prove anything. I think the books that try to do this are incredibly boring and tedious (how many "studies" can you quote?) I am just sharing my observations and thoughts. I will not challenge published research although I will at times, as I have already done, quote studies. And I am certainly not writing this book to cause any readers to fire their doctors and throw away their medicines. Please don't do that. And, by the way, remember; I'm not your doctor. I'm just a frustrated post modern philosophy fan who happens to earn a living as a psychiatrist. Again, I am trying to appeal to you, my readers, on a common sense level. I am not arguing in the science discourse and will not enter that "regime of truth" to make my points. In fact, I'm going to leave the language games of science and medicine behind completely in the next chapter because in chapter two we are going to take a journey to the land of Oz. Chapter two, coming right up is titled "Oil for the Tinman".

Chapter Two:
OIL FOR THE TINMAN

We all know the story The Wizard of Oz. The main characters are Dorothy, her dog Toto, the Scarecrow, the Tinman, the Cowardly Lion and, of course, the Wizard himself. It is such an imaginative story and entertaining movie. But I would bet that few of you have read the book on which the movie was based. It too is titled The Wizard of Oz and was written by L. Frank Baum in 1900 (Baum 1999). Billed as the first purely American fairy tale, it gained wide popularity at the time. In fact, L. Frank Baum wrote a total of fourteen books about the imaginary Land of Oz. As is always the case, the book is much more detailed than the movie. Of particular interest here is the story of the Tinman, because in the book we learn a lot more about the Tinman than was included in the movie.

In the movie we first meet the Tinman after Dorothy has already set out on her journey to the Emerald City to find the Wizard of Oz. She had rescued the Scarecrow from his pole in the farmer's field and they were journeying together when Dorothy heard a groaning sound coming from the woods. She and the scarecrow investigated the source of the sound and found it to be coming from a man made entirely of tin. This Tinman stood motionless, with his axe raised in the air as if he was about to take another swing at the partially chopped tree in front of him. He could not move but he could still speak and told the shocked duo that he had been calling for help for over a year but that "no one has ever heard me before or come to help me." Amazingly, all he needed was some oil from the oil can sitting a few feet away in his cottage. Following his instructions Dorothy and the Scarecrow soon had the Tinman well oiled and he was able to at last lower the axe and move about freely. The Tinman asked his rescuers how it was that they were in the area and they told him about their plans to seek help from the great Oz. After mulling it over for a few minutes the Tinman inquired whether they thought Oz could give him a heart. "I guess so", replied Dorothy so the Tinman decided to join them on their journey to the Emerald City. After making sure they had the oil can with them (in case it rained and the Tinman rusted again) they set off together down the yellow brick road.

The movie offers no background story on the origins of the Tinman. But the book does and it is a disturbing and tragic tale. In the book we learn that soon after freeing the Tinman all three set off on the road to Oz engaging in some friendly conversation. The Scarecrow and Tinman get into a disagreement about whether it's better to have a heart or a brain. Given a choice the Scarecrow would opt for the brain, the Tinman the heart. As he says: "But once I had brains, and a heart also; so, having tried them both, I should much rather have a heart." So now we know. The Tinman was once a human with a human brain and heart and now he is just a metal man with neither. What in the world happened to him? Here is the story he tells:

"I was born the son of a woodman who chopped down trees in the forest and sold the wood for a living. When I grew up I too became a woodchopper, and after my father died I took care of my old mother as long as she lived. Then I made up my mind that instead of living alone I would marry, so that I might not become lonely."

"There was one of the Munchkin girls who was so beautiful that I soon grew to love her with all my heart. She, on her part, promised to marry me as soon as I could earn enough money to build a better house for her; so I set out to work harder than ever. But the girl lived with an old woman who did not want her to marry anyone, for she was so lazy she wished the girl to remain with her and do the cooking and the housework. So the old woman went to the Wicked Witch of the East, and promised her two sheep and a cow if she would prevent the marriage. Thereupon the Wicked Witch enchanted my axe, and when I was chopping away at my best one day, for I was anxious to get the new house and my wife as soon as possible, the axe slipped all at once and cut off my left leg."

"This at first seemed a great misfortune, for I knew a one-legged man could not do very well as a woodchopper. So I went to a tinsmith and had him make me a new leg out of tin. The leg worked very well, once I was used to it; but my action angered the Wicked Witch of the East, for she had promised the old woman I should not marry the pretty Munchkin girl. When I began chopping again my axe slipped and cut off my right leg. Again I went to the tinner, and again he made me a leg out of tin. After this the enchanted axe cut off my arms, one after the other; but, nothing daunted, I had them replaced by tin ones. The Wicked Witch then made the axe slip and cut off my head, and at first I thought that was the end of me. But the tinsmith happened to come along, and he made me a new head out of tin."

"I thought I had beaten the Wicked Witch then, and I worked harder than ever; but I little knew how cruel my enemy could be. She thought of a new way to kill my love for the beautiful Munchkin maiden, and made the axe slip again, so that it cut right through my body, splitting me into two halves. Once more the tinsmith came to my help and made me a body of tin, fastening my tin arms and legs and head to it, by means of joints, so that I could move around as well as ever. But, alas! I had now no heart, so that I lost all my love for the Munchkin girl, and did not care whether I married her or not. I suppose she is still living with the old woman, waiting for me to come after her."

"My body shone so brightly in the sun that I felt very proud of it and it did not matter now if my axe slipped, for it could not cut me. There was only one danger—that my joints would rust; but I kept an oil-can in my cottage and took care to oil myself whenever I needed it. However, there came a day when I forgot to do this, and, being caught in a rainstorm, before I thought of the danger my joints had rusted, and I was left to stand in the woods until you came to help me. It was a terrible thing to undergo, but during the year I stood here I had time to think that the greatest loss I had known was the loss of my heart. While I was in love I was the happiest man on earth; but no one can love who does not have a heart, and so I am resolved to ask Oz to give me one. If he does, I will go back to the Munchkin maiden and marry her" (Baum 1999: 39-42).

Both Dorothy and the Scarecrow had been greatly interested in the story of the Tin Woodman, and now they knew why he was so anxious to get a new heart.

"All the same," said the Scarecrow, "I shall ask for brains instead of a heart; for a fool would not know what to do with a heart if he had one."

"I shall take the heart" returned the Tin Woodman; "for brains do not make one happy, and happiness is the best thing in the world."

So there you have it, the full story of the Tinman right from Baum's novel. While reading it I thought to myself that it's a good thing The Wizard of Oz movie was made in 1939. If it were made today we would no doubt be forced to endure gory, anatomically correct CGI scenes of the Tinman chopping his body to pieces with his own axe (with a video game to follow). But why am I telling this story in a book about psychiatry spinning out of control? I am doing it to illustrate by analogy how a superficial, surface analysis of a serious problem can and often does leave many complex and critical underlying issues unexamined and unaddressed. So here is the analogy I am proposing. The rusted and immobilized Tinman represents someone suffering from the "immobilizing" effects of depression and the oil is the antidepressant medication that alleviates his symptoms. (I want you to understand that I am not endorsing the idea that antidepressants actually do reliably cure what we have come to call clinical depression. The questionable validity of psychiatric diagnoses and effectiveness of medical treatment require careful critical analyses which I will do in chapters three through seven. But for the sake of this analogy and the points I want to make we will just consider the Tinman's immobility to be depression and the oil to be the "Prozac" that got him moving again).

Let us now ask this question: *aside* from the obvious rust related immobility, how should we define what is "wrong" with the Tinman? He couldn't move. Oil fixed that. Simple; he needs to be oiled. But are there any underlying issues to examine that his response to the oil might cause us to overlook, minimize or ignore? How about this one?

HE IS A MAN MADE OF TIN!

A formerly flesh and blood human being is gone and in his place is a...what? I guess you would have to call him a kind of cyborg, a walking and talking brain and heart-lacking thing, crafted by a tinsmith. And what happened to the flesh and blood human the Tinman used to be? An old lady paid off a Witch to assassinate him because he threatened her cozy lifestyle, an assignment she attempted to carry out in the most sadistic and heartless way imaginable. To show how this relates to modern psychiatry I will need to broaden the perspective under which we examine the Tinman's story by looking it at it in relation to both technology and sociology. We will start with technology.

Building a functional body out of metal is an impressive technological achievement but not an unimaginable one. We Americans talk about the wonders of technology all the time. Technology is invoked every time we discuss conquering barriers and solving problems in our daily lives. Technology is a large part of the proposed solution to the most terrifying problem in America today, terrorism. Few of us have any idea how those huge machines that our bags go through at the airport work but we are assured they are the "latest" technology designed to "sniff out" any explosives someone is trying to smuggle aboard. Technology will allow us to guard our borders, safeguard our shipyards and win wars in foreign lands we are told. And when we see images of drone planes, robot soldiers and smart bombs we tend to believe that. (Should we?) Technology, of course, also has many important applications in our everyday lives. Blackberries, cell phones, broadband internet, CAT scanners, computers and carpet sweeping robots, they simplify our lives, freeing us from tedious tasks and delivering us entertainment and diversions to keep us happy twenty-four hours a day. (Or do they?). Okay, let's be honest, we are all coming to realize that technology is truly the proverbial two-edged sword. Sure we have incredible technological superiority in the Middle East, so why are we still caught up in such a mess over there? Yes, the internet, the blackberry, cell phones and GPS are incredibly impressive devices, but has our quality of life really improved since they have come along or are we more stressed than ever, in part *because* of these new technologies? America has had a longstanding love affair with technology and breaking up *is* hard to do! In fact, it's impossible. Technology is here to stay and technological advances will continue to produce amazing products. But, it is time to examine this love affair, because, as we know, love can be blind, and we need to look more closely and critically at our relationship to technology because mainstream psychiatry so clearly and enthusiastically embraces and promotes a technological approach to mental healthcare. (As a for instance, one of the most active areas in addiction research is in laboratories where rat and other animal brains are being used to study the neurobiological basis of cocaine, heroin and alcohol abuse. The goal is to use the latest technologies to eventually create drugs, which we will call "medications", which will somehow prevent us from using recreational drugs, which we will continue to call "drugs").

To more fully examine our relationship to technology I need to introduce you to another philosopher, Martin Heidegger, generally considered to be a postmodern and/or existential philosopher, and very, very controversial (Guignon 1993). As discussed in chapter one, postmodern philosophy can, in very broad terms, be described as multi-perspectival, a basic belief that there are many different ways to explain or interpret what we experience as human beings and that the role of the philosopher is to analyze and understand the significance of *how* and *why* we interpret things the way we do. In contrast, the so-called modern or analytic philosopher seeks the *correct* way to interpret our experiences that will ultimately result in a clear understanding of the true nature of reality. To the modern philosopher technology is an essential tool in our search for truth while to the postmodern philosopher technology is a phenomenon to be understood as part of the lived experience of human beings. This doesn't mean that postmodern philosophers are anti-technology because (here comes another Roderickism) as Rick Roderick says "I would much rather have a toothache today than in the 14th century." Postmodern philosophy is more focused on the fact that along with stark physical reality there is a "lived" reality in which *interpretation* and *meaning* play a central role. Think about Christianity for example, and how the varying "interpretations" of the Bible have so concretely affected our lives for the last two thousand years. Here are a few more examples of what I'm talking about: The earth revolves around the sun, true or false, fact or interpretation? Of course, it's a true fact. But how much of a role does that bit of factual knowledge play in determining the quality of our everyday lives? Basically, none in the early 21st century. But there was a time when one's *belief* about the relative movements of the sun and earth was literally a matter of life and death. You could lose your life for even whispering your belief in the fact that the earth was not the center of the universe. Next example: Sex before marriage is wrong, fact or interpretation? I hope everyone will agree that this is an interpretation, an opinion, and that neither a yes nor a no answer is an indisputable fact. Clearly some facts are indisputable truths, a part of the brute physical reality of the universe (sometimes called "facticity" by post modern philosophers such as Heidegger) while others are clearly interpretations (e.g. sex before marriage being right or wrong). The important issue here is that BOTH affect us in our daily lives. The major problem that Heidegger focuses on, however, is not that this distinction exists, but that the power of the so-called objective facts derived from science are so compelling that we begin to believe that scientific thinking should be the basis for providing solutions to ALL human problems (a perspective that some postmodern philosophers label "scientism"). Heidegger calls this dominance of this perspective *Gestell*, a German word usually translated as "enframing", but for the purpose of this book I will simply call the "technological attitude." Let's look at what that means and how it is relevant to the Tinman and, by extension, psychiatry.

Heidegger's critique of technology is not (although it is often misinterpreted to be) an attack on technology itself. He too values the devices and advances that science and the scientific method have brought about. His concern is that as a result of the success of the application of science through technology humankind has developed a basic *attitude* about life *in general* that prioritizes and values technological thinking (sometimes called instrumental rationality) and technological achievement above all else (Heidegger 1971). This technological attitude requires that all issues, even ethical ones, be "problematized" into a form that has the potential for *solvability* by scientific means. Thus, a doctor cannot respond to emotional distress if told the source of distress is "my life" but can respond if the distress is appropriately "problematized" as a cluster of symptoms we can interpret as a "clinical depression." Similarly, the issue of sex before marriage can be problematized by choosing a variable such as divorce rate and then creating a study to compare divorce rates in people who engaged in sex before marriage versus those who didn't. But would this really be a valid result at any level? In actuality, an issue such as the positive versus negative impact of sex before marriage cannot be legitimately studied because, as I've said before, there are a near *infinite* number of *uncontrolled variables* distinguishing each couple being studied from every other couple being studied. There are, to me, obvious inherent and unavoidable barriers to "scientifically" studying complex social and psychological problems in human beings, but for some reason we are not deterred. Think about how many times you have heard some TV news reporter breathlessly announcing the "results" of this or that study "proving" something or other about our lives and how we should live them followed a week or two later by another study stating just the opposite.

Do you see how pervasive the technological attitude has become? Do you see how we have come to rely on first problematizing and then studying issue after issue to tell us how to run our lives? Have you ever thought that your out of control kid or your neighbor's kid could use a good spanking, like you used to get? What stops you? Well in large part it's been sentences starting with the words: "Studies have shown…". Well *whose* studies exactly? And *how* was it studied? And what exactly were the results and who exactly was *interpreting* the meaning of those results? (In my opinion, when psychiatric studies are subjected to this type of scrutiny, they can start to fall apart pretty quickly). Let's face it, no matter how much we would like to believe or have come to hope that some day there will be answers for every social and psychological problem we face, not every issue we face as human beings can be "problematized" into a question that can be scientifically studied without risking radically distorting the issue. We are just too complex, society is too complex and there are too many variables that cannot be controlled or accounted for. Let us return to the Tinman's story and look at some of the technology issues involved.

There are a couple of major modern technology issues in the story of the Tinman. The first has to do with the power of technology and who or what sets limits on that power. In the *Wizard of Oz* Frank Baum (in the year 1900) imagines a technological ability to rebuild a human body out of metal. Of course he takes it to the extreme by rebuilding the entire body, absent in his account, a brain and heart. The immediate dilemma that comes to mind here is one we are clearly facing today; just because you *can* do something technologically does that mean you *should*? I believe that everyone reading this would agree that the technological ability to build functional body parts is generally a good thing and that we are all in favor of continued research and progress in everything from artificial limbs to artificial retinas. But it becomes less clear when you start talking about technologically enhancing or improving human capabilities with, for example, some sort of a brain implant to make people more intelligent or talented (they are already talking about this in nanotechnology). Interestingly, we do seem to have made up our minds in some areas like, for example, using technologically developed supplements and chemicals to enhance the power, speed and endurance of professional athletes. We don't approve and make that clear by the word we choose to describe this behavior: "doping." On the other hand, prescribing powerful amphetamines to adults that report having trouble multitasking (so-called "Adult ADD") we've chosen to call "treatment". Interesting, huh? Overall, however, I think we remain very leery about mucking around in people's brains without knowing exactly what we are doing and what the outcome or long term effects might be. We may be leery, but I need to tell you we are already doing this on a wide scale basis. It's called psychiatry. So how is it that treating five-year olds with brain altering drugs with unknown mechanisms of action and unknown long term effects is okay, but it is not okay for athletes to take performance enhancing drugs?

The general observation then is that technology, no matter how "objective" it appears to be, is still a human grounded activity, in which human feelings, beliefs, desires, values and ethics play a role. But *whose* feelings, beliefs, desires, values and ethics matter most? It can't be everyone's because not every one agrees that medicating children is okay and athletes taking steroids is not. I've heard arguments on both sides. So it must be (hello Monsieur Foucault) that the opinion that matters most has something to do with the *power* of the person expressing the opinion and that sheds a whole new light on technology. Not only are decisions and policies guiding the use of our products of technology related to power, so is the rationing of economic resources that allow expensive technologies to be applied to solving one problem instead of another. No wonder we are always talking about how much some research experiment or technological achievement costs; it's not just about money, it's also about power.

The Tinman, in some ways, represents the pinnacle of technological achievement: resurrection and maybe even immortality: Do Tinmen die? That once again begs the question, just because we *can* do it, does that mean we *should* do it? Think about human cloning as a good example of this dilemma. Going back to Heidegger, his contention is that the "technological attitude" distorts important human concerns because in the "technological attitude" *utility, efficiency, ordering and control* are the dominant guiding principles. And I would add to this list: *profitability*. Heidegger conceptualizes human beings subjugated to the concerns of utility, efficiency, ordering, control (and profitability) to be nothing more than a sort of "standing reserve." (Foucault uses the term "biopower" while, in an even less flattering light, Nietzsche likens us to "the herd." Think about the massive layoffs in corporate America to get a sense of what these labels are referring to). In summary the question raised by the Tinman's story is just because we can build him, should we build him? Doesn't so easily rebuilding his body somehow shift the concern (or at least soften the concern) that his deplorable condition was brought about by the actions of others in their shared societal structure? This is not an easily solved dilemma and we won't find the answer within the technological attitude because from that perspective the rebuilding of his body was a technological triumph. We need to look elsewhere. Suppose we were to ask ourselves a different question; suppose we would ask what could be done that would prevent us from needing to face this dilemma in the first place? To do this we would need to look beyond the Tinman himself to the society in which he lives; a society that somehow has created the *conditions for the possibility of* inexpensive sadistic assassinations in the first place. (Are we not, in fact, having a debate about the limits of torture in our society right now?) Let's turn to sociology.

Sociology is a discourse mentioned in chapter one when we were discussing the humanities. It is an extremely complex and controversy filled discipline that tries to understand the workings of societies. It straddles the line between scientific and non-scientific approaches and both are found in its rich literature. Of importance to us in our Tinman analogy and critique of psychiatry is how sociology focuses on the impact of society, culture and cultural beliefs and values on the lives of individuals. I believe that this topic is nearly totally ignored by medical psychiatry. One of the major critiques of medical psychiatry by a number of postmodern thinkers is how it focuses exclusively on the individual and his or her symptoms, in a sense "locating" problems with anxiety, depression, phobias, compulsive behavior and the like *in* the individual, not *in* the society or culture itself. "Post-psychiatrists" Brackin and Thomas call this methodological individualism: "a focus on decontextualized aspects of a person's behavior" (Brackin and Thomas 2005, p.15).What would a context centered approach yield in our evaluation of the Tinman? It would at the least help us to recognize that if our friendly and hardworking woodsman did not live in a society where a lazy woman could so easily hire an assassin to mutilate and destroy him, then he would have never been made into a Tinman in the first place and his joint rusting immobilization and need to be rescued with the oil would simply never have happened. Put into the discourse of psychiatry we can frame the issue in the form of this question: Are more and more people getting diagnosed and treated for depression because there are more and more people that are, for some reason, developing chemical imbalances inside their brains OR are more and more people getting depressed because our culture is growing increasingly depressogenic? There is also a third part to this question that asks whether more and more people are getting labeled as depressed because the psychiatric and pharmaceutical industries are getting so good at marketing and the answer to that is clearly yes, but as you will learn, this phenomenon is simply part of what makes our culture depressogenic as a whole. For now, we need to look more closely at the word depressogenic.

The alarm goes off. Its 5:30 already? Bob gets out of bed, into the shower and then grabs some breakfast. Egg whites and rye toast, why the heck did he commit to that diet, especially now? He has to drive right past Burger King every morning, maybe today he'll get that breakfast croissant and hash browns, then just skip lunch to make up for it. Then it hits him, the cold panicky feeling he tries so hard to avoid. But once it hits, it hits. The merger rumors are getting louder. Especially worrisome was the meeting last Friday when the vice president gathered everybody together to announce in no uncertain terms that they were not selling out. "This is our bank, we built it from the ground up", he says, "and no faceless corporation is going to just march in here and swallow us up. Not in my lifetime." That's when Bob knew for sure that the merger was on. How had he gotten so cynical? "Fool me once, shame on you, fool me twice, shame on me." This caused him to chuckle quietly to himself as he recalled President Bush butchering this saying on TV. But his little laugh was short-lived. This was not funny! It would be his third takeover in ten years. Bob is getting older and his salary and benefits have built up. He knows all too well that his years of experience, his creativity and past successes will not protect him. He learned that harsh lesson during the last merger. "You're letting me go?" he had asked incredulously. "I created the mortgage refinance division from nothing. I made you guys a fortune!" "And we appreciate it Bob, but the company is going in a different direction now..you understand" they said. Yeah he understood..oh yeah, he understood..

Then the negative spiral just took over. His daughter was such a disappointment, dropping out of college to get married to that jerk. And now she won't even take his phone calls. Then there's his wife. Blaming him for having to move halfway across the country for this new job and now, after just two years, he was going to get downsized again. How could he even bring himself to tell her? And then it happened. It flashed through his mind. Suicide. God, that's scary. Oh he's thought about suicide before, hasn't everybody? But this time it actually felt like a viable option, a real choice to consider. That had never happened before. He actually felt tears starting to well up in his eyes. All of his hopes and dreams…how did it come to this? He was a good man, an honest man, a God fearing man. He decided to see the counselor at his church during lunch.

The counselor was a good man too. He saw the pain in Bob's eyes and listened closely to his story. He expressed his concern, especially about the suicide stuff. He pulled out a questionnaire for Bob to fill out. It was a Beck's Depression Inventory, a multiple choice questionnaire asking about his mood, his sleep, his appetite and his sex life. It also asked about suicide and Bob checked off the next to highest box, a 2 point answer that he "would like to kill himself." That wasn't quite true but it was the answer that was closest to describing the very complex feelings about suicide he was having. (Bob noticed that a lot of the questions had answer choices that were not quite right, so he just checked off whichever one was in the ballpark). The counselor looked over the quiz and added up the score. "You are suffering from pretty serious clinical depression Bob," he announced. "It's not your fault; you have a chemical imbalance in your brain. But don't worry, there are good treatments available." Bob expected the counselor to start talking to him about his job and marital issues because they didn't even ask about them on the questionnaire. Instead the counselor took out his business card and scribbled a word on the back. "I want you to take this to your family doctor as soon as possible. Tell her I'm recommending you be started on this medication right away."

Bob glanced at the card on the way back to his car. Written there was the word "Cymbalta". That sounded familiar. That's right, he heard about it on TV. "Depression hurts. Where does it hurt? Everywhere. Who does it hurt? Everyone." You got that right he thought to himself (what a catchy commercial). As soon as he got back to his office he called his doctor and the secretary fit him in at four o'clock. He looked up Cymbalta on the computer and read the testimonials and success stories on the Eli Lilly website. Amazing, he was starting to feel better already.

Yes I made up Bob's story but it is not far-fetched. What "caused" Bob to feel awful and start thinking seriously about suicide? Was it a coincidence that he developed "clinical" depression just when he was going to get downsized again? Of course not. No one would argue that sociocultural issues emanating from stressors such as corporate downsizing didn't have something to do with it. However, as I pointed out, the depression "test" he took didn't ask him any questions about that. There was no essay section at the end for him to fill in the details of his story, just multiple choice questions about his sleeping, eating, sex drive, mood and concentration. Just symptoms, as if he existed in some sort of vacuum, unaffected by the events of his life and the society in which he lives. That is exactly what Brackin and Thomas are referring to with the term methodological individualism. The Beck's Depression Inventory is a widely used diagnostic tool in clinical medicine and psychiatry. The method by which we make psychiatric diagnoses relies almost exclusively on decontextualized (removed from their context) lists of symptoms in individuals. They don't even ask if your dog died yesterday. What do the psychiatrists who are in control of formulating diagnostic practices have to say about this? Do they think we should be making diagnoses without considering the context?

Here is a 100% true story. In 1997 I was at a meeting that the AAPP (The Association for the Advancement of Philosophy and Psychiatry mentioned in the introduction) sponsored to gather scholars from around the world to address concerns about the DSM model of psychiatric diagnosis. (By that time we had moved up from DSM III to DSM IV). All the big shots from the DSM team were there. Among them was Allen Frances, M.D., the chairperson of the Task Force on DSM IV. You really couldn't find a bigger mucky-muck than that. He was on stage taking questions from the audience. I eagerly raised my hand because I had something IMPORTANT to ask. Finally it was my turn. Here was my question: "When I was in training we were very focused on the concept of reactive vs. endogenous (arising for no reason) cases of depression. The clinical implication was that it was the endogenous depressions that required medication while the reactive depressions should be treated in some sort of therapy. Whatever happened to that distinction?" I have to tell you that I expected my question to generate some real buzz because it was challenging the growing dictatorship of biological psychiatry. Talk about a letdown. Dr. Frances answered me with a dismissive statement that I can still feel the sting of today. "That's why we have Axis IV" he said, "next question." What he was referring to is that the DSM model of psychiatric diagnosis has five axes or sections that, when all are filled in, fully describe the diagnosis of the patient. The first, Axis I, is where you write down your primary psychiatric diagnosis. For example in Bob's case it would probably be Major Depression, Single Episode, Severe Without Psychosis: Code # 296.23. There is no distinction made on Axis I between reactive and endogenous depression. Axis IV is where you record what are called "Psychosocial and Environmental Problems" along with the qualifiers mild, moderate or severe. I will have a lot more to say in chapter three about the DSM but there is a point I want to make here. First, let me quote directly from DSM IV where the guidelines for Axis IV are described:

> A psychosocial or environmental problem may be a negative life event, an environmental difficulty or deficiency, a familial or other interpersonal stress, an inadequacy of social support or personal resources, or other problem relating to the context in which a person's difficulties have developed.
>
> (DSM IV pp.29-30)

Remember when I said that modern psychiatry is reductionistic and dehumanizing? Whew! How do you like that impersonal, cold and uncaring language? I guess living in an urban ghetto with drive-by shootings and presenting to your doctor with complaints of anxiety would earn you an "environmental difficulty" stressor while finding out that your husband fathered a child with another woman he met in an internet chat room would be a "familial or other interpersonal stress." You would still get your Axis I diagnosis of Generalized Anxiety Disorder (for our woman from the ghetto) or

Major Depression (for the hapless wife), but Axis IV would be used to record the "context" or stressors under which your disorder arose. The language of Axis IV is dismissive in and of itself but I need to explain to you why I felt that Dr. Frances' answer to me was so painfully dismissive. I work in psychiatry and I can tell you this for a fact: *No one cares what is on Axis IV!* Researchers don't care, doctors don't care, the courts don't care, insurance companies don't care and pharmaceutical companies don't care. All that matters is what is on Axis I. What that means is that you will be "treated" solely for your Axis I condition, and 99 out of 100 times that will be with medication. Maybe you'll be sent to "therapy", maybe not.

But here is what I consider the more insidious part. You will also be learning from experts with great authority that it isn't the ghetto or the cheating husband that is *causing* your deep pain; it may contribute, but it is your brain's imbalanced chemistry that is ultimately at fault and needs to be fixed. Again this is methodological individualism; it shifts the focus from social and interpersonal problems to problems located inside the individual and it is also scientism because we certainly cannot solve the problems of the ghetto just to alleviate this one person's anxiety or somehow wave a magic wand so that no husband will ever cheat on his wife just so this one lady will feel better. You must present your question in the form of a solvable problem or the scientist cannot help you. As you will learn in future chapters, this is leading to the development of standardized treatment protocols that, in essence, remove any individual interpretation of the facts by the doctor. Let's just say machine-like is a pretty good description.

But I don't really need to tell you this because no doubt you've already directly experienced this dehumanizing and reductionistic shift in all medical care from your family doctor to your hospital. How many of you who see doctors in busy primary care offices walk away feeling like the doctor (or most likely physician assistant or nurse practitioner) really listened carefully to your complaints and explained the diagnosis and treatment? Remember *Gestell?* Efficiency, order, control and profitability rule the day under the sway of this technological attitude. The so-called "thought leaders" in medicine are nearly 100% behind this standardized and codified delivery of medical care. In psychiatry it's called "evidence based" medicine, a concept I will deconstruct for you later in the book. For now though, back to our story.

By the time Dorothy and the Scarecrow meet up with the Tinman there was little they could do about the sociocultural factors involved in his mutilation and need to be remade out of tin. All they could see that there was to do was to solve the immediate problem by oiling his rusty joints. But here is what I find striking (I know this is just a fairy tale, but go with me), Dorothy and the Scarecrow did not seem the *least bit concerned* with what had happened to the Tinman. They didn't stop their journey and choose to march right down to city hall or the local newspaper to express their incredulity and outrage about what an old woman and Witch had done to this good hearted man. They didn't lobby for legislation to outlaw hired assassination. No, they had their own problems, their own agendas, and it was time to get on with their journey to Oz. But they did take the oil can to prevent any future episodes of rusting. (The analogy here to the practice of taking "prophylactic antidepressants" is obvious. We'll get back to the topic of choosing to use medication like an insurance policy against possible future emotional pain in later chapters).

I want to briefly mention a philosopher I've met who takes an even wider perspective on the sociocultural roots of depression. His name is David Michael Levin and he edited a book called *Pathologies of the Modern Self. Postmodern Studies on Narcissism, Schizophrenia and Depression* published by the New York University Press in 1987. Dr. Levin is a scholar who made, what I believe, to be strikingly true observations about how living in a modern western culture foments an unavoidable state of depression. Thus, the totality of the culture *itself* is depressogenic, i.e. it creates depression as the background mood of existence. I want to share some of Dr. Levin's thoughts with you before we move on with our story of the Tinman. He said:

> Our sacred traditions are almost gone, and now even our great secular traditions are rapidly disappearing; even the institution of the family is in fateful danger. We have very little security in an age that cannot forget the devastation of Hiroshima and the Nazi death camps in Germany, and now faces the risk of nuclear annihilation. What *is* constant, permanent, settled? We can depend on nothing. Is it surprising that depression be so widespread? (Levin 1987, p.493)

(*note: This was written in before global terrorism)

Okay, that's some pretty heavy stuff, "depressing" just to read. Is it true? Is Levin right when he goes on to say that we live in an age where "nothing grips us anymore, where no beliefs unite and motivate us", what he calls the "age of nihilism?" (Nihilism is the belief in nothing). You decide. But you can't deny that his thoughts deserve a place at the table when we are discussing psychiatry. And ask yourself; what are the psychological effects on individuals of terrorism, Darfur, crime, poverty, insecurity, gas prices, Enron and everything else we hear about on the news day after day? Should we really be "locating" an "epidemic" of depression, anxiety, obsessions, panic attacks and the like solely *in* the individual's brain chemistry or should at least some of our attention be turned to the social conditions we share? It's amazing to me how many of my patients report a total remission of their panic attacks, feelings of depression and other symptoms when they take a cruise or some other totally relaxing vacation. This is particularly true when they don't watch the news or pick up a newspaper the entire time. I think the most important clinical implication of what Levin has to say is that we are wrong if we set the bar too low in labeling individual cases as abnormal or "clinical" depression because collectively, as a culture, there is a background level of depression that represents the *totally normal* response to living within what he calls this age of nihilism.

How about the Tinman's culture? It seems pretty depressogenic too. There is plenty of violence and pain in Oz, a culture terrified and dominated by two powerful demagogues, the Evil Witches of the East and West. The Tinman, frozen in place needing oil to function, might have been the outcome of a singular event in that culture, but the sociocultural conditions for the possibility of such an event occurring at all were already in place. I think it is essential for us to recognize that the current domination of the medical model in psychiatry with its growing number of speculative diagnoses and wild combinations of medications also requires sociocultural conditions for the possibility of that domination to also be *already* in place. We will revisit this issue and more clearly define these sociocultural conditions (e.g. the "quick fix" mentality) throughout the book. To illustrate the phenomenon of using psychotropic medicine to alleviate the pain of intolerable overall social conditions we need look no farther than the use of the drug "soma" in Aldous Huxley's *Brave New World.* Here are a couple of quotes about "soma" from that book:

"All the advantages of Christianity and Alcohol, none of the disadvantages."

"…you do look glum, what you need is some soma."

That second one hits pretty close to home. It sounds a lot like what we are increasingly advising each other to do, especially since antidepressants started advertising on TV. Just substitute the word Zoloft or Paxil or Cymbalta for soma. This is what I tell my patients when I'm trying to educate them abut the potential impact of the emotional numbing properties of antidepressants: "If Prozac were around in 1775 we would still be singing God Bless the Queen and going to cricket matches." They laugh; they are antidepressant veterans and they get it. Sometimes dysphoria and anxiety and anger can be a good thing. (A lot more about this in chapter six).

It's time to get back once again to our friend the Tinman because his story is not yet over. When we left him he was on the road to Oz seeking a heart to replace the one he had himself chopped up with his enchanted axe. We will skip the details of the journey to Oz and jump ahead to the discovery that the great and powerful Wizard is a fake. The Wizard's secret was not discovered by our intrepid travelers until after they had fulfilled his command to destroy the Wicked Witch of the East. Apparently he did not expect them to succeed and had no idea how he would fulfill his promises he had made to each one of them, including giving the Tinman a heart. But even though he was described by Baum as a humbug, the Wizard was wise in other ways. He understood that often people already have inside them what they think is lacking, like courage, brains and a heart. All they need is some encouragement to bring it to the surface. Remember these insightful lyrics by America?

"Oz never did give nothing to the tinman that he didn't, didn't already have"

The Wizard decided to take advantage of a well known phenomenon, the placebo effect. Give someone a sugar pill and tell them it will have this or that effect and a percentage of them will report a response. I heard from my father-in-law that back in the days when doctors weren't scared to death of lawsuits he used to give some patients placebos for their "pain". (He was an orthopedic surgeon). In chapters six and seven I will tell you all about the amazingly high percentage of placebo responders in psychiatric medication studies, a percentage so high that it challenges the notion that there is any legitimate response to the actual medications. So the Wizard used placebos to deliver on his promise to the Scarecrow, the Tinman and The Cowardly Lion. Our friend the Tinman got a silk heart-shaped pillow stuffed with sawdust put into his chest. Did it work? Well the Tinman thought it did and, in fact, cried real tears when the Wizard flew away in his balloon.

The Wizard is described as a trickster, a deceiver, a humbug. And I suppose in relation to how he fooled a lot of people, including the subjects that he got to build the Emerald City, he was. But Baum describes the Wizard as a kind, goodhearted man and clearly the people whose lives he touched were the better for it. One might argue that along with some questionable ethics the Wizard also possessed great wisdom. Wisdom is defined as experience and knowledge together with the power of applying them critically or practically.

Wisdom has been an important concept in human life throughout time and in all cultures. There is a large body of literature which I like to think of as wisdom based literature in religion, philosophy, ethics…even medicine. In our technological age wisdom is being degraded and ignored and I am deeply concerned that we are all suffering because of it. A doctor being challenged by an insurance company for not discharging a patient from the hospital per the insurance company protocol can no longer say to the insurance company "Look, I've been a doctor for thirty years and I just have an uneasy feeling about this patient and want to keep an eye on him in the hospital for a while longer." That just won't work. Protocols, practice manuals, treatment algorithms, numbers and computers are running the show. This is in all branches of medicine but I believe that it is particularly destructive in psychiatry.

I'm dead serious when I say that psychiatry, as it is being practiced today, can do real harm to you, your family and society. I have used the story of the Tinman to illustrate my concern about the reductionistic and dehumanizing effects of medical model psychiatry. At the end here I am hinting at the solution being found in what I am calling wisdom literature and thought. So let us now embark on our journey together. First I will fully explain what is going on in psychiatry by looking at the flaws and weaknesses in how psychiatric diagnoses are currently being made in chapters three, four and five. We will then take a hard look at everything you need to know about psychiatric medications (chapters six and seven) and then fully examine the social and economic forces that have led to and sustain the current domination by medial model psychiatry (chapter eight). The rest of the book will be devoted to looking at what you can do to help yourself, your family and your society by learning to rationally judge how to respond to medical model psychiatry. We will look at when agreeing to a trial of psychiatric medication is a good decision and when it is a bad decision. We will look at how to decide whether or not you are having a legitimate response to medication. Finally we will examine alternatives to medical model psychiatry and what they have to offer in your pursuit of emotional wellbeing. There is a lot of material to cover here; some familiar, some not and some things that will shock you. I am not claiming to have the Truth on my side. I am simply a practicing clinician with an interest in post modern philosophy who wants to share his concerns about psychiatry with you and hopefully teach you a few things along the way.

OKAY...On to Chapter Three.

Chapter Three:
DIAGNOSTIC PRACTICES IN PSYCHIATRY: *Good Intentions...Bad Outcome*

> Let us further consider the formation of concepts. Every word instantly becomes a concept precisely insofar as it is not supposed to serve as a reminder of the unique and entirely individual original experience to which it owes its origin; but rather, a word becomes a concept insofar as it simultaneously has to fit countless more or less similar cases—which means, purely and simply cases which are never equal and thus altogether unequal.
>
> Friedrich Nietzsche – *On Truth and Lies in a Nonmoral Sense*

> It has 20 million faces but only one name...depression.
>
> Prozac advertisement

Don't worry if you don't fully understand what Nietzsche was trying to say. It will become clear while we explore how and why the DSM process of psychiatric diagnosis, (initially developed in an attempt to organize the discipline of psychiatry and create a foundation for research), has spun so totally out of control. To illustrate this we will look at how the *word* depression, formerly used to simply describe a common human feeling, has been transformed by mainstream psychiatry and the marketplace into the *concept* of depression as a mental disorder (or, if you prefer, a "serious medical condition" like they call it on TV). Here we will see how the "technological attitude" that is guiding psychiatry has resulted in numerous concepts (diagnoses) that do exactly what Nietzsche describes: roughly "fit" countless more or less similar cases (see Prozac ad) while at the same time lumping together (in the reductionism needed for "scientism") people whose problems are individually much more complex, nuanced and unique, or, in Nietzsche's terms, altogether unequal. This then is the dehumanizing impact of DSM diagnostic practices that we previously discussed. By the way, there is a part two to the Prozac ad quote, a part that I added in a paper I wrote. The full quotation is this:

> It has 20 million faces but only one name…depression
>
> Prozac advertisement
>
> It is time for the psychiatric profession to insist once again on 20 million names.
>
> Phillip Sinaikin MD
> (Sadler, 2005 p.327)

There are a number of books that have been written over the years critical of psychiatry at many levels. Often, the most serious criticisms leveled at psychiatry are about the limits it imposes on personal freedom through its practices of forced hospitalization and medication. There are those who argue that there is no such thing as mental illness and that the entire endeavor is merely a disguised form of social control. There are even social activist groups such as the Hearing Voices Network, (this is their real name), who fight against forced psychiatric treatment, choosing instead to celebrate their uniqueness. What most authors and others critical of psychiatry tend to focus on is what has for centuries been called madness. In today's psychiatry loss of touch with consensual reality, delusions, and hallucinations are called psychotic symptoms which can be associated with a number of disorders but is most diagnostically central to the mental disorder schizophrenia. Historically the major impetus behind the development of psychiatry as a distinct specialty arose from the social need to control people who were "mad" (although a lot of socially problematic people such as debtors and criminals used to be lumped in with psychotics in the past). I will mention psychotic illnesses and symptoms as part of this chapter on diagnostic practices, but I am electing not to deal in detail with illnesses such as schizophrenia in this book. (For a very readable account of how psychiatry has over the years dealt with psychotic illnesses I would suggest journalist Robert Whitaker's *Mad in America: Bad Science, Bad Medicine and the Enduring Mistreatment of the Mentally Ill*, published by Perseus Publishing in 2002).

The reason that I am focusing on non-psychotic conditions is because I believe that, in most cases, what is called schizophrenia is truly a brain illness and that the scientific method and medical model are well suited to explore a greater understanding of the causes of this illness. So I am not going to deal much with the conditions currently categorized in DSM IV as "Schizophrenia and Other Psychotic Disorders." Covering the controversies about appropriate medical and psychosocial treatment for schizophrenia will distract us from the focus of this book and the reasons why I am suggesting that you should be afraid of mainstream psychiatry. The focus of this book is the widespread intrusion of modern psychiatry into *our everyday lives* by its redefining of our emotional, cognitive and behavioral struggles as medical disorders.

There is a long and complex history of the practice of diagnosis in psychiatry with each school of thought issuing their own set of categories of pathologies consistent with their theories of the causes of mental and emotional suffering. It wasn't until around the time of World War II that psychiatry was forced to come up with some sort of reasonably organized list of psychiatric diagnoses. During and after WW II Western society, especially America went into hyper-drive in its project to develop a rationally organized, rule-driven and orderly economy and society. This seemingly endless process of the rationalization of society has itself spun out of control, resulting in a current level of complexity and stressfulness that affects every one of us everyday, and, as you will see, builds demand for pharmaceutical relief.

Have you tried to get a building permit lately or attempted to understand a new tax law or ballot referendum? Do you find yourself staring in disbelief at yet another quality assurance plan at work that has double the pages of last year's new plan? (Soma anyone?) When you are sitting in a hospital bed waiting for the nurse you summoned thirty minutes ago, do you know what she is doing? Chances are she is doing paperwork; filling out forms and charts takes over 40% of a nurse's time now. I just read in today's paper a new set of guidelines for teachers outlining "appropriate" vs. "inappropriate" contact. The gist of the new regulations: Don't ever be alone with a student and don't touch anyone, anywhere.

Time for a *Roderickism*:

Rick says that the world has become a kind of double world. While the world is as rationalized as it has ever been, it produces a kind of paradox because when the world is organized by instrumental rationality it produces a situation in which human beings themselves no longer feel rational.

Today most of us feel like we are literally drowning in a dense pool of rules and regulations; Almost every doctor over 50 that I know would retire in a second, not because they have lost their love of practicing medicine, but because there are so many regulations and barriers to providing even minimal quality of care that the doctors just burn out and give up!

Around WW II many forces outside of psychiatry played a role in applying pressure to the profession to look and act more "scientific" and for its diagnoses to conform more closely to the International Classification of Diseases (ICD) being used worldwide. Under these demands the first two diagnostic manuals were developed by psychiatry (DSM I, published in 1952 and DSM II published in 1968) but they were loosely organized hodgepodges of diagnoses that received little attention outside of the profession of psychiatry. DSM I and DSM II served their purpose at the time. Although not very scientifically rigorous, they did allow for diagnoses and numerical diagnostic codes to be attached to patients and the services provided. This served the needs of growing bureaucracies that required numbers and codes to provide payment for services, make decisions about life and health insurance and statistically track all sorts of things for all sorts of purposes. Other than that, however DSM I and DSM II remained rather obscure texts, used mostly in settings like state hospitals and, due to their relative invisibility, did not draw much critical attention. (This despite the fact that both DSM I and DSM II had some pretty controversial diagnoses in them such as homosexuality being defined as a mental disorder). But then along came DSM III, published in 1980 after having been in development since 1974. This was a complex text, requiring years of preparation, planning and approval processes. The American Psychiatric Association's official diagnostic manual was no longer going to be some obscure text sitting on shelves in state hospitals. **DSM III would quite literally change the world!**

Since the purpose of this book is to help you become a more educated and thoughtful consumer of what medical psychiatry and its pals in the pharmaceutical industry are selling, you need to learn how the DSM III and DSM IV came into being and are being used by today's clinicians. I cannot possibly cover every element in the controversies about the DSM's but if this intrigues you, here is the title of what I consider to be *the* book that comprehensively and fairly deals in detail with all sides of the debate. It is the previously mentioned *values and psychiatric diagnosis* written by John Z. Sadler M.D. It was published by Oxford University Press in 2005 and there is simply nothing better written on the topic of controversies in psychiatric diagnosis.

Okay, lets put ourselves into the position of the psychiatrists charged with the task of coming up with a new way to categorize and organize the myriad diagnoses that had historically emerged through the practice of psychiatry and psychology over the past hundred years or so. Where do you even start? At the time when DSM III was being formulated there was no clear-cut "regime of truth" running the show in mental health. In 1980, the year DSM III was published, I was in my third year of residency in psychiatry. To illustrate the wide range of theories and approaches in psychiatry back then all I have to do is list the various perspectives of the teaching faculty at that residency: The residency director was a pretty traditional Freudian psychoanalyst. Another analyst on the staff was more into object relations theory and called himself a "Kohutian" analyst. Another psychiatrist favored behavioral therapy while two others were rational-emotive cognitive therapy zealots. We had an adjunct professor who taught orthomolecular psychiatry, an approach based on vitamin and nutritional therapy. There was a large community of "Ericksonian" therapists in town who emphasized the use hypnosis in their treatment. Finally, my substance abuse rotation was two months at an orthodox 12 Step program of recovery where the use of psychiatric medications was rare and generally frowned upon. The point here is that psychiatry at the time of the publication of DSM III was highly eclectic; many points of view guided diagnosis and treatment. Although DSM II had been in existence for 12 years it was rarely discussed and used only for coding purposes. But DSM III was going to be quite different. Within a few short years of its release DSM III would be characterized by its supporters and critics alike as the BIBLE of psychiatric diagnosis and treatment.

So lets turn the clock back to the 1970's and see how this bible-to-be was born. There was initially little interest in devising a new diagnostic manual and I understand that the person chosen to lead the project was a relative unknown at the time. His name was Robert Spitzer (Spiegel 2005). He had previously been involved in the creation of DSM II but eventually came to strongly criticize its lack of reliability. To begin work on a new manual Dr. Spitzer enlisted help from five other psychiatrists he personally chose for the project. Apparently, what they all had in common was a desire for precision in psychiatric diagnosis. Most of the members of this inner circle were researchers and tended to favor a biological perspective. Were there also psychoanalysts, humanistic psychologists, cognitive therapists, existentialists, feminists or behaviorists in this group? No. Were there any non-MD's in this group? No again. These were doctors who clearly saw themselves as scientists. And their diagnostic manual would reflect the rigor and precision of science. This group of five psychiatrists charged with developing the new framework for psychiatric diagnostic thinking had a couple of nicknames: The "DOP's" (Data Oriented People) and the "Young Turks" (no explanation needed). They completed their initial drafting of the new manual in a year. It was then submitted to thousands of other psychiatrists and mental health professionals for comment and for reliability studies and it would be another four years until the final product would be released.

But there is something that needs to be made crystal clear. It was in that first year of development that the "Young Turks" would establish the basic form and content of this new manual. When it was released to a wider audience it was for refinement, not for a foundational critique of the basic model they developed. Even today, in the midst of development of DSM V and after years of controversy and massive criticism from all sides, the basic form of the manual and its grounding in what you have learned in this book is the "technological attitude" or "scientism" has, and never will change! That is why I am asking you to be afraid of psychiatry. Its "scientistic" foundation was set in place 36 years ago and despite revisions and modifications, its core reductionistic and dehumanizing perspective remains unchanged. Couple this with the meteoric rise of corporate influence and greed and...well you'll see.

Let's get back to Spitzer and his core group of allies in 1974. During the heady days of the development of DSM III (and later DSM III-R) nothing got into those books without Spitzer's input and approval. So really, in some sense, what you are continuously exposed to in your everyday life, what psychiatrists, counselors and psychologists tell you is "wrong" with you, your spouse your parent or child, is grounded in the vision of this one man, a man whose perspective was itself grounded in a core belief of scientism, the *possibility* of a rational and logical uncontaminated *objectivity*. That is why Dr. Sadler named his book ***values*** *and psychiatric diagnosis.* His goal was to carefully and convincingly argue that because there is no such thing as a value-free, uncontaminated view of reality, then the DSM III project was fatally flawed from the start. But let's look at how Spitzer and his colleagues tried to attain this objectivity and how it has resulted in the out of control psychiatric diagnostic practices we see today.

The foundational concept in DSM III was to create a manual that described the presentation of mental disorders while remaining absolutely neutral on the causes of them. The term often used for this is "atheoretical" but it is also sometimes described as "value-free." Now let us consider what DSM III was charged with categorizing:

1. Cognitive,
2. Behavioral and
3. Emotional abnormalities and disorders in human beings.

Implicit in any definition of "abnormal" is a pre-supposed clear-cut concept of "normal." So here is your first big clue as to why DSM objectivity is an illusion. Who (or what) determines what constitutes *normal* human thinking, behavior and emotions to set the standard by which *abnormality* is defined? Somebody is making a value judgment here, clear and simple. Let's look at an everyday example, the concept of a "workaholic." We've all heard this term being used. It is not a DSM mental disorder but it does describe a certain type of person. Is it normal or abnormal to be a workaholic? According to recently published data Americans take the fewest vacation days of any Western country and work the longest hours. Is that a good thing or a bad thing? Is it abnormal to be a country full of workaholics or is it an adaptive advantage? Can you see how there is not a neutral value and judgment free stance from which to figure out the answer? Whatever answer you give will clearly reflect the values and beliefs underlying that answer. So why should it be different when you or anyone else is asked to distinguish abnormal from normal behaviors or emotional states? You cannot categorize mental "disorders" without an underlying value-laden definition of mental normality. I'll bet you that some parents are already going "Aha, that's right" as they examine their struggle with the issue of whether the rambunctious and disruptive behavior in school by their son is just "boys being boys" or signs of a serious mental disorder; a tragic struggle that sometimes goes way beyond a mere difference of opinion when school officials insist that your child be medicated or suspended. Okay, we are already establishing that Spitzer and his colleagues could not be truly "objective" so let's examine how they tried and what that resulted in.

What Spitzer and his colleagues tried to do was develop a system of categorization (also called"taxonomy") that would be grounded in the description of observable clusters of "signs and symptoms." But what categories would be used in the classification scheme? Which signs and symptoms should be lumped together and what "disorder" would this define? These are tough questions. In fact it forces us to pause and ask; how exactly does *anyone* create any system of classification? Philosophers have thought about this a lot. Here is a contribution to the issue from Michel Foucault from his book, *The Order of Things* (Foucault 1970). As an example of a historically legitimate but clearly bizarre categorization of animals Foucault quotes a list he found in a Chinese encyclopedia:

- belonging to the emperor
- embalmed
- tame
- suckling pigs
- sirens
- fabulous
- stray dogs
- included in the present classification
- frenzied
- innumerable

- drawn with a very fine camel hair brush
- etcetera
- having just broken the water pitcher
- that from a long way off look like flies

Is this for real? Foucault says so. At the time it was written it probably paid to know which animals belonged to the emperor. It was dangerous not to. The primary reason Foucault cited this categorization of animals was to demonstrate that a certain degree of arbitrariness exists in any system of classification, it is inescapable. So an important question to ask is how a particular system of classification meets the needs of or promotes the point of view of the person or persons who develop it. What if I asked you to develop a *personal* set of categories for animals? Not "scientific", just personal. Would it be ridiculous or bizarre to come up with something like this?

- animals I would have as a pet
- animals I would definitely not have as a pet
- animals I know I'm allergic to
- dangerous animals
- animals I've never seen
- animals I'd like to see
- snakes…Brrrrr

No, there is nothing bizarre about this. This is a reasonable set of categories for an individual. In fact you might just run through a list like this in your head if your kids ask for a pet for Christmas or friends invite you to a whale-watching cruise. But what if you were asked to come up with a *scientifically valid* way to classify animals or, for that matter, mental disorders? That would be a lot more challenging and should clearly be left to the "experts." Remember, every "regime of truth" needs their cadre of experts. In pre-selecting his particular group of "experts" Robert Spitzer (unknowingly?) set the stage for the dominance of the biopsychiatry "regime of truth" that we see today.

There is a catchy phrase used in science. It refers to the process of classifying things in direct relation to "objective" reality. The phrase used is "carving nature at the joints", referring to a natural way to separate wholes into meaningful parts. Because DSM III was created by scientists, this was their idealistic goal as well. Separate mental disorders into syndromes and categories that reflect natural reality, uncontaminated by subjective judgment. In fact, in the ideal taxonomy, the necessity of human judgment would be reduced to the barest minimum. Right off the bat the framers of DSM violate this principle. Let me quote from the introduction to the book (actually from DSM III-R) where they address the problem we just discussed, distinguishing normal from abnormal in human emotions and behaviors:

> In DSM III-R each of the mental disorders is *conceptualized* as a *clinically significant* behavioral or psychological syndrome or pattern that occurs in a person and that is associated with present *distress* (a *painful* symptom) or *disability* (*impairment* in one or more *important* areas of functioning) or with a *significantly* increased risk of suffering death, *pain*, *disability* or an *important* loss of *freedom*. In addition, this syndrome must not be *merely* an *expectable* response to a particular event e.g. loss of a loved one. Whatever its original cause, it must currently be *considered* a manifestation of a behavioral, psychological, or biological *dysfunction* in the person (DSM III-R 1987, p.xxii, italics mine).

Perhaps you can see why I subtitled this chapter good intentions, bad outcome. As the saying goes Spitzer and his colleagues "gave it the old college try." But as you can clearly see in the words I italicized above, subjective value judgments infect every concept that forms the foundation of their entire diagnostic process, i.e. distinguishing the category of normal versus abnormal mental functioning, behaviors and emotions. It is simply inescapable. The terrible consequences of not openly acknowledging this is where the real problems with medical model psychiatry begin. Before I go further in elaborating these consequences (and supporting my warning for you to "be afraid") let me take you on a tour of DSM so you will understand more clearly the basis on which psychiatric diagnoses are made. I am going to shift over now to DSM IV because it is the diagnostic manual currently in use. It really doesn't differ that much from DSM III and DSM III-R even though Dr. Spitzer is no longer in charge. (If the history and politics of the development of the DSM's is of great interest to you I will have some references in the appendix for some really good books on the topic).

DSM IV was published in 1994. There is no "author" cited; it is simply "published by the American Psychiatric Association." This creates the appearance that the book reflects the collective wisdom of American psychiatry and lends great weight and authority to this text around the world. DSM IV is 886 pages long and costs $84.00. There are 365 separate mental disorders listed (DSM I, in 1952, contained 107). I'm sure it will be no surprise that each successive manual delineates a greater number of mental disorders than its immediate predecessor. (Name one thing that gets simplified as it gets revised in our "rationalized" culture). The book begins with a rather lengthy introduction that both justifies the manual while at the same time apologizing that it couldn't be better, i.e. even more scientifically rigorous. Each successive manual also goes to great lengths to argue that the current version is a vast improvement over the previous manual and a lot of science "power words" like empirical validation are thrown in to reinforce this claim. But to my eye there is actually very little change from one manual to the next. The basic concept of the existence of a discrete number of psychiatric illnesses that can be clearly identified by a characteristic set of observable symptoms *and* are separable from the context in which they appear, has not changed at all. The other thing that hasn't changed at all is something less tangible but still very real; it's how the sheer heft and physical appearance of the book along with its organization and content communicates a strong message of (to borrow a term from Steven Colbert) "truthiness." It's no accident that this text has been likened to the Bible and other canonical texts (even by its critics).

There are two cautionary statements in the introduction that merit our attention. The first is this: "The specific diagnostic criteria included in DSM IV are meant to serve as guidelines to be informed by clinical judgment and are not meant to be used in a cookbook fashion" (DSM-IV 1994, p.xxiii). I see two red flags here: The first is the recommendation for the use of "clinical judgment?" Okay, I'll bite; what the heck is that? What does the adjective "clinical" mean? We see this word used as an adjective frequently in psychiatric literature. Perhaps you've heard the term "clinical depression." Aside from lending the word depression a medical "feel" what makes a depression clinical? (Let me tell you, I am just getting started with this stuff. By the time I'm finished deconstructing medical model psychiatry you are going to see how it resembles Walt Disney World more than it resembles a medical science. Just hang on, we'll get there). Next question: *whose* judgment is clinical? What are the required qualifications to be able to make a "clinical" judgment? Do you see how these vague words loosen the edges of the DSM diagnostic system, allowing a certain freedom and flexibility to cover its deficiencies and lack of true scientific rigor? The second red flag in this statement is that the founders of the DSM model of psychiatric diagnosis felt compelled to warn us not to use it in a cookbook fashion. There can be only one reason to issue such a caution and that is that the DSM lends itself so perfectly to *being* used in a cookbook fashion. In fact, despite the admonishment by the authors, to call how DSM is being used today as a "cookbook" would be generous. Cookbooks require attention to detail and some recipes can be quite complex. With the proliferation of simplistic DSM derived checklists being so widely used to make psychiatric diagnoses today it would be more accurate to say that DSM is being used like a "2 minute microwaveable meal." Paradoxically, using truncated, cookbook-like checklist diagnostic assessment tools based on the DSM was pioneered by Robert Spitzer himself when he created Prime MD for Pfizer Pharmaceuticals to promote the use of the antidepressant Zoloft. How do I know about this? I was a speaker on that promotional tour with him (more about Prime MD later).

The second cautionary statement comes from DSM IV from a page titled, interestingly enough, "Cautionary Statement." I am not going to reproduce the entire cautionary statement here, just one sentence. It reads: "The proper use of these criteria requires specialized clinical training that provides both a body of knowledge and clinical skills" (DSM IV 1994, p.xxvii). I have seen a number of patients in my office who carry the diagnosis and are taking medication for bipolar disorder even though they don't agree with the diagnosis. Asked about this they invariably tell me that a doctor made the diagnosis without really explaining it in any detail and when they looked it up on the internet, did not think that the description matched their problems. Those who had the courage to request a clarification from the doctor were often shot down by a statement such as "I am the doctor" or appeased by some sort of explanation such as the one cited in chapter one that "you have mild bipolar spectrum disorder." You know what? This cautionary statement that only a highly trained professional could know how to utilize the DSM manual is a bunch of elitist hogwash. This truly *is not* rocket science. It is a proposed diagnostic system for emotional and behavioral problems that anyone with a decent education could understand and has a right to argue against when they are the ones getting the label attached to their name in some computer system. That is, of course, unless you are too young to understand the implications of a mental illness diagnosis, such as the schoolchildren getting diagnosed as bipolar by "experts" in the field.

DSM IV is a complicated book. After all you can't fill 886 pages with nothing. So there is quite a bit of information in this book ranging from complex instructions on how to use the five axis diagnostic system to an appendix listing the corresponding ICD 10 codes that fit DSM IV codes. Numbers, numbers, numbers; what would we do without numbers? Fortunately I can spare you about 95% of what the DSM IV text contains because what matters most to doctors and to you is simply the Axis I diagnosis. These are the "mental disorders" diagnoses (unless someone is diagnosing a personality disorder because that goes on Axis II). The diagnosable disorders are organized into 17 categories such as Sleep Disorders, Eating Disorders, and Anxiety Disorders and so on. Within each category there are a variable number of specific disorders that fit the category. For example Panic Disorder, Obsessive Compulsive Disorder and Social Phobia are among the specific disorders under the general heading of Anxiety Disorders. In each general category there is often a lengthy explanation of the shared features of disorders within that category. For example, the difference between drug abuse and drug dependence is fully explained before going onto specific drug abuse or dependence diagnoses. Same goes for mood disorders. It can get pretty complicated to really use this manual with precision. But don't worry, hardly anybody does. What are actually used in the everyday world are the diagnostic criteria that describe the symptoms of each mental disorder. I am sure this is getting a little confusing so before we go any further let me simply list the diagnostic criteria for Major Depression and you'll see what I am talking about. From page 327 of DSM IV here are the diagnostic criteria for an "episode" of Major Depression. Take a deep breath, it's pretty long:

Criteria for Major Depressive Episode

A. Five (or more) of the following symptoms have been present during the same 2-week period and represent a change from previous functioning; at least one of the symptoms is either (1) depressed mood or (2) loss of interest or pleasure.

Note: Do not include symptoms that are clearly due to a general medical condition, or mood-incongruent delusions or hallucinations.

1. depressed mood most of the day, nearly every day, as indicated by either subjective report (e.g., feels sad or empty) or observation made by others (e.g. appears tearful). **Note:** In children and adolescents, can be irritable mood.
2. markedly diminished interest or pleasure in all, or almost all, activities most of the day, nearly every day (as indicated by either subjective account or observation made by others)
3. significant weight loss when not dieting or weight gain (e.g., a change of more than 5% of body weight in a month), or decrease or increase in appetite nearly every day. **Note:** In children, consider failure to make expected weight gains.
4. insomnia or hypersomnia nearly every day
5. psychomotor agitation or retardation nearly every day (observable by others, not merely subjective feelings of restlessness or being slowed down)
6. fatigue or loss of energy nearly every day
7. feelings of worthlessness or excessive or inappropriate guilt (which may be delusional) nearly every day (not merely self reproach or guilt about being sick)

8. diminished ability to think or concentrate, or indecisiveness, nearly every day (either by subjective account or as observed by others)
9. recurrent thoughts of death (not just fear of dying), recurrent suicidal ideation without a specific plan, or a suicide attempt or a specific plan for committing suicide

B. The symptoms do not meet criteria for a Mixed Episode (see p. 335)
C. The symptoms cause clinically significant distress or impairment in social, occupational, or other important areas of functioning.
D. The symptoms are not due to the direct physiological effects of a substance (e.g., a drug of abuse, a medication) or a general medical condition (e.g. hypothyroidism)
E. The symptoms are not better accounted for by Bereavement, i.e., after the loss of a loved one, the symptoms persist for longer than 2 months or are characterized by marked functional impairment, morbid preoccupation with worthlessness, suicidal ideation, psychotic symptoms, or psychomotor retardation.

Whew! I'm tired from just typing that. And this was all on one page of an 886 page book! Now here is a surprise. If you are making a diagnosis of Major Depression you are not done yet, there are two more number blanks to fill in. The diagnostic numerical code for a Major Depression is 296._ _. If you submit a diagnostic code of just 296 Medicare and Medicaid and most insurance companies will send your bill back without payment because all five blanks are not filled in. Blank four is where you record the course of the "illness." You choices are single episode (coded as 2) or recurrent (coded as 3). The fifth digit is used to record severity, 1 for mild, 2 for moderate, 3 for severe without psychotic features, 4 for severe with psychotic features (mood congruent or mood incongruent), 5 for in partial remission and 6 for in full remission. So for Major Depression the code can be 296.23 or 296.33 or 296.34 and so on. Before we proceed with deconstructing these diagnostic criteria (you had to know that was coming) I want to take a little detour into the world of numbers. You know who (or perhaps I should say what) loves numbers? *Computers* love numbers. How nice that the DSM provides all these numbers so computers can track, evaluate, classify, allow services, deny services and make myriad other decisions without bothering with any sticky details about the particular patient being analyzed.

Perhaps you were a little surprised by the fact that insurance companies won't pay the doctor unless they get the full 5 digit diagnosis. Well here's an even bigger surprise. The doctor who sees you will not get paid AT ALL if you end up with a diagnosis that isn't covered by the insurance plan and that even applies to the FIRST VISIT to a doctor who has never seen you before. Here is a common example. Major Depression, single episode, severe is coded 296.24. But you might also go to a doctor (especially under the influence of all the hyperbolic TV commercials about antidepressants) to seek relief when you are grieving the loss of a loved one. Bereavement is in fact mentioned on page 684 of DSM IV but it is not considered a mental disorder so there are no diagnostic criteria. It does however, have a diagnostic code. Bereavement's code is V62.82. (Yes, the "V" means something; we'll get to it shortly). In its single paragraph on the topic DSM IV does acknowledge that "some grieving individuals present with symptoms characteristic of a Major Depressive Episode." There are some clinical features listed that can be used to separate Major Depression from grief by looking for symptoms that are not characteristic of a "normal" grief reaction. (The scare quotation marks around the word normal are in DSM IV. Even the DSM writers must have realized that defining what constitutes normal grief was really overreaching). Nevertheless "abnormal" grief (by default major depression), is suspected if there is 1) guilt about things other than actions taken or not taken by the survivor at the time of death; 2) thoughts of death other than the survivor feeling that he or she would be better off dead or should have died with the deceased person; 3) morbid preoccupation with worthlessness; 4) marked psychomotor retardation; 5) prolonged and marked functional impairment; and 6) hallucinatory experiences other than thinking that he or she hears the voice of, or transiently sees the image of, the deceased person. (Spitzer and company sure like to make lists). As usual DSM does not "personalize" their evaluation by mentioning incidental facts like how the loss of an eight year old child might lead to a different and more prolonged grief reaction than the loss of a 95 year old mother with a ten year history of Alzheimer's Disease; or how the nature of the pre-death relationship to the deceased might affect the degree of guilt and worthlessness felt by the mourner. I bet you that some readers have seen enough! "DSM is nuts!" they are saying to themselves right now. But stick with me because it only gets "better" and there is so much more you need to learn.

The next God-like pronouncement from our authors of DSM IV defines *how long* normal grief should last before it is considered to have converted to Major Depression, drum roll please...that number is two months. Yes, they give a precise figure. After two months of mourning you should be pulling it together or you have developed a mental disorder requiring treatment. (I remember when that figure used to be six months and don't know why they changed it, although I would suspect some pharmaceutical company influence was involved). I am not even going to comment here, just let this percolate in your mind a bit. Okay, there are two issues about this I do want to discuss. The first is spiritual. Maybe I'm truly old fashioned but I've always felt that the pain and suffering of the mourner, at least in part, is a marker of the love felt for the person who died. It honors their memory. Calling that state Major Depression (a brain dysfunction based medical condition) completely deflates that spiritual dimension of loss and grief by the reduction of the death of a loved one to simply a "stressor" that "precipitated" an episode of Major Depression (a lot more about spiritual issues later in the book). The second has to do with the aforementioned V codes. There are a lot of V codes in DSM IV's diagnostic system. They are listed under the general heading of "Other Conditions That May Be a Focus of Clinical Attention." Translation: Reasons you might come to a mental health provider other than having a psychiatric illness. This is a good thing! V codes include many common problems such as bereavement, parent-child relational problem, partner relational problem, adult antisocial behavior and so on. There are 25 V code diagnoses in DSM IV, including the diagnosis "No Diagnosis on Axis I" (code V71.09). That appears to be a very good thing, allowing healthcare professionals an opportunity to say "I examined this patient and find that there is no psychiatric disorder present." By the way, that doesn't automatically mean that the patient does not require or would not benefit from professional help. But it certainly most often has the result that they don't get any professional help because most insurance companies do not pay for ANY service if the diagnosis is a V Code. And, to reiterate, that even includes the very first visit when the mental health professional has no idea why that person made an appointment or what the problem is.

Okay, so let's be painfully realistic now. What do you think happens? Do you think everyone does the noble thing? Let me rephrase that: Do you think *anyone* does the noble thing, sticks to their conviction that there is no mental disorder, and submits a V code diagnosis while informing the patient that their insurance will not cover that visit so please pay your $200 on the way out? I remember one time when I tried it on a hospitalized patient; I diagnosed Bereavement instead of Major Depression as the reason for admission. Guess who hounded me mercilessly to change my diagnosis? The hospital! They were not getting paid and the patient didn't have the money to pay. Obviously the expeditious thing to do is just give a reimbursable diagnosis code. So you are officially saying the patient is mentally ill; big deal, at least the patient gets professional help and everyone is getting paid. Perhaps the framers of DSM III could not have anticipated this but the V code distinction remained unchanged in DSM IV when this dilemma was already well known.

Gwen (not her real name of course) was new to my practice. As I was writing this, I had only seen her on two occasions. However, I was lucky enough to get detailed psychiatric records on her dating back some fifteen years. She presented to me with a diagnosis of...try to guess...what could it be?...you got it...Bipolar Disorder! She was fifty years old and had just recently moved to the area. Her medications were a mood stabilizer (Lithium), an antidepressant (Effexor) and a second generation antipsychotic also approved for bipolar disorder (Zyprexa). I took my history. There was one brief psychiatric hospitalization 20 years ago. No arrests or incarcerations ever (this is an important question in assessing if someone has Bipolar type I disorder because when they are manic they usually end up in a hospital or jail. It's pretty tough to be as crazy as Bipolar I disorder patients get and escape public notice). All of her psychiatric care had been outpatient and included both medication and psychotherapy. Since I was in the midst of writing this book I asked her a couple of questions about the consequences of her bipolar diagnosis (since I already strongly suspected it was bogus and, surprisingly, so did she). Here were the consequences she reported: She had trouble getting life insurance and it cost more. She could not get *health insurance from the same HMO that was covering her when she got the diagnosis by one of their doctors. Talk about irony! She had gained 30 pounds since starting the Zyprexa about 2 years previous. (More about weight gain on psychiatric medications in chapter seven). Finally, I mentioned to her how some doctors tell patients that bipolar disorder is just like diabetes and that they will have to be on medications for life and she said "That's* ***exactly*** *what my doctor told me."*

I will come back to Gwen's case in chapter four when I get into the nitty-gritty about the bipolar diagnosis. For now, how about a little joke?

Q: How do you get mental illness diagnosis from a psychiatrist?
A: Make an appointment.

Not so funny when you think about how a cavalier or temporarily economically advantageous diagnosis of a mental disorder can come back to haunt you in places like, say for example, a court battle over child custody or application for health insurance. I was once the consulting psychiatrist for Embry Riddle University in Daytona Beach. A lot of people go there to train to be pilots. I rarely saw any consultations from Embry Riddle because a diagnosis of depression, especially if treated with medication, means no pilot license. I know that every medical license application I've filled out as a doctor asks specifically if I have ever been diagnosed with and/or treated for a mental disorder. All of a sudden that revision of the Axis I diagnosis to a reimbursable code doesn't look so benign anymore. But wait, we are not done with numbers yet! There is yet another list of numbers in DSM IV directly linked to reimbursement to the provider, indication for inpatient care, number of services allotted and even qualification for disability. It's called Axis V.

On Axis V we are asked to give the Global Assessment of Functioning or GAF score. The range is from 1 to 100; the higher the number, the higher the "level of function." I will not torture you with another wordy and confusing list from DSM. Here are a few highlights: 90 to 100 is a superior functioning person who is "sought out by others because of his or her many positive qualities" (Leonardo DaVinci, Oprah, George Clooney?) 0 to 10 is a "persistent danger of hurting self or others." 41 to 50 is "serious symptoms"; 51 to 60 "moderate symptoms"; 61 to 70 "some mild symptoms" and so on. I wish they had never invented Axis V or would just get rid of it because I am tired of being asked about GAF scores. Anytime I turn in a treatment plan, fill out a history and physical or answer questions on a disability form I almost always have to come up with three numbers: the current GAF, the GAF at the time of admission or on the first visit and the highest GAF for the past year. I've got to go shuffling back through my records to see what arbitrary number I picked on the first visit, totally make up a number for the "highest functioning" question and then look up the GAF page in the DSM to remind myself what they mean so I can fill out something reasonable for the current GAF. Of course I have to juggle all of this with my best guess as to the motivation of whoever is asking for the GAF score. What the framers of DSM III and the current head honchos seem to naively ignore is that when you give someone a number score, no matter how arbitrarily assigned, some bureaucracy is going to take those numbers seriously. Bureaucracies love numbers because you can just plug them into equations and arrive at decisions in a split second without any of those pesky humans who want "details" getting in the way. Of course this can backfire on the bureaucracy if the person submitting the GAF secretly learns about the rules of the game. True life story: Mental health professionals quickly learned that Medicaid would deem an inpatient hospitalization "medically necessary" (would pay for it) only if the admission GAF was lower than 40 (a step below "serious symptoms"). How long do you think it took the hospitals to "instruct" their admission staff to make sure admission GAF's were below 40 on all newly admitted patients? I am not saying the admissions staff was told to be sure that if, after careful and conscientious evaluation, the patient's GAF was above 40 then they should not be admitted and be referred to outpatient instead; I am saying that all patients admitted should have a GAF below 40…wink, wink. The GAF is terrible and should just be eliminated!

Let's turn now to a deconstruction of the diagnostic criteria for Major Depression. I am not going to insult you by reprinting the criteria and italicize all of the words requiring subjective judgment by the patient, the doctor, or both. It's just too obvious how values and beliefs infect every aspect of diagnosis to go over them sentence by sentence. You can see how the authors did their best to try to lend some "objectivity" to the diagnostic criteria by including time factors (two weeks), minimal numbers of symptoms (at least five of the following) and the severity adjectives "clinically significant impairment." (That's two of my favorite science obfuscation adjectives in a row, clinical and significant). Recall though that a deconstructive reading also looks at what wasn't said, what wasn't included in a text and why; so why these particular symptoms and not others? Why not uncontrollable bouts of crying for instance? Why not irritability? What about physical pain? (See Cymbalta in chapter six). Why two weeks, not one or three? Why five symptoms, not four or six? Why should weight loss or gain earn a place "at the table", especially in a society so preoccupied with eating and dieting? Of course I could go on and on. And finally, why is the description of the course and symptoms of a Major Depression in DSM IV essentially unchanged since DSM III published sixteen years earlier? We didn't have *any* breakthrough discoveries in sixteen years that could lend more specificity and accuracy to that diagnosis? Can you see how much clearer the problems and weaknesses of a text reveal themselves in a deconstructive reading?

I believe I can offer a reasonably comprehensive answer to all of the questions I've raised. The diagnostic criteria and diagnostic categories were derived and have remained essentially unchanged in the twenty-six years since the publication of DSM III because, basically, whether they are **valid**, i.e. *describe an* ***actual cellular mediated*** *human disease* is not the primary focus or concern of the DSM III model of classification of mental disorders. It never was! The framers and followers of the DSM III model of psychiatric diagnosis did not prioritize the question of the validity of psychiatric diagnoses, they prioritized reliability. Remember the list of the faculty in my residency and their widely divergent perspectives on mental illness? You'd be lucky to get that group to agree that the sky is blue, let alone what's wrong with a particular patient. This eclecticism was the state of psychiatry for a couple of decades after psychoanalysis lost its exclusive grip on the field. Psychiatry was losing its identity as a medical subspecialty. It didn't help when its lack of medical precision was displayed for the whole country during the trial of John Hinckley for his assassination attempt on President Reagan. The attorneys were able to find world-class forensic psychiatrists holding diametrically opposing views on whether John Hinckley was insane or not. It was time to get psychiatrists onto the same page. So the framers of the new DSM model focused on *reliability* by developing a strategy for diagnosis that would maximize what psychiatrists could generally agree about (descriptions of psychiatric symptoms) while minimizing what they disagreed about (the cause of those symptoms and how to treat them). The basic concern of reliability can be summed up this way: If you have the same patient assessed by one humdred psychiatrists, how many of them would come up with the same diagnosis? That is a measure of reliability. Now, whether there is something actually "wrong" with that person, that's a completely different matter.

Recall my example about the workaholic. I could easily come up with a list of diagnostic criteria for "workaholism", put it in DSM IV and then send a "workaholic" to 100 psychiatrists for a diagnostic assessment and find that my "workaholism" diagnostic category had a high level of reliability. Does that IN ANY WAY make it true that workaholism is a mental illness or disorder? No, of course it doesn't. Reliability has next to nothing to do with validity. But, as you will plainly see throughout this book, that by stepping around, stepping over and generally avoiding that crucial fact, DSM medical psychiatry has managed to attain a high degree of what could only be called pseudo-validity as a classification of brain based diseases that present as mental disorders.

But you know what? I care about validity. I care about it A LOT. I have to because I am not a researcher running studies on rat brains in a lab or doing university-based efficacy studies on some new drug. I'm on the front lines trying to figure out what to do about patients with their incredibly complicated life stories, long psychiatric histories, multiple failed treatments and painful emotional problems that are now looking to me for answers. That is where I crave validity and certainty as much as a gastroenterologist or cardiologist craves them. But I can't have them; because psychiatry isn't the same kind of science as gastroenterology or cardiology. In fact, in my eyes, psychiatry isn't a science at all. Karl Popper is a well known philosopher of science. (Not everyone agrees with him. There's never been a philosopher that everyone agrees with). But Popper is widely respected and I like his definition of what makes a science legitimate. In essence, he believes that what defines a discipline as a science is the potential disprovability of its hypotheses and theories (Popper 2002). Lacking the possibility of being disproven, then no finding can be said to be true with certainty. You can perform an experiment one thousand times with the same outcome and then on experiment one thousand and one something different results. Look, I even confuse myself when I try to explain this so let me tell you the illustrative story I tell my patients when I try to explain to them how and why psychiatry is not a medical science and that a diagnosis of bipolar disorder is not "just like a diagnosis of diabetes" even if their previous psychiatrist used those exact words. The story goes like this:

You get a phone call from school about your eight year old daughter's behavior problems. You meet with the counselor who suggests an evaluation by a child psychologist the school uses. You take your daughter to the psychologist and are pleased to see degrees from Emory University and Vanderbilt on the walls. This psychologist "specializes" in the evaluation of ADD in both children and adults. He spends half a day administering a battery of psychological tests and then calls you in to share the results. You are told your daughter clearly has ADD. You protest because you've never seen her bouncing off the walls like her male classmates but are reassured by the psychologist that ADD in girls often presents as merely inattention and daydreaming without any hyperactivity. He recommends a program of behavior therapy described in a book he has written as well as stimulant medication that her pediatrician can prescribe. But you are the cautious type and decide you want a second opinion before you just jump right into putting your daughter on Ritalin. Besides, you are a little concerned that because the psychologist was recommended by the school, he might have been prejudiced towards medication.

So you do your homework and get the name of a board certified child psychiatrist whose practice is in a nearby city. You check the board of medicine website and are pleased to see that this doctor is a woman (you are not sure why but somehow that feels "safer" to you). You are also very pleased to see that she attended medical school at Yale and did her child fellowship at Johns Hopkins. So an appointment is made. Two hours are scheduled for the examination which includes a family interview of you and your husband as well as a comprehensive examination of your daughter. The psychiatrist seems very nice and asks you and your husband a long list of questions and has you fill out a comprehensive questionnaire. (There seem to be an awful lot of questions about history of mental illnesses in any of your relatives). The psychiatrist also reviews the test results from the first psychologist. Finally, you are called into the office so the doctor can tell you what she has found. In a soft and soothing voice the doctor tells you that your daughter is suffering from bipolar disorder, also called manic-depressive disease. WHAT!!! Your head starts to spin. You are not 100% sure what manic depressive disease is but you know that you have a crazy brother who has been in and out of psychiatric hospitals and, although you haven't spoken to him in years, the diagnosis bipolar disorder sounds familiar. But that just can't be. Your daughter isn't crazy, she's nothing at all like your drug abusing lunatic of a brother. You gather yourself enough to ask the doctor why the other doctor did all those tests and diagnosed ADD and are informed that psychiatrists are just beginning to recognize that childhood bipolar disorder is often mistakenly diagnosed as ADD. Sometimes kids "have both."

The doctor then goes on to explain about the medications used to treat bipolar disorder but by now your head is spinning and you can't think straight. You ask the doctor for permission to think this over and make a follow-up appointment to discuss meds. The doctor agrees but warns you not to wait too long because untreated bipolar disorder is a dangerous condition and can result in suicide if not promptly and properly treated. "Jesus Christ", you think to yourself. You know your daughter tends to be moody and throws some pretty dramatic temper tantrums, but mentally ill, manic depressive, how can that be? But this doctor is from Yale and Johns Hopkins, she must know what she is talking about.

That evening you share your tale of woe with your sister-in-law and best friend. You are a little shocked to find that they've been hearing about a lot of kids being diagnosed bipolar but then your friend injects a note of caution. She says that her sister in Philadelphia has a seven year old daughter who the doctor also diagnosed as bipolar but that they sought a second opinion from a psychologist who specializes in family therapy and said that after about ten therapy sessions with him "everybody was better" with no medication at all. She promises to call her sister and tell her to ask her psychologist for a local referral. So the following week the whole family including your eleven year old son goes for a three hour appointment with a family psychologist recommended by the therapist in Philadelphia. You are pleased (but getting a little confused) to see he has degrees from UCLA and Emory. All of the professionals you're seeing are from top notch schools; how come they don't agree with each other's diagnoses? And this third doctor doesn't "disappoint" you either. "There is nothing wrong with your daughter", he announces. "I am so glad you didn't let them label and medicate her." He suggests a twelve session course in family therapy and guarantees a positive outcome. You again ask for some time to think it over. Yeah it's great to think that there is nothing wrong with your daughter's brain but what if the family psychologist is wrong and she should be on medication? If she has ADD then without meds she will not do her best in school. And, you've read, she will be more prone to drug abuse and sexual experimentation. (Where was that article; was it Ladies Home Journal or Reader's Digest?) But what about untreated bipolar? The psychiatrist warned that not treating early onset bipolar disorder could result in irreversible damage to her brain. What a mess. Well that's about all the thinking you can do about this today. You need some down time so you settle back to watch your favorite TV show: House.

You've watched House enough times now to pretty much know what's going to happen: exotic life threatening disease repeatedly mistakenly diagnosed and treated (often with a treatment that can kill the patient) until finally the moment of epiphany (usually when House is bouncing his oversize tennis ball) followed by racing down the hall to institute the life saving therapy just in the nick of time. House is never wrong, never. Sure wish you could find a doctor like that for your daughter. Just then YOU have an epiphany. House is wrong ALL THE TIME. He is the one who also makes all the mistaken diagnoses and institutes treatment that can nearly kill the patient. How does he realize his diagnosis is wrong and change course? Of course: it's when the lab results, biopsy, toxicology report or MRI results come in. Yet your daughter didn't have any lab tests or X-rays or biopsies. She had a lot of "testing", especially by the ADD specialist, but it didn't resolve anything. You are still sitting here anguishing about what expert to believe. Why can't they solve it? Maybe you can get them all in one room and force them to PROVE they are right or at least DISPROVE the others are right. The psychiatrist said that bipolar disorder is caused by a chemical imbalance in the brain, the ADD psychologist likened ADD to faulty wiring. Can't they measure the chemicals to see if they are in or out of balance? Can't they check the "wiring" to see if it's faulty or not?

Good questions and totally reasonable. The answer, in a word, is no! Psychiatry is not a science in the same way that gastroenterology is a science or that cardiology is a science because both of those (and all the other medical specialties) have something that psychiatry doesn't, a much clearer understanding of how the *structure* of the organ (heart, kidneys, liver) results in the *function* of that organ. As Dr. House busily scrambles around trying to pin down the diagnosis, all of those lab, X-ray and pathology reports he gets are telling him whether what he suspects is true or not. "Hmm, liver function tests are all normal, so this can't be hepatitis," he says. "Go CT scan her belly!" The liver function tests he ordered are a quantitative evaluation of how many liver enzyme molecules are in the blood. These enzymes are contained almost exclusively in liver cells so that if their levels are elevated, we know that liver cells have been damaged and spilled their enzymes in the circulating blood. And we also know what will happen if the liver fails. Because we know how the liver works! We know what the cells in the liver do and how they do it. We know how to evaluate the liver and have many options, from blood tests to ultrasounds to biopsies. And when someone has symptoms that look just like liver disease, we can also *prove* that the liver is *not* the cause (through those very same testing procedures) and look elsewhere for the cause of the symptoms. So in the definition of science we are discussing we can disprove the hypothesis that there is liver disease even if the symptoms strongly suggest it is. That is what makes gastroenterology a "science" in Popper's terms.

What our anguishing mother realized after visiting the three top-notch mental health specialists and getting three highly divergent diagnoses is that despite all the talk about chemical imbalances and damaged circuits, in psychiatry there is something REALLY BIG missing. And she is right. What is totally lacking in psychiatry is that essential understanding about the relationship of brain structure to brain function. I'm telling you, this is the truth! I don't care what you are hearing about the limbic system, the frontal cortex, the reptilian brain, PET Scans, functional MRI's, hunger centers, pleasure centers or religion neurons; it's true. And I can prove it to you right now. The subject matter of psychiatry is the higher level brain functions of cognition, motivation, emotion, perception etc. The general term that we use to describe the miraculous simultaneous operation of these higher functions is consciousness! I challenge you to find one person who can explain in clear terms HOW the billions of interconnected neurons firing off tiny electrical impulses results in what we directly experience as consciousness? You can look all you want, but you won't find anyone with the answer. Sure theories abound, educated guesses, highly complex stories of neural nets, quantum mechanics and parallel processing; those you will find. But those are just guesses, and so far, not very fruitful ones. (Just trace the history of AI, artificial intelligence, to see what I mean. I'll have some references for those interested at the back of the book. You can also read about consciousness and the brain in a well written series of articles in the January 29, 2007 issue of Time Magazine. In there you will see that the top scholars in neurobiology and cognitive science agree on one fundamental fact, we do not now and may never know how the brain produces consciousness. And these are the top scientists in the year 2007. Psychiatry has been doing it's "as if" thing since 1980).

For our purposes this is what I want you to understand: No matter how many times the DSM is revised, no matter how "reliable" it gets in the sense of describing clusters of "symptoms" that professionals will agree on and be able to "reliably" separate out and see in their patients, without VALIDITY, it is just a sophisticated guessing game subject to the whims of professional opinion and political agendas (one day homosexuality is a mental illness, the next day it is not), to professional rivalries and faddish beliefs (one doctor "sees" ADD in most of his patients, another "sees" Bipolar Spectrum), economic competition (between therapists, hypnotists, doctors, psychologists, fundamentalists, 12 Steppers and more), and most frighteningly (and also most clearly) subjected to the economic forces that shape our marketplace and control the "regimes of truth" that we are exposed to and come to believe. Remember discourse control from chapter one? That is what we are talking about here. Our frantic mother is trapped by the power and exclusivity of the medical model discourse into making life defining decisions for her daughter and no one can provide a shred of legitimate scientific evidence whether there is a physical brain disorder or not. I suppose she could take her daughter to one hundred highly trained mental health experts and choose the diagnosis and treatment plan that the highest number of doctors recommend. But she will not get to see a television image of an ulcer like she could at a gastroenterologist or see an X-ray image of a clogged coronary artery like she could at the cardiologists. So how is it that the general public and many doctors believe that a diagnosis of bipolar disorder IS like a diagnosis of a medical illness like diabetes? Because of a process I am going to describe to you right now, a process called reification.

Over the course of history human beings created words to describe their feelings. Among the many words used to describe unhappiness were words like melancholic, down, hopeless, demoralized, bummed out, sad, etc. etc. Depression was one of those words too. Then, as Nietzsche pointed out, words used to describe a person's unique individual experience can evolve into a "concept" that tries to capture shared elements of the original experience which "simultaneously has to fit countless more or less similar cases—which means, purely and simply cases which are never equal and thus altogether unequal." Here Nietzsche is focusing primarily on the evolution of language. But if we turn to the social function of language we can see that there is yet another step in the evolution of language and that is from a "concept" to a living, breathing reality. This evolutionary step is called reification, the most damaging dimension of our psychiatric diagnostic system's dissemination into our everyday culture and everyday language.

The dictionary defines reify as "convert (a person, abstraction etc.) into a thing; materialize." To expand on that, I like to think of reify as describing how a concept or idea in some person's mind becomes part of what we call reality. It is no longer perceived as an idea, it just "is", it exists as part of our shared, consensual reality. Just to prove that I am at least sometimes on the same page as the creators of the DSM model they too expressed concern about reification when they said in a paper published in 1991 that they were concerned with "the tendency for clinicians to apply the diagnostic system in a rote and religious fashion and force boundary patients into one or the other category" (Frances 1991).

Sadler defines the problem this way: "The idea with reification is that the abstract and hypothetical DSM categories are used as if they are 'real' genuine things in the world." "Within a reified practice of diagnosis DSM categories are assumed to be real things- diseases that are closely if not exactly analogous to pneumonia and myocardial infarction. Such a reified diagnostic practice wields diagnosis as a self-evident truth, and offers diagnosis as a salve of definitive knowledge. Reified diagnosis understands its object, the patient's disorder, only as a technological problem requiring a technological solution." And finally "the reified diagnosis is one that has penetrated into the everyday conceptual apparatus of the user…and appears without qualification in various and widespread social practices" (Sadler 2005, p.337). Do you recall the case history in chapter one about the guy diagnosed bipolar spectrum and ADD who ended up on sixteen pills a day? Then there was his overly involved mother who took him to his appointments, called his doctor, read his progress notes and occasionally had him committed involuntarily to the psychiatric hospital? All of the above mentioned aspects of reification are evident in this case. The patient was told he had a real disease (two actually) that accounted for all of his life problems and could be fixed by medications. This was, in Sadler's words, like a "salve of definitive knowledge", not to him, but to his mother. Further, this reified diagnosis *did* penetrate into the everyday conceptual apparatus of the user and into widespread social practices every time he obediently took his medication and also, more dramatically, when the police force and hospitals cooperated in the commitments initiated by his mother. Yes, you SHOULD be afraid. Because this is nuts! But it is real. You know I'm sure that communism looked like a really great idea at one time, on paper, as a concept emanating from some brilliant minds. But communism as an actual way to organize society, reified communism, a disaster! (See North Korea, Cuba and USSR).

So the framers of DSM express concern that their suggested diagnostic system not be used as if the concepts and hypotheses in it represent reality and that it be used as a guide by experienced clinicians to formulate individualized treatment plans, not as some sort of cookbook. Well guess what guys? TOO LATE! DSM *is* reified and it *is* used as a cookbook and the situation is getting worse by the day. Remember that the above mentioned patient was not diagnosed by his doctor as having bipolar disorder; he was diagnosed as having "mild bipolar spectrum" disorder. Well what the heck is that? It's not even in DSM IV. But I can tell you one thing with certainty; it is in MY MAIL nearly every day. Bipolar spectrum is one of the hot new topics in psychiatry today. It's in my mail in the form of invitations to conferences and article after article in various professional journals and papers. It's as popular a topic as Adult ADD. The number, scope and inclusiveness of reified DSM diagnoses is growing to the point that it is no longer hyperbole to speculate that there will be a mental disorder diagnosis for every man, woman and child in this country someday soon.

In the next chapter we will more fully examine the explosive growth and influence of medical model psychiatry by looking at how the growth in number and types of disorders is, in part, a necessity brought on by the medical model itself.

Chapter Four:
IF YOU ARE GOING TO LIE, MAKE SURE IT'S A GOOD ONE!
Diagnosis goes crazy

Every once in a while I like to watch the TV show *Cops.* What is especially amusing on that show is when one of the addicts, robbers or prostitutes they are busting tries to lie about what they were doing. The cops are used to this and are very good at asking more and more specific questions until the initial lie just falls apart. Although I find *Cops* to be more sad than funny, I do have to admit that the lies that are told to cover the other lies can get pretty far-fetched and amusing. In the title of this chapter I am metaphorically alluding to the medical model of psychiatric diagnosis as a sort of "lie" because I want to show you how the initial "lie" (that psychiatry is a medical science) keeps forcing psychiatry itself deeper and deeper into a corner where there is no choice but to keep coming up with more and more (often increasingly far fetched) "lies" to hold it all together and keep the whole system from collapsing. Only in this case, it is not the least bit amusing.

I'm not sure anyone involved in planning DSM III during the 1970's could have fully anticipated the impact and power this text would come to have. Some of the statements made by Robert Spitzer, however, presage the course things have taken. In working out the definition of a mental disorder Spitzer favored the concept of mental disorders being defined as a "subset of medical disorders" (Mayes 2005). He apparently wanted to include this precise language in the DSM III but non-MD mental health professionals vehemently protested and did manage to keep it out. So the words aren't there but the impact of this underlying principle has been the direct source of the growth and power of biopsychiatry. In the language you have learned in this book, what DSM III did was to attach the floundering and unfocused specialty of psychiatry directly to the *awesome* power of the "regime of truth" we call medicine. But, keep in mind, as we all learned in the movie Spiderman One: "With great power also comes great responsibility." It is in attempting to fulfill those responsibilities and meet the demands and requirements of a being a true medical science that psychiatry has spun so wildly and dangerously off course.

I am going to present a case history to illustrate my concern but first, a little personal information: During my eleven years in private practice (1997-2008) I had slowly but surely withdrawn into my own insulated world. I no longer saw hospital patients, stopped doing consults at medical hospitals and didn't accept capitated contracts with any HMO's. Eventually I no longer accepted any new Worker's Compensation or chronic pain patients and in my last year I severed my ties with two organizations, the Impaired Nurses Program (IPN) and the Physicians Resource Network (PRN).

I gave up many areas of my psychiatric practice because I didn't want anyone outside my practice judging me or telling me what to do (like when that hospital pestered me to change the diagnosis from bereavement to major depression). I found that in contrast to my perspective, nearly all doctors, non-MD mental health professionals and every agency, institution and bureaucracy inside and outside of psychiatry subscribe to the model of mental disorders as a "subset of medical disorders." Therefore, they naturally and *rightfully* expect psychiatry to act like any other branch of medicine and give pretty definitive answers to questions such as: What's wrong with the patient? They expect a description of the course, duration, treatment and prognosis that goes along with that diagnosis. They want definitive answers to questions about disability, about return to work dates, about whether they are safe to carry a gun (police officers) or perform surgery (physicians). That's part of the responsibility of belonging to the discourse of modern medicine, a responsibility that doctors, their patients and our society take quite seriously. That is why I withdrew from the above-mentioned areas of practice; I simply could no longer in good conscience give the definitive diagnoses, treatment plans, prognoses and assurances of safety that those institutions and agencies required. Let me share an actual case history with you that fully illustrates this problem. It involves a patient I took care of for four years and who had for the bulk of that time been monitored by PRN, the Physicians "Resource" Network. This case clearly shows how psychiatry attempts to fulfill its responsibilities as a medical science and what an incredible mess that can result in, even when, quite literally, lives are at stake. Understanding my goals in writing this book and having gone through what he did, my patient has graciously given me permission to share his story with you. I will, of course, protect his identity.

We'll call him Bill. I first saw Bill as a referral to me from the Physician's Resource Network in October of 2002. I got involved initially by receiving a phone call from the hospital in which this doctor worked. A "PRN certified" physician was required to render an opinion on this doctor's return to work status. Since his work involved delicate and dangerous surgical procedures and prescribing some pretty heavy-duty medications, this was not some minor or frivolous decision. It was a responsibility that I needed to take very seriously. And I did.

The event that triggered the need for a PRN evaluation had occurred about two months earlier. This doctor presented to the emergency room of his own hospital accompanied by his wife who was very concerned about his emotional and mental state. According to ER records the patient's chief complaint was exhaustion from lack of sleep after a weekend on call where he had gotten only two to four hours of sleep per night. He was evaluated and discharged from the emergency room after receiving clearance from the staff psychiatrist and getting treatment for elevated blood pressure. As he seemed to be deteriorating both mentally and physically his wife brought him back to the emergency room and he was then admitted to psychiatry. The emergency room records I have report that the patient was "calm and cooperative" and that his speech was "clear-coherent." His mood and affect were described as "flat-'exhausted'-guarded" while his thought process was "organized but with some paranoia re conspiracies against him." Finally, it is noted that he was having auditory hallucinations, hearing "the voice of God." So he was admitted to the psychiatric unit but only for a day because his treating psychiatrist felt that it would be best for him to be further evaluated and treated at a hospital in which he was not a staff physician. The diagnosis from this psychiatrist was bipolar disorder, manic with psychosis. That was on a Wednesday.

At the new hospital Bill started to experience chest pain and was put in a telemetry bed for monitoring so the staff psychiatrist initially saw him as a consult on the medical floor. I would have to surmise that he was not flagrantly psychotic or agitated since he was kept on an open medial unit. By Friday acute heart disease was ruled out and the consulting psychiatrist came by to inform the patient he was being transferred to the psychiatry unit. That psychiatrist told him that a different psychiatrist would be on call that weekend but, according to the wife, thought that would be good because "he didn't know exactly what was going on with Bill." Surprisingly, the weekend covering psychiatrist discharged Bill on Sunday. The psychiatric medications he was discharged on were Zyprexa (an antipsychotic medication used for bipolar disorder) and Depakote (an anticonvulsant medication also used for bipolar disorder). The discharge diagnosis, however, was not bipolar disorder. At that hospital the discharge diagnosis was

Generalized Anxiety Disorder and possible prescription medication withdrawal. (I know, I know; then why did they discharge him on medications for bipolar disorder? Welcome to Psychiatryland folks!)

It was after that hospitalization that I got the call about Bill needing a "PRN certified" psychiatrist to decide whether he could safely return to work. Having been around the block a few times, I knew that I could not do the comprehensive evaluation needed on an outpatient basis and since his two day evaluation as an inpatient at the above hospital didn't sound too comprehensive, I recommended he go to a hospital in a nearby state that I knew did a good and thorough job. He agreed. (It's amazing how cooperative people can be when their job and license are on the line). *But for some reason, at that hospital the admission staff elected to focus on my future patient's possible addiction to prescription medications.* (Oh, I didn't mention that? Well this is what psychiatric cases are like in the real world, complicated; very, very complicated!).

Bill had been on prescribed "controlled" medications for a long time prior to his "breakdown." His outpatient psychiatrist prescribed anti-anxiety medication and he was on opiate pain medication prescribed by a neurologist. Being on controlled substances got a lot of attention at this hospital, well-known for its "dual diagnosis" (addiction plus an underlying psychiatric disorder) treatment unit. According to the wife's typed recollection the patient was "bullied" into saying he misused his prescription medications. The fact is that when he was forced to stay in a motel overnight before getting admitted to this hospital he "borrowed" two Xanax pills from his wife to help calm his nerves and get some sleep. This showed up in his records more than once as evidence supporting diagnosing him as a drug abuser. It also came out during that hospital stay that he had some past problems with alcohol. I don't know precisely what happened in admissions but he was indeed admitted to the dual diagnosis unit to be detoxed from his controlled meds and treated for his "manic" condition.

He was kept in the hospital 13 days and discharged on three medications for bipolar disorder and no medications for pain. The improvement in his mental status was interpreted as directly related to his bipolar medications. His discharge diagnoses were Bipolar I disorder and Polysubstance Dependence. He was not cleared to return to work and it was recommended that this difficult and liability laden decision should be made by his outpatient psychiatrist. Guess who? Me. And I hadn't even met the man yet.

Things might seem pretty clear-cut at this time and you might be wondering why I am telling this story. I would need to evaluate and monitor his bipolar disorder and drug abuse and somehow judge whether he was "safe" to return to work. But I have to tell you that I was a little disappointed that the hospital I had recommended to evaluate Bill was reported by him as a pretty negative experience with an outcome that neither Bill nor his wife agreed with. So I started over, taking my own comprehensive history, asking the questions I believe needed to be asked before I accepted any other doctor's diagnosis. (I've learned to never accept someone else's diagnosis at face value, an unfortunately far too common practice). Over the next couple of weeks I spent about three hours with the patient and also had a two hour session with him and his wife together. Finally I made my monumental diagnostic decision. Here is an excerpt from the letter I wrote in November of 2002 to the hospital regarding his return to work status:

"...my conclusion is that no firm diagnosis of either a psychiatric or substance abuse problem can be made at his time."

Why did I say this? Well, I'll tell you. Despite all the previous diagnostic decisions and immediate initiation of intensive medication therapy, I did not find that Bill met the DSM IV criteria for Bipolar I disorder nor did he meet the DSM IV criteria for substance abuse or dependence. I took an extremely detailed and careful history from both Bill and his wife and I thoroughly reviewed all the records I could obtain and it simply wasn't there. (Okay. I know; I am writing a book critically deconstructing the DSM model of diagnosis but here I am citing DSM criteria as the basis for disagreeing with the previous doctor's diagnosis of bipolar disorder and substance abuse. Why? Because this case had important LEGAL implications and whether I or anyone else likes it, the Bible of psychiatry is the reference text that is used in court). *So what did I have? Sure there was an episode of a possible psychosis but he was so heavily medicated from that point on, how was I to know if he would have remained symptomatic? I had also learned long ago that ER doctors and psychiatrists tend to describe the patient's behavior with general labels that imply a diagnosis. I frequently see medical records where the patient is reported to be "manic" or acting "manicky" but that is a non-specific and biased description. I want to know what is seen. Is the patient agitated, euphoric or excessively irritable? Is there rapid pressured speech and flight of ideas? Are there grandiose delusions, excessive energy and a lack of need for sleep or rest? These are the symptoms of mania. That is what a "manicky" person looks and sounds like. So I paid a lot of attention to the ER report where, in an unmedicated state, he was described by the nurse as calm and lucid. That didn't jive with my experience of manic psychosis. Mania is about as opposite to calm and coherent as one could imagine. His "mania" also did not last seven days, another diagnostic criterion for Bipolar I disorder. Also, on very close questioning I could not elicit from Bill or his wife any evidence of previous full blown episodes of mania or depression (which one would expect to see in Bipolar I disorder, where the age of onset is typically much younger).*

What he was seeing a psychiatrist for prior to his "breakdown" was difficulties with anxiety, a problem he'd had since his father died when Bill was thirteen. That is why he was on anti-anxiety medication, one of the controlled substances he was ostensibly addicted to. He also had a long history of sleep problems for which he occasionally needed sleep medication. As for the more worrisome substance, the pain medication, I received documentation from his neurologist that this was prescribed for him and he never requested early refills or "lost" his prescription (thus no evidence of abuse). So what can I say? Something happened in August of that year but I don't know what. And just because he was taking controlled substances and had a past history of some alcohol problems, that didn't make him an addict or dangerous to practice. (Just to be safe, I checked; there were no reports of this doctor having any problems at the hospital, no patient complaints, no disciplinary actions and certainly no lawsuits despite his practicing while on these medications for years). So I took a deep breath and cleared him to return to work. But he remained my patient and I needed to submit reports to PRN and he was still on a boatload of bipolar medications. Where to go from here?

Rationally, if I didn't think he had bipolar disorder then why would I keep him on bipolar medications? Just to be safe? I suppose that would be a reasonable (and certainly self protective) compromise but as you will learn in chapter seven, medications for bipolar disorder are far from benign compounds free of risks or serious side effects. Besides, I reasoned, with all those emotion numbing medications on board how would I ever know whether he got manic or hypomanic again? Since I planned to carefully follow him for at least two or three years (under the requirements of the PRN contract) I figured that if he was going to go manic (or suffer a major depression) I could see it with my own eyes. So we slowly tapered Bill off of all of his medications. And I watched…

In the meantime PRN was doing its own thing. They did not seem satisfied with the completeness of the diagnostic assessments to date and arranged for Bill to be evaluated by a couple of top guys at the University of Florida. One was a general psychiatrist, the other a specialist in addiction. These guys did a thorough job and submitted lengthy, detailed typewritten reports. Here is the diagnostic conclusion reached by the general psychiatrist: "By history he has had anxiety symptoms for the past 10 years. Rule out Generalized Anxiety Disorder." He then goes on to say that he cannot make any definitive mood disorder or substance abuse or dependence diagnosis. The addiction specialist submitted this diagnosis: "Probable alcohol, sedative and opioid abuse. Cannot rule out sedative and opioid dependence. Anxiety disorder by history. Psychotic Disorder Not Otherwise Specified." End of story for the University docs. PRN got the consults and made their decision in June 2003. He would be allowed to take opiate pain medication as prescribed by his neurologist but no other controlled substances and no over the counter cold or allergy medicines containing benedryl or pseudoephredine (huh?). There would be ongoing urine drug screen monitoring and he was ordered to enroll in a cognitive-behavior therapy program to learn to "calm himself without drugs." (You know I could have sworn this case was about a putative bipolar disorder and that the use of controlled substances prescribed by his doctors wasn't at issue. But he was under the auspices of PRN and this addiction focus was their familiar territory. Not a word about the bipolar disorder and he was now fully off all mood stabilizers for four months).

Bill kept working with no problems. He took his opiate pain medications and still seemed to somehow manage to function. I continued to see him monthly and saw no evidence of any mood disorder. Everything was going just swimmingly. That was (insert foreboding music here) until August 2005.

Apparently the folks who design urine drug tests had fixed a major flaw in urine drug screening which was the inability to detect the use of alcohol except when the testee is acutely intoxicated. In other words, an A.M. urine screen did not reveal if the testee drank the previous evening. But they developed some new technology which could detect whether even small amounts of alcohol had been ingested in the past 18 hours and Bill got popped. Remember this was August 2005, two years from the original psychotic episode. He had been working as a doctor without problems and I had him off all psychiatric meds for about 18 months and there were no signs or symptoms of depression, mania or psychosis. But PRN oversees physicians with substance abuse and/or psychiatric problems and they keep up the monitoring for a long time. I was not in the decision making loop at PRN; in fact I wasn't even informed that they ordered Bill to have another comprehensive evaluation by a substance abuse treatment program. Nobody asked me to do this evaluation because if I had, I'm sure I would have diagnosed "no big deal" and that would have been the end of it (the guy can't have a drink?). But the "Resource" Network wanted a more intense and comprehensive (and unbelievably more expensive) evaluation of this (for the first time in 24 months) urine drug screen that found evidence of ingestion of alcohol. Since his license and career remained on the line, he had no choice. The evaluation itself required a ***five day stay*** *at the facility. A very detailed report resulted from that evaluation, as did a very emotionally traumatized patient.*

The program he was required to attend for his five day evaluation was out of state. The only record I have is of his "neuropsychological" evaluation. He was interviewed and given a comprehensive battery of psychological tests. It was noted in the report that Bill was anxious and guarded throughout the interview and testing and expressed concern regarding how what he said would be interpreted by the tester. Gee, I wonder why? (Let me back up a bit before reporting the results of his evaluation. Previously, PRN had required Bill to undergo psychological testing to establish whether or not he was "cognitively impaired" by his use of pain medication. He was tested by a PhD psychologist and found to have an IQ of 131 and no evidence of cognitive impairment whatsoever). The results were not the same by the neuropsychologist at the substance abuse program. In fact he found Bill to have an IQ of only 93! WHAT? I think we can hazard a guess at how his IQ dropped from genius level to below average during this test. He was scared to death of that place. Here is something I found in the report; it says: "At one point during testing, he said that he needed to call his wife and insisted it was very urgent that he speak with her. He was informed that it was against the policy during his evaluation period for him to make such a phone call, which he accepted without difficulty." Cut off from phone calls to his wife for five days. Nice. I wonder how any of us would do on an IQ test under those circumstances. Think you could put forth your best effort?

You have probably guessed that the results of this evaluation would not be too favorable and you would be right. Here is what it said: "The results of the evaluation indicate that ("Bill's") attention/concentration and verbal learning abilities are currently moderately to severely impaired... yada yada yada...test results seem to reflect his significant anxiety and possibly a withdrawal syndrome. His cognitive abilities will likely improve when his anxiety and possible substance abuse is better controlled...yada yada yada...It is noted that he was previously diagnosed with bipolar disorder. (Be afraid!) *...yada yada yada...the overall impression is that he likely has a significant history of substance abuse, which he is minimizing...yada yada yada...it is not recommended that he return to his medical practice at this time...yada yada yada...It is recommended that he be admitted for inpatient dual-diagnosis treatment."*

Need a minute to digest this...Admitted for a four to six week dual diagnosis program? What are the dual diagnoses? Bipolar disorder and drug addiction? What evidence is there of either of these? He has been symptom free for two years after his brief psychotic episode, most of that time on no meds, and has been closely monitored by PRN urine drug screens. Why it's almost as if you can say anything you want to in Psychiatryland. (That's right...Be very afraid!). *Okay. Good news. Bill didn't get admitted. Instead he got a lawyer to, ahem, "negotiate" with PRN and that was the end of the recommendation for inpatient treatment. The trauma of that "evaluation" experience, however, exacted a price. I met with Bill and his wife a few days after he was discharged from his five day stay. After that experience (quoting from my notes) "he could barely sleep and now he is showing some mood lability, paranoia and sense of desperation." He wasn't manic or overtly psychotic. His wife and I concluded that under stress with high anxiety and sleep deprivation, Bill can get a little psychotic. You know, we might have been able to figure that out a couple of years before and saved everybody a boatload of grief, pain, expense and trauma. But that might have been a little tough to pull off. You see there isn't a described psychiatric disorder that correlates with Bill's particular symptom package. But remember the point of all of this, that, as a medical science, psychiatry accepts the responsibility of acting like a medical science, making diagnoses and rendering treatment. Since Bill didn't display the classic symptomatology (nor meet the diagnostic criteria for) any DSM IV Axis I disorder and since he was agitated and hearing voices, then a best guess or closest approximation would have to do. Over the course of his evaluation and treatment these "best guesses" would ultimately come to include:*

1. *Generalized Anxiety Disorder*
2. *Schizophrenia*
3. *Bipolar I Disorder*
4. *Bipolar II Disorder*
5. *Substance Induced Mood Disorder*
6. *Opiate Abuse*
7. *Opiate Dependence*
8. *Benzodiazepine Abuse*
9. *Benzodiazepine Dependence*
10. *Acute Drug Withdrawal Syndrome*
11. *Psychotic Disorder Not Otherwise Specified*

He would be treated at one time or another with antipsychotic medications, mood stabilizers, antidepressants, anti-anxiety drugs and sleeping pills. PRN finally let Bill go and I continued to see him once every three months to refill his sleeping pills and keep an eye on him. Aside from the ups and downs of daily life, he did fine.

I feel that I can still make some sense out of being a psychiatrist by seeing myself as undoing the damage done by other doctors. Here is a real case in point because I will guarantee you, with near 100% certainty, that if I hadn't been involved in the case that Bill would have retained his bipolar disorder diagnosis, would still be on medication (probably more than one) and he himself, his wife, his fellow physicians, friends and the hospital would be monitoring his "moods" for any evidence of the emergence of bipolar disease. I wrote in a paper once that it doesn't matter anymore whether or not there is something **actually wrong** with your brain; when you are diagnosed bipolar you **become** bipolar. This is what is meant by reification. I hope Bill's case has brought that concept to life for you.

One last thing before we move on. Out of curiosity I had my secretary go into the computer to find out how much I had been paid for the services rendered to Bill. This includes intake evaluations, medication checks, emergency family visits, phone calls, filling out forms, and writing letters (although there is no formal reimbursement for the last three services). The total I was paid over four years by insurance and patient co-pays was $2631.00. There were 56 formal billable services performed. That averages out to about $47.00 per service. I only mention this here because in later chapters we are going to discuss how the low reimbursement to psychiatrists is also fueling the biopsychiatry frenzy. (I think I'll ask Bill one day how much he had to pay his lawyer).

In Bill's case there are eleven different diagnoses mentioned one time or another. I have looked all over for it but can't find the chart on another patient I wanted to tell you about because she held the record for the most diagnoses *at the same time*: nine. That's right; she presented to me with records from her previous psychiatrist listing nine separate Axis I diagnoses for this young woman. Now how could something like that happen? I will tell you. It's based on a central organizing principle in medical model psychiatry called "comorbidity." One of the first of the many dilemmas faced by *clinical* psychiatrists utilizing DSM involved having patients who displayed symptoms of more than one of the disorders delineated in it. What should you do then? Simple, just make more than one diagnosis. Apparently in America its starting to look like having two or more mental disorders is perhaps more common than having just one. For example, in a recent article about Adult Attention Deficit Hyperactivity Disorders (ADHD) it says: "In ADHD, comorbidity is more likely to be the rule than the exception.... Bipolar disorder, substance abuse, depression, anxiety, and personality disorders can intermingle in the ADHD patient's life, making diagnosis a challenge. One study showed that 70% of adults with ADHD had concomitant psychiatric disorders..." (Minde 2003). Imagine, ADHD, bipolar, depression, anxiety, and personality disorder symptoms all intermingling and overlapping, making diagnosis such a *complex challenge*. May I say in response to that: BALONEY!! In actuality the concepts of comorbidity and concomitant disorders makes diagnosis a snap...easy...a near mindless act where you can speculate whatever you want and never ever be "wrong" (if any new or unrelated symptoms emerge just add another diagnosis). To help you understand how and why this came about I am going to need to introduce you to another philosopher of science. His name is Thomas Kuhn.

Perhaps you have heard of Thomas Kuhn. He is famous for introducing the concept of paradigms into our everyday language. Kuhn was a philosopher of science who focused on the social aspects of science, scientific research and scientists (Kuhn 1962). He recognized that the way science worked in the real world was to have a large number of individual scientists who generally agreed upon and followed a particular theoretical framework called a paradigm. In this book we are critically examining the paradigm I've labeled medical science, looking particularly at psychiatry's utilization of that paradigm. What Kuhn found was that once a guiding paradigm is established then all of the specific research work arising from that basic paradigm is a phenomena he calls "normal science." What that means for us is that in relation to the paradigm that mental diseases are ultimately rooted in brain cell pathology (just like heart disease is ultimately rooted in heart cell pathology) then all the thousands of psychiatric studies published each year on drug trials, genetic studies, brain imaging and the like represent psychiatric researchers doing "normal science."

What is the purpose of "normal science?" Pajares says: "Initially, a paradigm offers the promise of success. Normal science consists in the actualization of that promise. This is achieved by extending the knowledge of those facts that the paradigm displays as particularly revealing, increasing the extent of the match between those facts and the paradigm's predictions, and further articulation of the paradigm itself. In other words, there is a good deal of mopping-up to be done. Mop-up operations are what engage most scientists throughout their careers. Mopping-up is what normal science is all about!" (Pajares)

The paradigm we are tracing here in this book, that mental dysfunction is an expression of organic brain dysfunction, actually has quite a long history. As I mentioned earlier, even Freud, with his sometimes bizarre sounding theories of childhood sexuality and his basic premise that unconscious conflicts produce "symptoms", truly believed that a neurobiological basis for what he identified as psychopathology would be found. But his taxonomy (categorization of disorders) was imprecise and strange and could never be married to the medical science model. What DSM III did was give this paradigm a language with which to communicate, so that researchers and academicians and clinicians engaged in the business of "normal" science within this paradigm could feel that when they talked about clinical cases and research findings, they were talking about the same thing. That is why reliability is such a highly prized achievement in medical research. Earlier, I distinguished reliability from validity. The paradigm concept promises, however, that through reliability-grounded research ("normal science") the validity will come. That is what keeps medical psychiatrists focused and allows them to deflect criticism. They have their proverbial "eye on the prize", a firm belief that eventually, with the emergence of increasingly sophisticated technologies and continued research, the actual physical connection between neuronal function and mental dysfunction will be discovered and incontrovertibly proven.

However…in the meantime…after decades of research that has yielded not a single definitive biological marker connecting brain dysfunction to mental disorders here we are; we humans who happen to be living (and sometimes emotionally suffering) in this, the historical era *before* these promised monumental breakthroughs in neurobiology. And yet we are being evaluated, labeled and treated *as if* they have already been achieved. This is the terrorizing magnitude, in my mind, of the dissemination and unquestioned acceptance of seemingly innocuous unproven ideas such as depression being caused by a "chemical imbalance." That is why we are looking so closely and critically at the text undergirding this phenomenon and affecting so many lives, the DSM IV. We are now going to examine *how* the unwavering support of what I have called the fundamental "lie" that psychiatry is a medical science, is forcing psychiatry to continue to elaborate increasingly far-fetched "lies" (diagnostic expansions and revisions) to manage a problem faced by all scientific paradigms, the dreaded *anomaly.*

Okay. Next definition; what is an anomaly? An anomaly is an unexpected finding, a fact, a phenomenon or experimental outcome that does not fit neatly or easily into the guiding paradigm. Anomalies threaten the paradigm and, by extension, all those guided by the paradigm, i.e. all of the hordes of researchers engaged in "normal science" as well as other interested third parties, (see chapter eight). This is what Kuhn and others have identified as a powerful political side of science. Changing a paradigm threatens the livelihoods of all those involved in doing "normal science" within the paradigm and all the others who benefit from the domination of that paradigm. So, paradigms *resist* change on many levels. But anomalies must be dealt with and every branch of science has dealt with and continues to need to deal with them. That, by the way, can be a good thing. Take the case of Mad Cow Disease.

This is a horrendous disease that slowly eats away at the brain until it ends up looking like a sponge. (Hence, the scientific name of the disease: bovine spongiform encephalopathy). Under the medical science paradigm it was pretty clear that this disease was the result of some sort of an infection. However, when our sophisticated technology was used to search for the infectious agent, no bacteria or viruses could be found. But the paradigm kept pointing to an infectious process; was there a flaw in the paradigm? The researchers kept searching diligently. Finally, they found their culprit, an extremely primitive form of life called a prion. A prion is actually simpler in structure than bacteria or viruses and yet the damage it does is profound. So here is a case where an anomaly forced a more diligent research effort that paid off with invaluable findings that supported, strengthened and expanded the paradigm. (And saved lives).

The Mad Cow example showed a positive outcome generated by working within a paradigm. But sometimes so many anomalies accumulate that the only way to fix the problem is to change the paradigm itself. As you might guess, this doesn't happen easily. When it does, Kuhn calls it a "scientific revolution." A well known example of major paradigm changes has occurred over the course of hundreds of years in the field of physics. First there was a long period when physics was Aristotelian (based on refinements of the thinking of Aristotle). Then it shifted to Newtonian physics and finally, in the 20th Century to a paradigm based on the work of Einstein. So scientific revolutions DO occur and in general, we are better off for them. (Of course it was Einstein's theories that lead to the atomic bomb, so...)

There are two other options in dealing with anomalies. They can simply be ignored. This has been done. Or, somehow the anomalies can be, lets say "persuaded" to fit the paradigm by some tinkering with the anomaly or making some "adjustments" to the paradigm itself. We have identified the paradigm guiding modern psychiatry as Spitzer's basic concept that mental disorders are a subset of medical disorders or, stated differently, that psychiatry is a branch of medical science. We have further identified the DSM III (and beyond) model as providing the fundamental language and basis for categorization in that science. What kind of anomalies might arise in medical model psychiatry?

Bracken and Thomas, (post modern theorists who are also psychiatric clinicians) say that medical model psychiatry "simply cannot account for the sort of problems we encounter in our day-to-day practices." I could easily add a hundred more quotes from *practicing clinicians* critical of the reductionistic and dehumanizing aspects of diagnosis and treatment in medical model psychiatry. Okay, so exactly what are the anomalies in today's psychiatry? If I could resurrect Charlton Heston I'd ask him to answer the question because I can still recall his inimitable delivery of the final line in the disturbing science fiction movie *Soylent Green*. Mr. Heston, you're on: **"IT'S PEOPLE!"** he said. Yes, the answer to the question of what the anomalies are in psychiatry is *people*, those indescribably complex beings who defy simplistic categorization, who have the audacity to *not* respond to the most rational medical treatment plans and keep living complicated lives with all of life's ups and downs right in the middle of treatment. ("I was really starting to feel better on the medication doctor but then my daughter called telling me she is getting divorced and I got depressed all over again. I don't think the medication is working anymore. Should I be on a higher dose?"). Just think about Bill. There was really something at stake when psychiatry was asked to evaluate him. Do you want someone who is getting audio messages from God picking up a scalpel and coming towards you with it? On the other hand, should that single event end his hard earned career as a doctor? (Besides does hearing God talk to you even qualify as a hallucination?) So how complicated was Bill's case? Was his an exceptionally unusual situation? Not at all! Psychiatric cases are by their very nature incredibly complex, every one of them. Because that's the way it is with emotional and mental problems in human beings. The deeper you go the more you get. As I have frequently said to my patients, we are not dealing with an infected hangnail in psychiatry; we are dealing with personhood, the whole package. Just ask yourself...what makes you tick?? How often are you misunderstood? How deep should someone go if you start having panic attacks, phobias, crying jags, or paranoia? Do you really want to just take a multiple choice test, get diagnostically labeled and sent home with a bottle of pills?

Okay, you're convinced. We are indescribably complex creatures that no system of categorization can encompass. But what about suffering people? Do you just step back and say...sorry, too complicated. Nothing we can do here! Of course not. But whatever you choose to do needs to *acknowledge* this inherent complexity and work *within* it. As you will eventually see in this book, within this complexity medical psychiatry can have its place and its role to play. But run the show? Be the "only discourse in town?" You see what's happening.

In its effort to make psychiatry more scientific DSM III chose to create a *categorical* system of diagnosis. In such a system diagnostic categories have rigid boundaries that define black and white situations. Either you fit the diagnosis (have the disorder) or you don't, no in between. This aligns psychiatry more closely to other medical diagnostic systems. For example, you either have streptococcus pneumonia that is causing your cough and fever or you don't; you either have a malignant brain tumor causing your headaches or you don't...categorically. When used as intended the same black and white separation is also true for DSM defined mental disorders. Recall that for a diagnosis of major depression at least 5 of the 9 listed symptoms had to be present for at least 2 weeks. What if your 5 out of 9 symptoms lasted just one week, then you felt better for two weeks but then you felt real depressed for three days and then woke up the fourth day feeling great? What do you have? Following the rules of our categorical system of diagnosis you'd have to be diagnosed as having Depressive Disorder Not Otherwise Specified (code 311). But this tells you nothing. If all the treatment studies and protocols were formulated using subjects with "full-blown" DSM defined Major Depression, then what about you? I guess you are an anomaly. Being diagnosed as Not Otherwise Specified (NOS) is a cop out. Yet in DSM IV there are NOS choices for nearly all the diagnostic categories. This certainly lends no credence to the diagnostic system and weakens its claims to "cut nature at the joints" (accurately delineate and describe what occurs in nature). In terms of our discussion of anomalies I'd have to characterize an NOS diagnosis as an example of simply ignoring an anomaly. A second option is to fit the anomaly into the paradigm by "tweaking" the data (by skewing and shaping the history of the presenting complaints or symptoms) or "tweaking" the paradigm. And that is exactly what is going on in psychiatry and what is literally causing this medical specialty to swing so wildly out of control that I felt the need to write this book to WARN you to BE AFRAID of the profession of which I am a member. As a first example, let's look at how the categorical boundaries of bipolar disorder have been loosened, making it easier and easier to "shape" a patient's history to conform to these expanded diagnostic requirements.

In my private practice, at any one time I would generally have about a dozen patients with Bipolar Type I disorder. I treated them aggressively with medication and saw them often to insure compliance and give supportive therapy. Most didn't need any other help in therapy because between episodes of mania and depression they had always been pretty normal. Bipolar I disorder is a very serious condition and even though we don't know what causes it, I have no problem calling it a mental illness. The categorical diagnostic criteria for Bipolar I Disorder in DSM IV has the characteristic structure of "at least" X number of symptoms lasting "at least" X period of time and causing marked impairment. Like it did for Major Depression, DSM IV lists the diagnostic criteria for an *episode* of mania and then offers a number of qualifiers to more clearly define the particularities, e.g., recurrent vs. single episode etc. Bipolar is a bit more complicated diagnostically because there must be both episodes of major depression and episodes of mania (the two poles of bipolar). Let's look at the criteria for a manic episode, (DSM IV, p. 332):

Criteria for Manic Episode

A. A distinct period of abnormally and persistently elevated, expansive, or irritable mood lasting at least 1 week (or any duration if hospitalization is necessary).

B. During the period of mood disturbance, three (or more) of the following symptoms have persisted (four if the mood is only irritable) and have been present to a significant degree:

(1) inflated self esteem or grandiosity

(2) decreased need for sleep (e.g. feel rested after only 3 hours of sleep)

(3) more talkative than usual or pressure to keep talking

(4) flight of ideas or subjective experience that thoughts are racing

(5) distractibility (i.e., attention too easily drawn to unimportant or irrelevant externalstimuli

(6) increase in goal-directed activity (either socially, at work or school, or sexually) or psychomotor activity

(7) excessive involvement in pleasurable activities that have a high potential for painful consequences (e.g., engaging in unrestrained buying sprees, sexual indiscretions, or foolish business investments)

C. The symptoms do not meet criteria for a Mixed Episode (see p. 335).
D. The mood disturbance is sufficiently severe to cause marked impairment in occupational functioning or in social activities or relationships with others, or to necessitate hospitalization to prevent harm to self or others, or there are psychotic features.
E. The symptoms are not due to the direct physiological effects of a substance (e.g., a drug of abuse, a medication, or other treatment) or a general medical condition (e.g., hyperthyroidism).

I don't and neither would any of you have any problem identifying Bipolar I Disorder in someone currently suffering from a manic episode. They truly act crazy. A number of my Bipolar I patients had a tendency to take all their clothes off in public when manic. Some love to "spread the word", preaching religion in rather unorthodox and sometimes very dangerous places. They are usually euphoric, although can become rapidly irritated (and even violent) if their irrational manic beliefs are challenged. Manic episodes are often tragic, destroying and bankrupting people and families. I don't know if DSM IV has all of the diagnostic criteria just right, but I truly do believe that this diagnosis does "cut nature at its joints". Treatment often works quite well and once insight is established and the need for chronic use of medication accepted, people with bipolar disorder can do okay. If you'd like to learn more about what I'm calling real bipolar disorder, i.e. Bipolar I Disorder, you should read the book *An Unquiet Mind: A Memoir of Moods and Madness* by Kay Redfield Jamison, published by Alfred J. Knopf Inc. in 1995. Or you can see realistic portrayals of acute mania in the movie *Mr. Jones* starring Richard Gere or on the television series "Six Feet Under" where Brenda's brother is suffering from Bipolar I Disorder. Or watch the movie *Michael Clayton* starring George Clooney, also a very accurate portrayal of untreated bipolar I disorder in the senior partner Clooney is assigned to help. I'm sure you will understand why, despite it being a treatable illness, people would rather not have it. But at least the price they pay is a lot better than it used to be because in the past bipolar patients were often diagnosed as schizophrenic and tragically ended up on the back wards of state hospitals. (Fortunately, modern medicines are also sparing schizophrenics this fate but their overall outcome is still often discouraging and tragic. Some observers are rightfully arguing that the penal system has replaced the state hospital system and that a large number of schizophrenics are now "housed" in jail rather than hospitals. As I said at the beginning, the psychotic illnesses are not really germane to the topic of this book. Clearly psychiatric researchers have their work cut out for them in developing a greater understanding of the causes and treatment for schizophrenia).

So Bipolar I disorder is rather easily diagnosed when the patient is manic. However, practicing clinicians will often see patients who are not overtly manic but who carry the diagnosis of Bipolar Disorder from a previous physician (often without the type I, II, NOS etc. qualifier). As I mentioned before an unfortunate (but time-saving and "efficient") trend is for the new doctor to just accept the reported diagnosis at face value and simply continue medication treatment. I have seen quite a few patients who were (both correctly and incorrectly) diagnosed as bipolar by a psychiatrist at some point in time but then, for cost saving and convenience, would continue to get their medications from their primary care physicians without anyone ever questioning whether the medications were helpful or necessary. A typical worst case scenario was an elderly woman referred to me for an alternative medication for her "bipolar disorder" because the particular medication that a string of PCP's had prescribed for over thirty years had caused kidney failure (you don't want to trifle with bipolar meds!). When I took a history I found no evidence of Bipolar I disorder and simply took her off the offending medication. But, of course, the damage had already been done. An even more terrifying trend is for PCP's to make the initial diagnosis of bipolar disorder and start treatment, a practice that has been promoted (heavily) by pharmaceutical companies. We will discuss this in detail in chapter eight.

This brings us to a very sticky dilemma in diagnosing bipolar disorder (and many other psychiatric conditions), and that is the need to retrospectively reconstruct the "history of the illness" by asking patients to accurately recall past episodes of mood problems. After all, to make a diagnosis of a cyclic mood disorder you need to know about past episodes of high and low mood states. Here is my approach to patients presenting to me for the first time that carry a diagnosis of Bipolar Disorder (and let me tell you, that percentage is skyrocketing). My first question is to ask whether the patient has ever been in a psychiatric hospital or jail. If the answer to this is no, my concern about misdiagnosis increases. A true Type I manic can rarely if ever escape public notice and some action by society to protect itself and the patient. Beyond that first question, however, things start to get a little fuzzy.

I want you to honestly ask yourself a question. If someone asked you to look back on your entire life and recall if there was ever an episode of an abnormal or painful mood state that stands out in your mind, could you do it? Would it be an accurate reporting of an actual event in your life? I think many of us might recall periods of what might be labeled "depression", usually related to the loss of a loved one, getting fired, divorced or other trauma. But could we then accurately recall how long the episode lasted, what the "symptoms" were and how and when it went away? How about trying to recall if you ever got depressed for no reason and what the symptoms, severity and duration were then. Now, here is an even tougher question: Can you recall any time in your life when you felt excessively happy, optimistic and confident, when you felt you didn't need much sleep and perhaps went on a spending spree or engaged in casual sex that you later regretted? How would it be to try to answer that question? And yet that is exactly the question you *must* answer during a psychiatric evaluation for bipolar disorder, especially Type II, cyclothymic and the other categories that don't involve full blown manias. Obviously you don't have a videotape to rely on or anything else for that matter except your memory and the memories of your loved ones. It is here that you are most vulnerable and medical psychiatry has its best opportunity to "shape" your presenting complaint into something that fits its medical paradigm. Here is where your presenting complaints and history can be "tweaked" so that any "anomalous" data can be either discarded or squeezed into the paradigm.

For example the fact that you were using various recreational drugs during that "hypomanic" period can either be ignored (as it often is) or listed as a "co-morbid" condition interpreted as an effort to "self medicate" your bipolar disorder. (I will show you in chapter eight how the pharmaceutical industry and medical model psychiatry has created, among other things, checklist diagnostic instruments to efficiently "guide" you to an acceptable and medically treatable diagnosis, whatever your presenting complaint or problem is). "Tweaking" the history can also be a handy tool when the DSM diagnosis you are working with isn't leading to a positive response to medication. You can "review" the history and maybe "pick up" on something that was missed before. Remember Gwen, the lady with the diagnosis of bipolar disorder who had trouble getting life and health insurance I mentioned in the last chapter? I have her medical records dating back fifteen years. So I can tell you exactly when the above mentioned maneuver occurred in her case.

In the first note written by a social worker in 1991 Gwen's chief complaint was recorded as "I am a workaholic and I want to change that." She goes on to describe chronic problems in her work life, her love life and with life in general. She gave a history of a brief psychiatric hospitalization in 1986 when she had a bit of an alcohol problem and expressed some suicidal thoughts (no attempts). The social worker diagnosed her as having an "Adjustment Disorder." She also noted a history of a difficult childhood with probable alcoholism in the father. She suggested some reading material and scheduled Gwen for further psychotherapy. In the follow-up session the therapist recommended that Gwen continue her readings and cognitive therapy but added a recommendation to attend 12 Step meetings for co-dependants called CoDA. On the next visit Gwen reported that "I haven't felt depressed for a week. I've decided not to depend so much on my boyfriend."

(She probably learned that at a CoDA meeting). The therapist maintained her diagnosis of adjustment disorder and recommended some stress management work and to keep up with CoDA and her cognitive therapy. (I like this therapist so far. She didn't just jump right in to the medical model).

Unfortunately it is often the case that when someone starts to feel a little better they stop their therapy, returning again only when in crisis; Gwen no-showed for her next appointment with her therapist. She showed up again, in crisis, 8 months later. Her boyfriend was moving to Mexico for a job. Her father had died but left nothing to his five girls. The words hopeless and suicide came up. Gwen was referred to the psychiatrist who diagnosed Depressive Disorder NOS, rule out cyclothymia, and started her on Prozac. He also added on Axis II: Consider Borderline, Paranoid, Dependent, Passive Aggressive or Histrionic Personality Disorder. (Five possible personality disorders; love this job!)

Gwen remained pretty stable in therapy and under psychiatric care for the next two years. She went off Prozac for six weeks but didn't like how she felt so restarted it. The diagnosis remained unchanged, Depressive Disorder NOS. On most visits the psychiatrist described her mood as euthymic (normal mood). In the winter of 1994, however, Gwen reported not doing so well. The psychiatrist raised the dose of Prozac. (This is what I was talking about when I mentioned that while you are treating the patient life goes on, with all of its ups and downs, pleasures and pains. Somewhere along the way nearly all chronic patients report that their medication is "no longer working"). *So Gwen's psychiatrist raised the dose of Prozac but it didn't help. On the next visit the psychiatrist made his move. Since she was no longer responding as expected he elected to revisit the diagnosis. He dug deeper into her history, specifically searching for evidence of bipolarity and, by jove, there it was. Here is what he recorded that he found: "Used up her money, spends to cheer herself up. Buys clothes, furniture. Had $10,000—now $2000 left." A spending spree!! The psychiatrist started Lithium, the drug used to treat bipolar disorder (he diagnosed cyclothymia, a milder version).*

Gwen "responded" to the new medications but then, down the line wasn't doing as well. Antidepressants were changed and then changed back. She tried going off lithium for a while. In 1998 she was re-diagnosed again, this time as co-morbid adult ADD. She was put on a new antidepressant and Ritalin. She went to individual therapy. She went to group therapy. She had therapy for eating disorders. She did well for periods of time and then not so well. She got a lot of treatment.

I don't have all the details of what happened since 1998. All I know is that by the time she came to see me in 2006 she was on two medications for bipolar disorder (lithium and Zyprexa) and a different antidepressant than the ones mentioned in her previous records. I "undiagnosed" bipolar disorder and took her off her bipolar meds. She has managed to lose 24 of the 30 pounds she had gained.

She is starting therapy with a psychologist in my office. The last time I saw Gwen she looked nervous and expressed a lot of worries about just about everything. She told me she actually had never stopped thinking about suicide but her strong religious beliefs stop her from doing it.

So what IS wrong with Gwen? Forgive me if this sounds uncaring (it isn't) but who the hell knows? It's complicated! I was reasonably certain, however, that it was not Bipolar I disorder and was comfortable taking her off her bipolar meds. I'm also pretty sure it was not Adult ADD. I expect Gwen will be a chronic patient in both psychotherapy and under psychiatric care. She will continue to do well for a while then backslide. My plan was to get her onto the least potentially harmful medication regimen and keep her there. If that doesn't satisfy her, she will probably seek a medication change from her PCP or another psychiatrist. (Many of my patients have).

So clearly, the history can be "tweaked" so that the patient's condition conforms to a DSM diagnosis. I've also mentioned that the paradigm itself (or at least elements derived from the paradigm) can also be "tweaked" to deal with anomalies. It's especially helpful in psychiatry that the possibility of falsifiability, an element that Popper said *must* be present in a true science is not at issue here. As you will see in the next chapter, this unchecked freedom to theorize and alter diagnostic criteria has unleashed a terrifying new trend in psychiatry that officially justifies and sanctions the application of medical model psychiatric diagnosis and medication treatment to almost *any possible* manifestation of problems in living and emotional distress in you, your family and everyone you know.

Chapter Five:
CASES IN POINT
Bipolar Spectrum & Adult Attention Deficit Disorder

In DSM III-R published in 1987 there were only three official bipolar disorder diagnoses: Bipolar Disorder, Cyclothymic Disorder and Bipolar Disorder Not Otherwise Specified. There were severity and symptom qualifiers and a choice of "manic", "mixed" or "depressed" to describe the current episode. In DSM IV, published in 1994, a new diagnostic category was added, Bipolar Type II Disorder. Although mentioned in DSM III-R, the inclusion of the diagnosis of this second type of bipolar disorder in DSM IV officially sanctioned the syndrome *hypomania* as a distinct diagnosable expression of bipolar illness. (As a fortunate side effect this also separated out Bipolar I, what I like to call real bipolar disorder, into a separate diagnostic category). As the name suggests, hypomania is an attenuated form of mania that according to psychiatrist David Dunner (Dunner 1998) "was defined as including all of the symptoms of a manic episode but the syndrome not resulting in hospitalization, characterized by psychosocial disability or psychotic features." (Uh oh. There goes my jail and/or hospital diagnostic question). The duration necessary for a hypomanic episode to qualify for a Bipolar Type II diagnosis was arbitrarily set at only four days. Now many more patients could be guided to this less stringent diagnosis and be fit into the paradigm.

*[*NOTE*: I know that there are a hundred different ways to interpret the meaning and significance of a phenomenon like the emergence of a new psychiatric diagnosis, including the most common way, as a step forward in scientific knowledge. My basic guiding perspective, however, is that the explosion*

of diagnoses and qualifiers in psychiatry represents increasingly desperate attempts to address anomalies and maintain the integrity of the medical paradigm, lies covering lies. Remember that I said from the get-go that this book represents my observations and interpretations, not an argument about "truth". I just thought this would be a good time to remind you of this because this bipolar stuff is pretty serious business].

The next modification introduced in DSM IV is a course qualifier that does not get a specific diagnostic number but can be added to an existing five digit bipolar diagnosis. The qualifier is with **"Rapid Cycling."** I remember reading about the rapid cycling concept way back in my residency. DSM IV defines it as I remembered it being originally defined: "At least four episodes of a mood disturbance in the previous twelve months that meet criteria for a Major Depressive, Manic, Mixed, or Hypomanic Episode." Dunner actually calculated the maximum number of episodes of mood cycling in bipolar disorder based on the minimum number of days required in the criteria for manic, hypomanic and major depressive episodes. He said: "By definition, the greatest number of episodes per year would be twenty for bipolar II patients." (Four-day hypomanic episodes and two week depressive episodes equal eighteen days per cycle or twenty cycles per year.) Similarly, about seventeen cycles per year would be the maximum number for bipolar I patients.

I need to tell you that this is tickling my funny-bone again just like on "Cops". The "lies" are getting so outrageous. The "lie" in this instance is that we can historically recount with precise accuracy the day a hypomania ends and a depression begins; that it's just that simple.

Time for another *Roderickism*

In discussing the incalculable depth of complexity of the modern world Rick critiqued the populist message delivered by the then independent candidate for president, Ross Perot. He said that Perot's appeal was that he would take the most complicated social and economic issues and then propose a concrete (but totally unrealistic) solution followed by his famous catch phrase: "It's just that simple."

On a related topic I need to acquaint you with an appendix in DSM IV. It's Appendix B, pages 703 to 762. The appendix is titled "Criteria Sets and Axes Provided for Further Study." In English that means proposed diagnoses that we haven't made up our minds about yet. For example, Pre-menstrual Dysphoric Disorder (PMDD, a.k.a. real bad PMS) is in this appendix. Also parked in Appendix B are a number of proposed diagnostic categories that I would label "anomaly handlers." One such diagnosis is Recurrent Brief

Depressive Disorder whose criteria are basically the same as major depression except that the episodes "last at least two days but less than two weeks." So now we have a diagnosis that would require counting precisely how many days of major depression you have and do it retrospectively for the last year because the other diagnostic requirement is that "the depressive episodes occur at least once a month for twelve consecutive months and are not associated with the menstrual cycle." And, you know what? "It's just that simple!"

Getting back to the rapid cycling issue, I was proud of myself for accurately remembering the original definition because I was getting confused and seriously concerned about a diagnostic trend I was watching develop in patients under the care of other psychiatrists. They were being diagnosed as "rapid cycling" bipolars only their "cycles" were not the full syndromal severity and duration required in the DSM IV rapid cycling qualifier. Their mood "cycles" were being measured in minutes, hours or days. You know "I'm feeling great one minute and then the next minute I feel like killing myself and I don't know why." These patients were actually calling themselves rapidly cycling bipolars and sometimes presented me with little journals (handily supplied by the pharmaceutical industry) where they had been tracking their moods on an hourly basis. They were, of course, on psychiatric medications, at least three or four at a time, but few would report that the medications (often frequently changed) helped very much and seemed to fully expect me to try something else. Often the only medication they ever felt any relief from was Xanax, Valium or other anti-anxiety (controlled) medications. And, oh yes, did I mention that quite a few of these patients had current or past problems with drug or alcohol abuse?

WHAT WAS GOING ON IN PSYCHIATRY? WERE THEY KIDDING ME? WHAT THE HECK KIND OF "DIAGNOSIS" WAS THIS?

Apparently the idea of attenuated, (or, as they are officially called, "truncated"), episodes of depression and hypomania, (with the possibility for clinical presentation as almost any irritated emotional state), was catching fire in psychiatry. Clearly the doors of medical model psychiatry were being flung wide open to cover any and all comers. Dealing with these patients in my practice was becoming a nightmare. They would do some incredibly self-destructive thing (e.g. relapse on drugs, suddenly break off a relationship, or make a suicide gesture) and then instead of suffering the consequences of that behavior and learn and grow from the experience, they'd be at my door seeking a medication change. It was difficult to fight this because, as I learned, the process of reification of "moodiness" and "impulsivity" and "immaturity" into a mental disorder was apparently already well advanced. You heard its name in one of my case histories in Chapter one. This all encompassing syndrome is called Bipolar Spectrum Disorder and let me tell you, it's all the rage in psychiatry. To get some quotes I could use I googled Bipolar Spectrum Disorder and found an article written by Arnold L. Lieber, MD titled "Bipolar Spectrum Disorder: A Practitioner's Overview of the Soft Bipolar Spectrum" (Lieber 2002). I decided to let Dr. Lieber teach you what Bipolar Spectrum Disorder is. (I'm not crazy about citing just one source but I'll need to ask you to just take my word for it that this article pretty accurately reflects mainstream psychiatry's thinking on this diagnosis).

Dr. Lieber describes himself as a "clinical psychopharmacologist" and he has held some powerful and influential chairmanships and other positions in psychiatry. The fact that he calls himself a clinical psychopharmacologist rather than simply a psychiatrist is actually a trivial matter; except for rare exceptions every psychiatrist earning a living today is doing so by making diagnoses and prescribing psychiatric medications which is precisely what a clinical psychopharmacologist does. Remember this "joke?"

Q: How do you get diagnosed as suffering from
a mental illness by a psychiatrist?
A: Make an appointment.

We can append this by adding:

Q: How do you get a psychiatrist to put you on psychiatric medication?
A: Make an appointment.

Right now I'm going to sit back and put my mental feet up on the chair and relax. The general topic here is an exploration of how psychiatry's medical science paradigm deals with anomalies. I made the remark that psychiatry's anomalies are people. Well now I can just chill out and let some direct quotes from Dr. Lieber's article support my point and then move onto the dizzying topic of controlling anomalies by simply making up diagnoses that, combined with the existing concept of comorbidity, can cover ALL clinical bases. We'll start with some scary numbers.

Dr. Lieber scoffs at the idea that the prevalence of bipolar disorder is the mere 1% figure traditionally quoted (about 3 million people). Even the 3% to 4% prevalence rate arrived at by including the DSM IV subtypes of Bipolar II and cyclothymic disorder are still way off. He says that "a much larger group of patients demonstrate milder and/or atypical forms of episodic mood disorders." Add in these guys and we get a prevalence rate of "5% to 8%." Now you're talking! Based on a U.S. population of 300 million we are talking about anywhere from fifteen to twenty-four *million* bipolars out there. Now that's what I call a market, oops I mean a worrisome number of people suffering from some variant of this terrible mental illness. So what knuckleheads came up with that 1% figure that was so way off, missing a good twelve to twenty-one million potential customers; rats…there I go again, …I mean sufferers. Obviously these were people from (in Dr. Lieber's words) "academic consortiums", who, not being practicing clinicians, don't understand what its like to deal with real live people and struggling with fitting all of them into the medical model paradigm. Practicing clinician Dr. Lieber understands. He says: "Any experienced practitioner of clinical psychopharmacology will attest to the fact that a ***majority*** of patients presenting in office or outpatient settings with symptoms of mood disturbance, anxiety and/or depression ***do not meet DSM diagnostic criteria***. Their symptoms often do not conform to the time constraints required and they tend to fluctuate over time. Anxiety and depression are likely to have atypical manifestations. Hypomania, when present, tends to be of the dysphoric (irritable) variety rather than the euphoric hypomania described in the DSM" (italics, mine).

Okay, I want to make sure I got that last point right. In DSM IV defined Bipolar Type II disorder the diagnostically required abnormal mood state of hypomania is defined as four consecutive days of feelings of extreme wellbeing, confidence, energy, racing thoughts, decreased need for sleep and excessive happiness but Lieber is telling us that if we follow that definition we are going to miss properly diagnosing the majority of Bipolar II patients because their hypomania is "dysphoric" (and the presentation of dysphoric hypomania is what exactly, being irritable ? Is that right?)

Lieber then talks in glowing terms about a world famous psychiatrist that I have met myself on a couple of occasions. His name is Hagop Akiskal, MD and he is best known for his work on psychiatric diagnosis. Dr. Akiskal is also well aware of the anomaly problem in the medical psychiatry paradigm and is working to correct it by expanding the diagnostic categories to better fit what clinicians are seeing. According to Lieber (quoting an article by Akiskal in *Psychiatric Clinics of North America 22:#3, September 1999)* Akiskal is proposing six types of bipolar disorders and subtypes within each type. Now that is getting kinda scary. Remember, all this is going on without any grounding in demonstrable physical pathology or, in other terms, NO PROOF! Why it's almost as if these hard core biopsychiatrists were like a cult or something. Okay, I admit, I set you up for this next quote from Lieber. You'll need a little background first. In the late nineteenth century lived "The great German neuropsychiatrist" (Lieber's words) Emil Kraepelin. Kraepelin is often credited as being the father of a descriptive approach to madness which involved close and careful observation and description of the signs, symptoms, duration, severity and other aspects of mental illness. Through this careful observation a diagnostic system would then naturally evolve (as opposed to starting with a theory and then diagnosing illness based on the theory). Sometimes modern psychiatry is characterized as Neo-Kraepelinian. Let's look at the word Lieber chooses to use when discussing the debt modern psychiatry owes to Kraepelin. He uses the word "master." Brrrrr...(Yoda anyone?)

Like the Time magazine article in chapter one I could spend a whole book critiquing Lieber's article. It's so rich with "deconstructables." Here is a very brief summary of what else he has to say. First he lists and describes the range of initial presenting clinical symptoms and complaints in bipolar spectrum disorder. There can be complaints of "episodic mood instability" with no minimal duration or specific symptoms required. Mood episodes can last hours to days and can include "depression, euphoria, irritability, rage, paranoia and/or anxiety." Other presentations can include episodic atypical depressions (including, among others, the "winter blues" and PMS), euphoric and/or dysphoric hypomanias, and if all other possible descriptions don't fit, "mixed states." Now that's what I call an all encompassing list. Do you see how far from DSM IV Lieber seems to feel he needs to stray to account for the actual people he sees in his office? Just to be certain that no outliers remain he also lists common co-morbid conditions in bipolar spectrum patients. This list includes: Thyroid disorders, Substance Abuse, Attention Deficit Hyperactivity Disorder, Borderline Personality Disorder and the catch-all concept of "other" Personality disorders.

In the next two chapters we are going to take a hard look at psychiatric medications. I am sure that by the end of those chapters you are going to find yourself asking the same question that I've been asking myself for years. What is all the fuss about?? Because you are going to see how all of this diagnostic complexity and controversy has almost nothing to do with what the "clinical psychopharmacologist" has to offer in terms of FDA approved medications for psychiatric disorders. I'll give you a preview...It aint much. But before we wrap up these three chapters on diagnosis I need to acquaint you with one more important phenomenon that affects psychiatric diagnostic practices, something that I like to call the "Oprah Effect."

Thus far we have been dealing with how medical psychiatry has handled challenges to its legitimacy, i.e. anomalies, by expanding and loosening the criteria for what one might call the "classic" psychiatric disorders such as manic depression. But there is a second path by which new diagnostic categories and trends can emerge which is through the impact of popular culture. I'm sure most of you remember the famous first successful weight loss by Oprah

Winfrey, immortalized by a video of her dragging out a wagon loaded with 67 pounds of fat, the amount Oprah lost on her liquid diet. That singular cultural event launched an industry that dominated the multimillion dollar weight loss business until the dangers of the liquid Very Low Calorie Diets (VLCD's) emerged. This is what I am calling the "Oprah Effect". Of course it doesn't require the involvement of Oprah Winfrey; a book, a movie, a TV show, a news story and just about any celebrity can launch a trend in America today. Are there trends and fads in medicine too?

George Bernard Shaw once wrote that:

> *medical practice is governed not by science but by supply and demand...the grossest quackery [cannot] be kept off the market if there is a demand for it. By making doctors tradesmen, we compel them to learn the tricks of the trade; consequently we find that the fashions of the year include treatments, operations, and particular drugs, as well as hats, sleeves, ballads and games.*

I borrowed this quote citation from an excellent book written by William Bennett, M.D. and Joel Gurin titled *The Dieters Dilemma* published by Basic Books in 1982. In that book Bennett and Gurin radically critique the diet industry with its rash of miracle plans and potions and products, each one claiming to have the secret ingredient for success: guaranteed to work where all others have failed. (Well it's nice to see that some things haven't changed in the 28 years since that book was written). In the chapter they call "Waist Products" there is a section titled "How to Write Your Own Diet Book" where they lay out 10 guiding principles to insure a successful book. (You understand, they are being bitingly sarcastic). As I was planning how to approach the final topic in this chapter, the diagnosis Adult Attention Deficit Disorder (AADD), Bennett and Gurin's book came to mind as I was reviewing the structure and content of a book that I believe played a significant role in the genesis and subsequent explosive growth of this diagnosis, one that doesn't really exist in DSM IV, even in Appendix B. The name of that book is probably familiar to you. It was very popular. It's called *Driven to Distraction. Recognizing and Coping with Attention Deficit Disorder from Childhood through Adulthood.* It was written by Edward M. Hallowell, M.D., and John J. Ratey, M.D. and published by Simon and Schuster in 1994. (Incidentally, you might recall, this was the same year DSM IV was published).

Let's first go to DSM IV and see what it has to say about ADD in adults. The diagnostic criteria for ADD is contained in a section of DSM IV called "Disorders Usually First Diagnosed in Infancy, Childhood, or Adolescence" (I guess that tells us something right there). Traditionally, the (always highly controversial) condition called ADD was theorized to have its onset in childhood but then remit by late adolescence. That is how ADD was treated for years. Stimulants such as Ritalin would be prescribed during elementary and middle school years and then be discontinued sometime in high school. There was no such entity as adult **onset** ADD and there still isn't. (I will show you how easily enthusiastic "Adult ADD" seeking clinicians and customers, er..patients, can sidestep this potential little glitch). In DSM IV the only mention of adults having ADD is in two sections where the childhood disorder is fully described. In the section titled "Specific Culture, Age, and Gender Features" it says: "In adulthood, restlessness may lead to difficulty in participating in sedentary activities and to avoiding pastimes or occupations that provide limited opportunity for movement (e.g. desk jobs)" (DSM IV p.82). On the same page, in the section titled "Course", DSM IV says: "In most individuals, symptoms attenuate during late adolescence and adulthood, although a minority experience the full complement of symptoms of Attention Deficit/Hyperactivity Disorder into mid-adulthood. Other adults may retain only some of the symptoms, in which case the diagnosis of Attention Deficit/ Hyperactivity Disorder, In Partial Remission, should be used." And that is it! That is all that the official diagnostic manual, the psychiatric Bible, DSM IV, had to say about ADD in adulthood when published in 1994. Now let's jump ahead to today. I previously quoted a recent statement about Adult ADD having co- morbidities in an estimated 70% of cases. But how many cases are we talking about? Well prepare yourself for some really "accurate" statistics. In a recent review article on ADD (Baron 2007) it is stated that this condition "persists into adulthood in approximately 10 to 60 percent of individuals diagnosed in childhood" (I am still stunned at times that psychiatrists have the 'cahoneys' to make such ludicrous statements in allegedly scientific articles; anywhere from 10 to 60 percent? Why not just say that we think a "whole bunch" of adults have ADD?) Based on what data I could find, in particular a recent NIMH report, I'm guesstimating we are talking about a prevalence of around 15 million adults having ADD. (The estimates for the number of children and teens with ADD are all over the map; I found estimates ranging from 3% to 16%). So how is it that an alleged mental disorder, barely mentioned in DSM IV, has become such a hot diagnosis today? My belief is that this is primarily a socially constructed disorder whose "popularity" is in part linked to the bestselling book mentioned above, *Driven to Distraction*. (I will have a lot more to say about the concept of social constructionism and look at a compelling critique of ADD called *Ritalin Nation* in later chapters). What is fascinating about this is to look more closely at that book and see how parts of it so closely resemble the formula laid out by Bennett and Gurin in their critique of popular diet books (and how very, very far it strays from any semblance of actual medical science).

Principle #1 by Bennett and Gurin is "Say what you are. Needless to say, it helps to be a physician." (check). Principle #2 is "Pick a catchy title." (check). Principle #3 is "Get them into the tent." This means you have to attract readers by expressing sympathy, telling them that it's not their fault and then promise to help them with a plan based on newly discovered scientific findings. (As you will see shortly, double check!) Principle #4 is "Present the master plan." (check). #5 "Pad, pad, pad. Fill the book with case histories, lists and diet aids such as recipes and meal plans." (check). Hallowell's book has list upon list, ranging up to one hundred items. For example there are the "Fifty Tips on the Management of Adult ADD", covering seventeen pages of text and the list of "Twenty-Five Tips on the Management of ADD Within Families" adding another six pages to the book. And as will be discussed below, there is the one hundred item self assessment questionnaire adding another six pages. This helps the book look thicker and more authoritative. Not every principle to design a bestselling diet book will be precisely relevant to designing a bestselling psychiatric disorder book but you get the point. I would add a few other keys to bestselling psychology or medical books of any kind. One is to offer glowing testimonials by patients, and, even better, the author's own personal testimony of salvation, I mean successful treatment. The "cure" for the previously unrecognized, misunderstood and disabling condition needs to be something simple…like a pill. Finally, as Bennett and Gurin also point out, cover your butt (I think I mentioned that in chapter one when I was covering my butt). Make sure you shift the ultimate decision-making and liability to that famous sage and guru popularly called "your doctor."

Let's take a brief look at *Driven to Distraction* to see how it fulfills the popularity guidelines we just laid out. The book opens with a preface "A Personal Perspective." The first line of the preface: "I have attention deficit disorder (ADD)." This is Dr. Hallowell speaking; he did all the writing. Then the first of many zingers: "I discovered I had ADD when I was thirty-one years old, near the end of my training in child psychiatry at the Massachusetts Mental Health Center in Boston." Whoa Boston; credibility central: Harvard, Boston University, Mass General, New England Journal of Medicine etc. (By the way, I went to Boston University School of Medicine). This next quote might surprise you as coming from the mouth of someone who somehow managed to get through undergraduate school, get into and successfully complete medical school and five years of internship and residency *before* what he describes as "one of the great 'Aha' experiences of my life." Hallowell recounts: "So there's a name for what I am! I thought to myself with relief and mounting excitement. There's a term for it, a diagnosis, an actual condition, when all along I'd thought I was just slightly daft." (We are now three paragraphs into the book and we already know that this physician's presentation on the unproven and highly controversial diagnosis of Adult ADD has about as much chance of being "fair and balanced" as a political story on Fox News).

In the remaining three pages of this short preface Hallowell manages to introduce as *inarguable* the theory that ADD is a purely physical, genetically transmitted "neurological syndrome." This is an interesting choice of wording. Perhaps he chooses the word "neurological" to distance himself from the sticky controversies about the biological basis for "psychiatric" disorders. (Isn't deconstructive reading fun once you catch on to how to do it?) So ADD is an inherited neurological syndrome passed on from generation to generation. Boy, so far he is making this sound very *scientific, medical and factual.* That must mean that none of the "symptoms" of ADD are my fault or my responsibility. By the way, what exactly are the symptoms of this biological derangement? Hallowell summarizes this in a short list (the first of *many, many* lists to come) as: easy distractibility, low tolerance for frustration or boredom, impulsivity, and a "predilection for situations of high intensity." Of course these are just the type of "symptoms" that can get people in trouble in their relationships, in school, on their jobs, and maybe even with the law as one pursues one's "predilections." Fortunately (by the way, we are still in the preface) Hallowell tells us that "Now with a name rooted in neurobiology I could begin to make sense of, in a forgiving way, parts of myself that had often frustrated or scared me." How nice for him

How about a real life story?

One of the things you will learn about me in this book is that I have been involved in (and paid rather handsomely for) marketing of psychiatric medications to fellow physicians. I'll get into this in detail in the next few chapters, but for now I just want to share a personal anecdote germane to our current topic. I was giving a drug company sponsored lecture at a doctors' dinner in Gainesville Florida. In the course of that lecture I made a sarcastic remark about diagnosing ADD in doctors, citing my incredulity that we could possibly theorize that successfully getting through medical school, an ordeal that demands focused attention, a sharp memory, thinking on your feet and absolutely no tendency to procrastinate, could be achieved by people with an unrecognized and untreated neurobiological defect in memory, concentration and staying on task. I delivered this concern in a somewhat sarcastic and flippant manner, expecting that any doctor would agree with the irrationality of such a theory. As soon as I finished my statement, however, two doctors in the audience rose to their feet and preceded to hand me my proverbial butt on a platter. They both stood up, an unusual move at a doctors' dinner meeting, to make sure everyone there understood just how off base my remarks had been. I was pretty much floored by the magnitude and thinly disguised anger of their responses. As I'm sure you have guessed, both of them were diagnosed as AADD, the diagnosis being made after they had finished medical school and residency.

Dr. Hallowell directly addresses the issue of achieving success despite unrecognized AADD by first stating that there can be an upside to AADD which includes "high energy, intuitiveness and enthusiasm." He then goes on to simply factually state without explanation that: "The disorder didn't keep me from becoming a doctor, and it hasn't kept many others from far greater success in a wide variety of fields." (This reminds me of some advertisements for medications for bipolar disorder in which they speculate about what major historical figures might have suffered from that disease. The list usually includes, among others, Abraham Lincoln, Isaac Newton,Vincent Van Gogh, Beethoven and Winston Churchill. But I'm never sure what the drug company is trying to say. Is it that these great men suffered and what a tragedy it was that they could not be diagnosed and treated with the medications we have today or is it that their greatness was somehow rooted in the depth and intensity of their cyclic mood disorders?)

Still in the preface, Hallowell then does what Bennett and Gurin called "get them into the tent". He says: "It has become clear to me that while ADD is hard to define exactly and while it almost never occurs in pure form—that is, without some accompanying problem, such as learning disability or low self esteem—it is a distinct syndrome, greatly in need of detection and treatment. Untreated, it leaves millions of children and adults misunderstood and unnecessarily floundering, even incapacitated." Well I guess that just about covers it. Any problems in life, any lack of success in relationships, job or school problems or just plain not feeling good about yourself might well be a marker of your underlying, ill-defined and unprovable yet very, very serious genetically inherited neurobiological defect manifesting as some or all of the symptoms of AADD. Just to prove there is such a wide range of potential real life expressions of this brain disease Dr. Hallowell provides a *one-hundred item* self quiz, laying out the various manifestations of ADD ranging from #3: Are you moody? (*Wait a second, isn't that a symptom of Bipolar Spectrum Disorder?)* to #19: Do you smoke cigarettes? to #26: In intimate relationships is your inability to linger over conversations an impediment? to #37: Are you particularly intuitive? to #47: Do you find it hard to be alone? to#55: Are you beset with irrational worries? to #69: Are you the life of the party one day and hang-dog (*huh?*) the next? to #88: Do you have many allergies? to #95: Do you love to travel? to #99: Do you love to laugh? to #100: Did you have trouble paying attention long enough to read this entire questionnaire? (*My answer to #99 is yes, I love to laugh and found myself nearly falling out of my chair laughing at the subtle irony of question #100. Doc, you got me. Yes, I got bored with your list of 100 questions and found my mind drifting off after about 50 questions. Can I make an appointment?)*

To me this is not a legitimate book about the discovery of the prevalence and impact of a previously unrecognized medical illness. It's a pop psychology book full of the types of unsubstantiated testimonials and anecdotes you see in most bestselling diet and self help books on the market. So why is this one bothering me so much? It's because I'm seeing more and more patients coming to me carrying diagnoses of AADD from other doctors, most diagnosed for the first time as an adult. If you think that the pre-requisite that you cannot diagnose AADD in someone without a history of childhood ADD would somehow keep the speculative diagnosing of AADD in check, think again! (Shame on you if you've gotten this far in the book and still think that any "fact" or "diagnostic requirement" would limit diagnostic speculation in the psychiatrist's office). You just need to "tweak" the history a bit and uncover "evidence" of unrecognized ADD in your adult patient's past history. And of course, as always, you can't be wrong. As Hallowell clearly states: "there is no definitive test for ADD, no blood test or electroencephalogram reading, or CAT scan or PET scan or X ray, no pathognomonic neurological finding or psychological test score." So why is there all this psychological testing used in diagnosing kids with ADD? As far as I can tell it's to support the supposed validity of the diagnosis by showing that Johnny can't concentrate during the testing. (Plus, sorry to say, it's a big moneymaker for psychologists "specializing" in ADD). Now here's one for the books! Hallowell says that an inability to concentrate ***not*** showing up on psychological testing of concentration does not rule out a diagnosis of ADD. But let Dr. Hallowell tell you in his own words. "Even professionals who know about ADD can miss the diagnosis if they rely too heavily on psychological testing. While psychological testing can be very helpful it is *not definitive.* Children who have ADD can appear *not* to have it when psychologically tested. This is because the structure, novelty and motivation associated with the testing procedure can effectively 'treat' the child's ADD. The child may be focused by the one-on-one structure of the testing, focused by the novelty of the situation, and be so motivated to 'do well' that the motivation overrides the ADD."

Hmmmm......What to say? ......I think I'll just let this quote stand on its own merit and move on. But I will make this general statement. In the light of how diagnostic thinking is moving in psychiatry we are seeing that the clinician is given free range. The clinician is the only one with the deep knowledge of secrets like how an ADD child can have normal scores on ADD detecting tests and STILL have ADD. The clinician is the only one who knows that an emotionally distraught person with multiple symptoms and complaints ranging from drug abuse to violence is really suffering from bipolar spectrum disorder. Of course…diagnosing and treating mental disorders is also how the clinician makes a living…Put simply: **TODAY'S PSYCHIATRISTS CAN DIAGNOSE JUST ABOUT ANYTHING THEY WANT!** I have personally known practicing psychiatrists who tend to "see" ADD in their patients and thus most of their patients are diagnosed ADD. Hallowell said: "Once you catch on to what this syndrome is all about, you'll see it everywhere." The same can be said for depression, bipolarity and anxiety disorders. That's why I chuckle when someone tells me they went to a specialist in ADD to evaluate him or her for ADD. What do you think this "specialist" will find? C'mon, just use your common sense!

I don't treat children. (Thank You Lord). So I don't deal with diagnosing and medicating kids and teens with any psychiatric medications, including stimulants, an increasingly hazardous professional responsibility. But as the Adult ADD diagnosis has caught fire I am having to address this stimulant medication issue in more and more of my adult patients. I practice in Florida. A lot of people move to Florida. Most of my "new" patients were under the care of a psychiatrist before they moved here. When they make an appointment with me not one of them ever gives the slightest thought to the possibility that I might not agree with the diagnosis and treatment provided by their previous psychiatrist. Really, why should they? They believe the first psychiatrist, who, in many cases the patient had been seeing for a long time, had done the medical science, established the diagnosis and, perhaps after a few false starts and some recent revisions, came up with an effective medication treatment plan. They have no inkling that another psychiatrist might hold a radically different view on diagnosis and treatment. So they drag in their paper bags full of prescription bottles, expecting me to unquestioningly endorse the current diagnosis and refill their current meds or make a few minor adjustments. I mentioned previously how exhausting it can be to try to educate the patient about my perspective, get some understanding if not agreement on their part, and then start to simplify and modify the diagnosis and medication treatment all in a one hour intake exam. For some patients, this simply is not achievable and when I realize this I will sometimes just surrender and endorse the diagnosis and fill the desired prescriptions. ("Choose the hill you want to die on" Dr. Laura once said). But this is why I have a particular beef with the new diagnostic trends because Bipolar Spectrum Disorder and Adult ADD patients are often on medication regimens that I cannot simply ignore and refill to ease the pressure on both of us. Because they are often on what I refer to as "heavy duty" medicines and that issue needs to be addressed, if for no other reason than it will now be my name plastered all over the prescription bottles. Add to this the pressure that my new patients are usually almost out or totally out of pills because they delayed making an appointment until their prescriptions from "up north" had no refills left and some of their medicines can be dangerous to stop abruptly. I will go over these issues in much greater detail in the next two chapters, but I do want to share a case history from my files. I have chosen a case where Adult ADD is among the diagnoses because the general treatment of choice for ADD (in children and adults) is from a very problematic class of drugs called psychostimulants. For ease of understanding, you can just call these medications by their more familiar name: amphetamines (a.k.a. SPEED)! As we will discuss more fully in the next chapter the government has created a multi-level schedule of a medication's abuse and addiction potential. The highest is Class One, the schedule for illegal drugs with no approved medical application, drugs such as LSD, Heroin and Cocaine. The next most dangerous is Class Two. Guess what most of the "stimulant" medications used to treat both child and adult ADD are scheduled? Bingo, you got it, Class 2. High abuse potential and, incidentally, high street value. So "welcome new patient that I have never met with one hour to evaluate who presents me with a list of medications they are about to run out of that usually includes one or more controlled substances including class 2 stimulants provided for a diagnosis I don't believe in from another doctor I never met…Welcome. Have a seat."

We'll call her Pam. She was a 60 year old divorced female referred to me from a fellow psychiatrist who was leaving private practice. This lady looked frazzled, disorganized and presented as very needy. I can never figure out what causes psychiatrists to take a particular interest in one of his or her many patients and go above and beyond but her psychiatrist had apparently chosen her. She saw him for both counseling and medication management. The psychiatrist had personally assisted her in getting Social Security Disability and Medicare; she said he even accompanied her to court one day. She, of course, spoke of this previous psychiatrist in glowing terms and understandably so. It was apparent from the beginning that her previous psychiatrist had set a standard of care that I could not possibly come close to matching. On top of that she had the feel of an hysteric, a type of female patient I don't do well with. As soon as I figured this out I stated to try to slowly introduce the concept that we might not be a good doctor/patient match. She seemed genuinely surprised and disturbed because her previous psychiatrist (Freudians would call him the idealized father figure) had spoken so highly of me. Then the "you know what" really started to hit the fan when I began to express my discomfort with her medication regimen. (By the way, she had already shared her diagnosis with me, Rapid Cycling Bipolar Disorder).The problem was her medication regimen included seven different medications that added up to seventeen pills a day. She had not brought her pill bottles with her and had no idea what pills she was running out of…except one! On that one she was very clear. She was going to need a prescription right away for Ritalin. I've mentioned Ritalin before without explaining it because it is such a well known "branded" name, kind of like Kleenex or Ketchup. Ritalin is the brand name for a drug called methylphenidate, or for our purposes here we can just use the previously mentioned familiar definition, speed (or "pharmaceutical cocaine" if you prefer). It is the amphetamine family of drugs that is used in most cases of AADD. They are Class Two; they are abusable, potentially addictive and have legitimate street value if you want to sell them.

So in my door had walked this clinical disaster who, by the way, was telling me that she didn't think the medications were working anymore as she started crying and shaking. I am no saint. I wanted this patient out of my practice. But that day, I was it, the only show in town. I had to deal with her medications on a medical level, i.e. decide what medicines it would be dangerous for her to stop abruptly. She claimed to have no other medical doctors established yet in the area and her previous psychiatrist was long gone. Three of the drugs she was on had painful and possibly dangerous withdrawal symptoms. Fortunately she said she remembers still having some refills on two of them. This was plausible. Only Class Two drugs require a new handwritten prescription for each month. No phone-ins and no refills written down in the corner of the prescription. A new prescription every month was the rule. Coming off Ritalin can be tough and dangerous. So I just decided I had no choice and gave her a prescription for a 30 day supply of three times a day 20 mg pills. This is a high dose of Ritalin, but there I was, giving her 90 pills. Was she going to take them as prescribed? Was she going to crush them and snort them to get high? Was a friend waiting outside to share them? Was she planning to sell them for some desperately needed cash? I told you I'm not a saint and I am also not Superman. I could not devote any more of my day to figuring out her current medication situation, locate and call her previous doctor or call around to pharmacies. We were already thirty minutes over the scheduled one hour as I tried to gently urge her to leave. When she finally realized that I was "rejecting" her as an ongoing patient, she did leave after telling me to go f— myself and slam the door. But she did get her Ritalin.

So this is a personal experience for me as a doctor but one that might help you understand why even from a totally self serving perspective I'm enraged at what is happening in my profession. Ten years ago I would never have had to ever deal with a new patient like her. Not that I didn't ever get borderline/hysterical personality disorders in my practice or at the hospital. That's been going on since time immemorial. But I wouldn't have gotten them pre-interpreted by a fellow psychiatrist as medically ill with Bipolar Spectrum and Adult ADD. Nor would they be on a dangerous combination of meds that I was ethically and legally compelled to deal with. Nor would the patient have been so self-assuredly confident that she had a neurobiological condition requiring complex medication management and frequent medication adjustments. Perhaps then she would not have been so falsely "empowered" to judge me and what I was saying as simply wrong and then curse and slam the door behind her. Remember this book is only my opinion but I am simply not seeing any evidence that the emergence and growing popularity of these seemingly "made-up" disorders is doing anybody any good…except maybe… we'll save that for chapter eight.

To sum up these three chapters on diagnosis: I believe that the growing number and wide range of mental disorder diagnoses (the covering "lies") often preemptively and carelessly made by M.D.'s, psychologists, therapists, ARNP's and PA's (physicians assistants) has become a frightening and dangerous situation. Further, I have argued that the reason diagnostic standards are deteriorating is because of the false presuppositions that lie at the foundation of the psychiatric diagnostic process (the "big lie"). I have drawn on the thinking of two philosophers of science, Karl Popper and Thomas Kuhn, to help us understand that the unchecked anything goes speculation going on now in psychiatry relies heavily on its inherent lack of falsifiability and is fueled by psychiatry's desperate attempts to maintain the appearance of an intact medical paradigm in the face of an ever-growing number of critics and anomalies.

Here I need to do something very important. When I have stated my opinions in the past I have been asked a very fair and reasonable question that goes something like this: "Fine, you have convinced me, medical model psychiatry and DSM IV are severely flawed systems of thought. But if you could wave a magic wand and make it all go away, what would you put in its place?" My answer: The simple truth. The simple truth that the doctor or therapist admits to the patient this way: "The simple truth is that my profession does not know anything with certainty. But we've learned some things through trial and error that might be of value to you. So you and I are going to work *together* and decide *together* what we can try to do to help you." This type of approach by the therapist is called a "knowing not knowing" by philosopher and clinician Ian Parker (Parker 1999). Kirk and Kutchins, the authors of two excellent books critical of DSM diagnostic practices put it this way when discussing how we might have escaped the DSM created dilemma of psychiatry appearing like a science only to find out over time and through experience that it clearly is not:

> One tack would have been to argue that diagnosis in the medical

> mode was premature for the mental health professions, that knowledge about human problems, about the interaction of the mind and body and about the person and the environment were too elementary, too unrefined to fit into a rigid classification of discrete disorders. Further, the argument could be extended to suggest that knowledge of effective treatment was much too loosely tied to diagnostic categories to provide much help for treatment planning. Therefore, the argument would go, diagnostic imprecision was neither troubling nor particularly harmful to therapeutic activity at its current stage of development. The reliability problem could have been discarded as trivial. (Kirk and Kutchins 1992)

What a great proposal for a saner psychiatry. Here is another from psychiatrist Michael Alan Schwartz, M.D. and philosopher Osborne P. Wiggins, PhD. They write:

> We cited as the clinical need to which the DSM was designed to respond: doctors' need for established lists of diagnostic categories in their day-to-day work. This clinical need, we think, is entirely legitimate and should be addressed adequately. We simply contend that because of the current limits of psychiatric knowledge the DSM pretends to a precision and complexity in its classifications which are neither scientifically justified nor practically necessary. We would like a diagnostic manual that more faithfully reflects the present limits of psychiatric knowledge. In this manual the categories would be few in number, and they would have the logical virtue of what in other publications we have called 'ideal types'. That is to say that they would be general concepts with broad coverage. The categories should be viewed as flexible; they should be adjustable in order to be useful for a wide variety of purposes. They should be so general as to remain open: they should lack specificity so that clinician's and researchers fill them in with whatever specificity they needed. The tentative and provisional nature of the categories should be acknowledged and recognized so that features of the disorders they indicate would not be reified or essentialized (Schwartz and Wiggins 2002, p.208).

These both seem to be well thought through and reasonable proposals asking us to, in a sense, start over and redo and simplify the psychiatric diagnostic manual to more honestly reflect what we do know and admit to what we don't know and have not discovered in the 30 years since the publication of DSM III. It would be like psychiatry saying: "Okay, we took at shot at scientific rigor but, much to our chagrin, that wondrous and mysteriously complex object, the brain, has so far refused to yield up its secrets to us." So now all we need is for the power elite behind DSM medical model psychiatry to own up to their mistake, apologize for leading us so far astray, and then reunite with the various mental health disciplines to develop a reasonable, useful and honest diagnostic manual. Is that too much to ask? You are not really going to force me to answer that are you? Clearly Kuhn is on to something is his description of how ***and why*** paradigms resist change. And what is the source of that resistance? Charlton Heston…you're on: "IT'S PEOPLE!"

Thousands of people, some quite powerful, as well as institutions, bureaucracies, organizations and wealthy corporations are supportive of (*and supported by*) the medical model paradigm in psychiatry. Many of them are employed in the massive "mop up" operations, engaged in the business of "normal science." Other interested parties have a lot tied to the medical model and DSM and stand to possibly lose a lot of money and power if the paradigm were overthrown or radically revised as suggested above. As a whole, one could say that the common factor that holds these diverse interest groups together and fuels their shared resistance to paradigm change in psychiatry is summed up best by a famous saying from the Clinton administration: "IT'S THE ECONOMY STUPID!"

What Kirk and Kutchins' and Schwartz and Osbourne's reform proposals do not acknowledge is that medical model psychiatry has moved down two separate paths since its inception in 1980 as DSM III. The first path is the one we have been discussing thus far in this book, the path to medical legitimacy. I have proposed that the progress along this first path has been basically zero, if not even a bit backwards. (Of course, that is not the view held by most others). But it's that second path we need to look at now because as much as a failure that medical model psychiatry has been (in my eyes) on its journey down the path to medical legitimacy, it has been an unprecedented knockout success on its journey down this second path, such a success in fact that it has rendered its failure on the first path irrelevant. What lies at the end of this second path that is so powerfully important that the failure to attain medical legitimacy doesn't even matter? Commodification! I'm not going to even try to explain what I mean by this until I first give you an example. So here it is:

There are 365 separate disorders listed in DSM IV, some well known and frequently diagnosed like "depression" but some less well known and more rarely used. One such diagnosis is listed under the general heading of Anxiety Disorders. It is a condition called Social Phobia (diagnostic code #300.23) but I'm sure you know it better by its more popular name Social Anxiety Disorder. In the early 1990's there were three second generation medications FDA approved for the treatment of depression: Prozac, Paxil and Zoloft. The company that makes Paxil picked up on the little noticed diagnosis Social Phobia and decided to run some drug trials. Using the DSM criteria, a study group who met the criteria for the disorder was identified and treated with either Paxil or placebo. The result of the drug trials was that the people on Paxil had a "statistically significantly" greater improvement in "symptoms" than those on placebo. Paxil got FDA approval for the treatment of Social Phobia. That's how it works. The DSM diagnostic system provides diagnostic criteria for the identification of discrete psychiatric disorders. This provides a study group (stated as something like "one hundred people with DSM diagnosed Social Phobia were divided into two groups") who can then be treated and the results of that treatment statistically analyzed to determine whether the treatment had any effect on the condition. Do you see how this could not be done if we had a diagnostic manual that was truly honest about what we don't know and just gave the kind of "general categories with broad coverage" that Schwartz and Osborne proposed? What would that study look like? One hundred people with vague and diffuse complaints of fearfulness and worries were divided into two groups. Sorry, but that just doesn't work. The drug companies and the FDA need *disease entities* to work with or the research is meaningless. That the DSM model of diagnosis *provides* just such a categorical list of discrete psychiatric disease entities is the only way the drug company and FDA economic machinery can turn in their direction. I am saying that in terms of the big picture, then, this is much more important than academic arguments about whether these diagnoses are valid or not. Sure, people criticize the diagnosis of Social Anxiety Disorder as a "pathologizing" shyness and making a disease out of a normal human problem but these tiny voices of protest are drowned out by the screams of joy and ecstasy heard... where? ...**ON WALL STREET!**

Much more responsible for the lasting success and unassailable dominance of the medical model in psychiatry than its clinical usefulness or theoretical validity is its commodifiability (I think I might have made up that last word, no matter). We live in a competitive market economy that has grown from a regional to a global economy. What anchors this world economy is the buying, selling and trading of commodities. Many things have been commodified in this new revved up world market. Information is a commodity bought, sold and traded on the open market. Of course commodities (physically tangible things) are still commodities. One such physically tangible thing is Paxil, a medicine. The competition in the economy dictates that the goal is to sell as much Paxil as possible. Rules and regulations and laws require that medicine can be sold only if approved by the government for a particular application (treatment of a disease). So that makes DSM a commodity because it provides the disease names needed for the approval process. (FYI: DSM IV itself is also a "commodity"; it sells millions of dollars worth of copies and associated learning materials every year). One way to sell more Paxil then (remember the goal is to maximize sales) is to expand the DSM disease entities Paxil can officially be sold to treat. And that is exactly what Paxil did after some very clever person or committee recognized that Social Phobia "wasn't taken." So Paxil got there first. (Since then other antidepressants such as Zoloft and Effexor have also been FDA approved for the treatment of Social Phobia). But getting there first has its advantages, especially if you have a lot of money to launch a public marketing, oops, I mean "education" campaign so that all those suffering from this formerly under-recognized debilitating disorder can get treatment. That brings us to the final commodity without which none of this would be possible. And what is that final crucial commodity? OK Charlton, one more time… **IT'S PEOPLE!** Yes indeed! The one irreplaceable commodity in our global economy is people…well, sort of. Not really "people" people, but CONSUMING people, also known by the flattering shortened title of just plain "consumers." Someone has to consume the commodities by exchanging capital for them. But that isn't the consumers' only role in this equation. We also need to consume the information that tells us what disease we have and where to go and what to ask for to fix it. This we do very well. Believe me, I know. Back in the 90's when Paxil was "the one and only medication approved for the treatment of Social Anxiety Disorder" thousands of consumers were self diagnosing and presenting to their doctors with their requests for Paxil. Today I'm hearing three things: 1. Do you think I'm bipolar? 2. I think I have ADD. 3. What about that new drug Cymbalta? The names change but the story stays the same. Finally we need people to convince other people to consume. For example, Paxil took the football players Terry Bradshaw (depression) and Ricky Williams (Social Anxiety Disorder) on tour to tell others how Paxil changed their lives. Remember I told you that I have also been paid to promote the use of various psychiatric medications at dinner talks and other lectures. (That will probably dry up if this book is published. What do you think?) The point here is that everyone needs to be in the consumer mode or it doesn't work. Sitting around feeling serene and content like some Buddhist monk just isn't going to cut it!

Earlier in the book I mentioned the term Nietzsche used to describe people in their everyday mode of existence "the herd." Then I mentioned Heidegger's conceptualization of people as "standing reserve." Not very flattering terms are they? But, believe it or not, these philosophers were not putting us down. They were merely observing people in what Heidegger called our mode of "average everydayness." You cannot just choose to walk away from your embededness in your culture and choose to be something totally different. (I realize this every time I get the urge to shop even though there is nothing I need. I too am a "consumer"). But you *can* rise above average everydayness when something important is at stake. I am hoping to convince you that something very important is at stake when you turn your consumptive eye towards psychiatry, because this isn't like choosing what car to buy or what new diet to go on or what to watch on TV. Once you turn down the "chemical imbalance" road there is often no turning back.

THIS ISN'T DISNEYLAND.
YOU PAY A REAL PRICE, MUCH MORE THAN JUST MONEY, FOR YOUR ADMISSION TO PSYCHIATRYLAND.

In the next two chapters I am going to educate you about psychiatric drugs, the good, the bad and all the ugly truths you need to know. I am going to draw the majority of the information I share with you from mainstream textbooks and the pharmaceutical company's own statements in the Physician's Desk Reference (PDR). This is not going to be some hatchet job because you will need a true "fair and balanced" understanding of these medicines and other medical options when and if you decide to seek psychiatric help or change the type of help you are getting. When you find yourself forced to make these potentially life-defining decisions about yourself, your family and friends; that is when you really do need to ***stand above the herd.***

Chapter Six:
SEROTONIN: The "X" Factor

> To believe that we can conquer depression, despair, anxiety with modern technology is the height of hubris and bad faith, a mere childish fantasy, unworthy of any thoughtful person who has their eyes open to human history and modern culture.
>
> David Kaiser, M.D.
> *Psychiatric Times.* February, 1997

I want to start this first of two chapters on psychiatric medications by focusing on antidepressants, by far the most widely used class of psychiatric drugs. In chapter seven we will explore the other four classes of drugs used in psychiatry: sedative/hypnotics, antipsychotics, mood stabilizers and stimulants. I will show you in these chapters how the same imprecision, arbitrariness and pseudoscience that characterizes current psychiatric diagnostic practices is mirrored by current psychiatric treatment practices, only in this case it involves more than merely writing down a diagnosis in a medical chart; it involves putting chemicals with unknown mechanisms of action and a wide range of side-effects and toxicities into your body and the bodies of your spouses and children. I will begin this chapter on antidepressants with a couple of recent case histories from my former private practice that illustrate the personal impact that medical model psychiatry's stubborn insistence that "depression" is a medical disorder has on people in emotional pain who elect to present to a medical doctor for help. After that, I will explain why I titled this chapter the "X" factor and then examine the antidepressant class of drugs in detail.

Where I lived while I was in private practice, Volusia County, Florida, I think we had generally decent medical care. We suffered from the same cost-containment and quality control issues as all of the rest of the states. North on Route 95 however, about ninety minutes from Volusia County was a pretty impressive medical facility, the Jacksonville, Florida branch of the Mayo Clinic. From what I could see the Mayo Clinic offered patients something they were having a harder and harder time getting in a managed care environment, a comprehensive and fully coordinated medical evaluation. I saw a lot of elderly patients in my practice, many of whom had complex medical problems. Occasionally some of them decided to go to the Mayo Clinic for an assessment. I usually received their medical records from Mayo and found that they did do an impressive and thorough job. In particular, it was noteworthy how all of the various specialists involved cross communicated and coordinated their findings, all documented in a comprehensive final report. They have consulting psychiatrists on staff at Mayo as well and occasionally they saw my patients even though psychiatric problems were not the primary reason any of my patients had gone there.

One of my patients, we'll call her Clara, went to Mayo for a work-up of her numerous medical problems. She was my patient because she was suffering from so-called "treatment resistant depression." (I don't think I mentioned this label in the last chapter. I see it as another "anomaly cover-up" which I will fully explain when we get to a surgical implantation treatment procedure for depression called Vagal Nerve Stimulation later in this chapter). On top of Clara's complaints about physical problems she also complained to her PCP about a sad mood, tearfulness, anxiety and a general lack of ability to enjoy her life the way she used to. The PCP "diagnosed" depression and ran her through a slew of antidepressant trials (something I like to call the "antidepressant merry-go-round"). She was ultimately referred to me because of a lack of response to medication, hence "treatment resistant." You need to understand that neither Clara nor her doctor were looking for or expected a psychosocial diagnostic reformulation of the case because she was not considered misdiagnosed, just not as yet responsive to medication. She was referred to me because I allegedly "know more" about antidepressant medications than her family doctor. Typically when this happens psychiatrists, who, in fact, believe they do "know more" about psychiatric medication than family doctors, will display their "special knowledge" by getting more medically aggressive. Drugs will be added, recommended doses exceeded and augmentation strategies employed. I liken this to "Chinese Menu" treatment: One from Column A, one from Column B etc.

Just to let you know that my metaphors are not merely "metaphorical" I want to tell you about one of my private practice patients. She was 48 years old and was seeking an opinion on her medications prescribed by another psychiatrist.

The reason I am mentioning her is because her case so neatly fits into my Chinese Menu model. She listed her medications for me: Luvox, Lithium, Abilify, Librium and Ambien.

Shown another way her meds are:

Column A	***Column B***	***Column C***	***Column D***	***Column E***
SSRI Antidepressant	Mood Stabilizer	Antipsychotic	Tranquilizer	Hypnotic
Luvox	*Lithium*	*Abilify*	*Librium*	*Ambien*

Back to Clara:

Unbeknownst to the patient and her PCP, however, is that I didn't do Chinese Menu treatment and psychosocial reformulations of cases are exactly what I do when confronted with "treatment resistant" patients. Although I deal with each patient on a case-by-case basis, Clara was among the many elderly antidepressant non-responders I saw who I "treated" by working on undoing the erroneous perspective about "depression" they had been taught by their doctor and others. I find that this "mental illness" label is frequently misapplied to the very common and totally normal (though undeniably unpleasant) psychological response to the accumulated traumas and losses and the growing number of health problems that accompany aging. You are all familiar with my "existential" diagnosis in these cases: "life." As I will explain later, that doesn't mean that I won't use antidepressants, even if just for what they symbolize, but I will try to help the patients see that they were misled if they expected these drugs to deliver what they had hoped. What had they hoped for? I can't tell you how many times I've heard these words: "I JUST WANT TO BE HAPPY…LIKE I USED TO BE."

Clara certainly had enough trials of various antidepressants (five in all) to prove that this class of drugs just wasn't going to do anything more than they had already done. So I decided to just keep her on her current drug and work on her accepting that the effect it had was as good as it was going to get. We could then work on her "depression" which in cases like hers I like to call by the more precise name, *demoralization*, a diagnosis proposed by psychiatrist Donald Klein (Klein et al. 1980). Loss of morale (*de*moralization) as an effect of accumulated traumas and stresses is very common. Some unfortunate people walk around with the sword of Damocles hovering above wondering what's going to go wrong next. A lot of my patients with chronic pain get demoralized, especially after two or three operations fail to relieve the pain, or make it worse. I'll guarantee you that antidepressants NEVER make chronic pain patients "happy." I'm not sure they do much of anything but numb them (more on numbing by antidepressants shortly) Nor do they ever do much for the elderly who are feeling demoralized near the end of that long and difficult journey called life. You've heard the joke: Inside every older person is a younger person wondering what the hell happened. I'm not saying that the demoralized patient cannot be helped; they can be helped in many ways. But lumping them into the category of biological depression and running them through med trials is not the way to do it.

That medicine was not the solution isn't exactly what Clara wanted to hear, of course. Nor did her husband and I understand. He had no idea what to do about her mood. Clara went to the Mayo Clinic for medical reasons but while she was there, as part of the comprehensive evaluation, she did have a psychiatric consult regarding her complaints of depression. When I saw her I asked about Mayo and whether she had seen a psychiatrist there. "Yes" she said, and then pulled his card out from her wallet. "The doctor told me to give you this and for you to read what he wrote on the back. He said you would understand." She handed over the business card with such a sense of awe and drama that you would think that I was about to receive instructions from God. I looked at the front. There was the psychiatrist's name and, as would be expected from a Mayo doctor, very impressive credentials. I turned the card over. There, written in ink was a single word:

CYMBALTA

I must admit, I was half expecting that "advice" to be on this Mayo psychiatrist's card but was still very disappointed when I saw it. Think about it, this highly trained specialist had four years of medical school, four years (or more) of a psychiatric residency and tons of clinical experience and what does this Mayo psychiatrist, *in essence,* recommend I do? "Try her on that new antidepressant that just came out since the other ones haven't worked." I could have figured that one out watching TV commercials. The real reason that I was disappointed is because I knew that it was once again *my job* to let this poor woman down, to re-educate her about the realities of antidepressant medication treatment. I was not a consultant; I was responsible for her ongoing care. I could not, in good conscience, join her in Psychiatryland and endorse fairy tales and magic wishes. No, that's the job of the pharmaceutical company's marketing department. The presence of the word Cymbalta on that psychiatrist's card only served to remind me how really, really, really good they are at their jobs. Like I needed any reminders!

What motivates the continued development of "new" antidepressants like Cymbalta is that there is a market out there hungry for new choices because, in simple terms, antidepressants simply don't "work" that well. (Later in this chapter I will show you the results of a recent $35 million government sponsored study on the effectiveness of antidepressants and I think you will be forced to agree with me). So despite all the initial hype and hoopla about Prozac, after over twenty years of clinical experience and the development of about nine new antidepressant drugs, more and more patients and doctors are faced with the same dilemma as Clara and me; antidepressants are not delivering the goods. They are not cure-alls and certainly not "happy pills" that we can use to alleviate the painful moods that are part of everyone's life. But they are not inert compounds either. I have seen very positive results from antidepressants and I have seen absolutely no response to them and every shade of response in between. If anything, the adjective I'd use to describe antidepressants is **disappointing.** They kind of remind me of what a real day on a vacation is like compared to our fantasies about the vacation before we actually go. Have you been to Rome? Rome is amazing but it is also crowded, expensive and tiring to tour. On my one-day tour of Rome you could see St. Peter's Basilica *or* the Sistine Chapel but you couldn't see both because the lines were too long. By the time I got back to the hotel I couldn't wait to shower and put my feet up and watch a little TV. Wait a second; the TV shows are all in Italian, nuts! And the tour bus leaves at 7AM tomorrow; that means getting up at six. Why did I try to cram so much into my first vacation to Italy?

Its time to take a realistic look at antidepressant medications and see what they are really all about. We are going to start by (forgive me Duke Ellington) taking a ride "on the X train."

As you may or may not know, "X" is shorthand for an illegal drug usually called Ecstasy. In truth the drug is MDMA, (I'll spare you the multi-syllabic chemical name), an amphetamine derivative first synthesized in 1912 by the German pharmaceutical company, Merck. It more or less sat on the shelf alongside numerous other synthetic compounds drug companies traditionally patent without a clear-cut application in mind. MDMA resurfaced in the 1960's when a group of psychotherapists started to tout its astounding ability to assist patients in making progress in therapy. These therapists gave MDMA the nicknames: "Window" and "Empathy." Its capacity to induce a four to six hour state of open-mindedness, well-being, and empathy (the ability to put oneself into the other person's shoes) allowed for, the therapists claimed, six months to a year's worth of therapeutic growth to occur in one session. "Empathy" made you feel connected, cared for and compassionate; it made you feel *terrific.* (Uh oh, I smell trouble). Naturally, it didn't take long for non-patients to discover this new euphoria inducing drug. It was re-nicknamed Ecstasy or Extasy or just X and spread like wildfire into the club and party scene. Due to its capacity to produce a period of near boundless energy, the all night dance parties called raves became a national phenomenon, catering to the sky rocketing numbers of teenage "rollers" (slang for ecstasy users). (Uh oh, I definitely smell trouble). Naturally, people began to overdo it and people began to die. You see Ecstasy had a rather unusual side effect, it made you forget to drink. It somehow blocked the sensation of thirst so some all night ravers, dancing and sweating, got severely dehydrated. One teenager in England died from water intoxication, drinking too much water when trying to compensate for the thirst blocking side effect of X. This is a strange drug. It also causes painful jaw clenching, a problem ravers solved by using pacifiers. I remember the first time I saw a video on raves and wondered why all these kids had pacifiers in their mouths. A lot of them had surgical masks on as well; apparently a dab of Vick's Vaporub inside the mask prolongs the high on X. "Partying" kids are nuts and they started to die. No water, too much water, getting dangerously overheated, taking too much X and taking other drugs with X...the party was over. MDMA was declared illegal in the mid eighties despite some therapists still arguing its value to mental health professionals and their clients. That's not to say, of course, that this stopped the use of MDMA. Ecstasy is currently one the top four drugs of abuse in the United States. The others are cocaine, heroin and marijuana.

OK, this is an interesting story Dr. Phill, but isn't this chapter supposed to be about antidepressant medications like Prozac and Zoloft; why the detour into the world of illicit drugs?

I took this detour because I want to show you how the way we think X works its "magic" is so similar to how we think antidepressants work theirs. It has to do with a brain chemical you've all heard about: serotonin.

All euphoria producing drugs of abuse are believed to work in part by causing a massive release of the chemical molecules used by the brain to transmit messages between cells (technically called neurotransmitters). They do this by causing the nerve cells to release their stored reserves of neurotransmitters all at once instead of in the tiny amounts usually released to transmit messages from one cell to the next. The "user" experiences the impact of this flood of neurotransmitters as a "rush" or "buzz" or "high". Among the many neurotransmitters (with many more yet to be discovered) are three that are of great interest to psychiatry: dopamine, norepinephrine and serotonin. What is relevant about this to our exploration of antidepressants is the fact that what distinguishes the intoxication people experience on ecstasy from the highs produced by other drugs seems to be because of its selective effect on the neurotransmitter serotonin. While it also induces a release of dopamine, ecstasy literally floods the brain with serotonin. Contrast ecstasy with less serotonin specific drugs of abuse like speed, cocaine and heroin and you notice a very interesting distinction; no group of psychotherapists has ever, as far as

I know, touted the benefits of using heroin, cocaine or speed to help therapy patients gain a greater sense of open-mindedness, empathy and compassion that could be used to speed up emotional growth and insight in therapy. No, wait a second, wasn't there something about LSD and insight and spiritual growth and Dr. Timothy Leary? As a matter of fact there was. LSD was also used extensively in psychotherapy before being declared illegal. LSD also works by affecting primarily serotonin. (Here is a little interesting aside. The antidepressant Serzone, which worked primarily in the serotonin system, had a unique side effect in some patients; some Serzone users saw "trails." These are afterimages, often in intriguing colors, that occur following something passing through your line of vision, created most often by swiping your hand in front of your face. This particular effect was one of the phenomena that LSD users used to enjoy).

The point is that serotonin is a remarkable neurotransmitter with myriad effects in both the brain and the rest of the body. In trying to more scientifically explore the precise function of serotonin, you begin to get a glimpse into the incredible complexity of the brain. Serotonin, like all neurotransmitters, sends messages from one cell to the next. The effect of serotonin therefore depends on the function of the cell receiving the message. But wait, there is more. The particular effect serotonin has on a receiving cell will also depend on what type of serotonin receptors (message receivers) are on the surface of the receiving cell. There are at least 15 types of serotonin receptors that have been identified, each apparently responding in its own unique way to serotonin stimulation. (Welcome to the indescribably complex world of neurophysiology) Okay, let's summarize: Serotonin, widely distributed in the brain and body, with multiple types of receptors having varying effects on a wide range of nerve cells, each with their own specific function.

STOP!! TOO COMPLICATED!!

You are right, way too complicated, so let's simplify. Let's look at what we already know. What does MDMA (and LSD) teach us about serotonin? It apparently is involved in brain circuits having to do with some very high levels of the expression of human consciousness; with spiritual issues such as feelings of belonging, of one-ness with the universe, compassion, empathy and love. It is impossible to summarize the effect of serotonin but I think there is one conclusion we can draw that is central to understanding the widespread use of antidepressants and, as we'll discuss shortly, the wide range of psychiatric disorders the serotonin drugs are currently indicated to "treat." There just HAS TO BE a felt effect from increasing brain serotonin activity, no matter whether you are "ill" or "normal." It's simply inconceivable to me that increasing activity in the serotonin system of the brain, by whatever means, would not have ANY effect on someone with a "healthy" brain. So rather than continuing to buy into the myth that only sick brains respond to serotonin, let's look for other examples of serotonin effects that are known to occur from drugs less powerful than ecstasy or LSD because clearly people don't usually report hallucinations or rushes of euphoria from using antidepressants.

Do you remember a product used in obesity treatment called Fen-Fen? It was a very successful but short-lived treatment option due to the unfortunate emergence of very serious heart and lung damage cause by this combination of medicines. The notorious Fen-Fen was actually a combination of two drugs, phentermine and fenfluramine. Phentermine is still on the market; it is simply an amphetamine appetite suppressant. Fenfluramine (also sold as a stand alone weight reducing drug called Redux) was a serotonin stimulant that didn't really block appetite; it quickened and enhanced the sense of satisfaction from eating. In a way you could say that Redux chemically calmed the negative feeling state we call being hungry. The reason this assisted weight loss was because it induced this sense of satisfaction with less intake of food. This effect occurs in the hypothalamus, a primitive system buried deep in the part of the brain that we share in common with many animals. After all, something needs to stimulate any organism to feed and then reward that adaptive behavior. But let's look at human eating because things are always more complicated with us.

Hunger is a negative and painful physical and emotional state demanding action. But there is a big difference between responding to hunger by inhaling a fast food meal during a ten minute lunch break and responding to it by eating slowly, like when dining at an elegant restaurant. In the first instance stretch receptors in the stomach wall deliver the message to the brain that more than enough food has been consumed while a second pathway from the brain instructs your hands to unbuckle your pants. At the elegant restaurant the meal is delivered in courses at a leisurely pace. For many people after the appetizer, bread and salad have been consumed and before the entrée arrives something happens. You feel satisfied. Not full or stuffed, satisfied. You are no longer hungry, you are **content**. The reason we don't experience this when eating rapidly is that there is a time delay of about 15 minutes for the messages from the intestines, where food is absorbed, to reach the brain and stimulate the serotonin system to shut off hunger. That is why all diet programs emphasize eating slowly. We'll call this effect of serotonin activity **contentment**, referring to the now *absent* stress and pain of hunger.

The reason I'm going into all of this detail here is, as mentioned above, to build my case to debunk the assumption that the serotonin stimulation caused by antidepressant drugs will have a *felt effect* and an impact on your mood only if your brain is sick (i.e. chemically imbalanced), otherwise a dose of Paxil, Prozac, Zoloft and the like will have no effect; it would be as if you'd taken nothing at all. The serotonin connection to ecstasy and LSD is not controversial while the idea that the more subtle serotonin stimulation caused by antidepressants will *not* impact a "normal" brain is nearly accepted fact. Why?? I think there are some clear-cut reasons for this. Psychiatry often argues that what **validates** the theory of a biological basis for conditions like depression and ADD is the curative response to medication. I will take up this topic in greater detail later in the book (by looking at how the same "logic" is applied to the even less tenable idea that the positive response to pharmaceutical amphetamines proves that both childhood and adult ADD are true biological illnesses). For now, I just want to make the point that is, I believe, inarguably apparent; i.e. that the felt effects of the serotonin stimulating properties of antidepressants don't require a sick brain any more than the alerting properties of coffee requires a caffeine deficient brain or the mood altering properties of alcohol requires an alcohol deficient brain. Since there are not a plethora of studies on the impact of antidepressants on "normal" brains I will simply offer my clinical opinion (that has some support in the literature) that one of the chief felt effects of antidepressant induced serotonin stimulation on the brain is state of "contentment" where stress simply feels less stressful. My evidence for this (outside of the literature) is the hundreds upon hundreds of patients who have described this to me.

In my clinical experience this reduction of the felt stressfulness of stress is one of the most predictable and reliable effects of serotonin antidepressants on the human brain. In the literature and PDR there is what philosophers like to call a "gesture" towards this in the reporting of a "side effect" usually labeled emotional blunting. My patients will almost always report feeling less stressed by stress and therefore often much less irritable (the spouses love it). You'd be surprised how many people come to psychiatrists because of difficulties controlling their temper, walk away with a diagnosis of "depression" but have a "good response" reported as less temper outbursts. But some patients complain that they don't like the emotional numbing because they also don't feel desired emotions as strongly either. They report being unable to cry even when they want to or to feel particularly giddy or any other welcomed emotional states like "horny" (more on that shortly). That doesn't mean, however, that they insist on coming off the medication. In fact, that almost never happens!

The "medical" term emotional blunting has a negative connotation, implying that this is an unwelcome and undesirable effect of medications. I don't agree. I think the emotional blunting by antidepressants has both a positive and negative side. Let me propose some alternative more positive "labels" for emotional blunting: How about "Que sera sera", or "don't sweat the small stuff man", or "live and let live I always say" or my favorite (that I read somewhere but can't remember where) describing emotional blunting as the "what the hell effect"? I hope you can see my point. This conceptualization of the emotional "blunting" from serotonin stimulation shows how it might very well be experienced as a positive and welcome relief to what psychiatrist David Kaiser describes as the state of today's typical patients: "discontented, unhappy, fragmented, and confused by an increasingly frantic, alienating and violent society" (Kaiser 1997).

PROBLEM	**SOLUTION**
Unbearable increase in pressure at work	*The "what the hell" effect*
Watching the 11:00 O'clock news	*The "what the hell" effect*
Raising children in today's world	*The "what the hell" effect*
Your teenager becoming a disrespectful brat	*The "what the hell" effect*
A marriage falling apart	*The "what the hell" effect*
The death of a loved one	*The "what the hell" effect*
General helplessness and rage	*The "what the hell" effect*
Four Dollar a Gallon Gasoline	*The "what the hell" effect*
Sarah Palin	*The "what the hell" effect*
Big Brother is Watching	*SOMA! (Whoops)*

With this in mind let's move on to look at information about the individual antidepressants and then examine the results of a recent $35 million government sponsored research study on the effectiveness of antidepressant treatment of depression.

I had originally intended to list all of the currently available antidepressant medications but that would unnecessarily complicate this chapter because the only drugs in wide use now are Prozac and the antidepressants released since Prozac. This includes the following medications (if the drug is no longer on patent I will list the generic drug name in parentheses):

1. Prozac (Fluoxetine)
2. Serafem (Fluoxetine)
3. Celexa (Citalopram)
4. Luvox (Fluvoxamine)
5. Paxil (Paroxetine)
6. Paxil CR
7. Zoloft (Sertraline)
8. Lexapro

9. Wellbutrin SR & XL (BuprprionSR & XL)
10. Effexor (Venlafaxine)
11. EffexorXR (Venlafaxine XR)
12. Serzone (Nefazadone)
13. Remeron (Mirtazapine)
14. Cymbalta
15. Prestiq

This list makes it look like there are a lot of antidepressants to choose from but that's a bit of an illusion. Some of them (all of the CR's, SR's, XR's and XL's) are simply slow release versions of the same drug (these are generally patent-extenders, see chapter eight). Also, if we break this list down into *hypothesized* mechanisms of action, (the *actual* mechanism of action is ***not known*** for all psychiatric medications), we will see that this lists reduces to just three categories:

1. **Serotonin antidepressants**: Prozac, Paxil (and CR), Zoloft, Luvox, Celexa, Lexapro, Serzone, and Remeron
2. **Serotonin/norepinephrine antidepressants**: Effexor (and XR), Cymbalta and Prestiq
3. **Dopamine/?norepinephrine antidepressants**: Wellbutrin (SR and XL)

You might be wondering right off the bat; why so many drugs that work the same? To answer that I want to introduce you to a book and author that I will be referring to frequently when discussing drugs and the companies that produce them. The book is titled *The Truth About Drug Companies. How they deceive us and what to do about it.* I'm sure you are not surprised that there is a book like this. There are many books about deception and corporate greed in the pharmaceutical industry. But I am choosing to use this book because of the author. Her name is Marcia Angell, M.D. The book was published by Random House in 2004. Before writing this book Dr. Angell had a pretty impressive job. She was the editor in chief of *The New England Journal of Medicine* which is among the most prestigious medical journals in the entire world. If Dr. Angell tells me what is actually going on at the drug companies and in drug research I am going to totally trust her and hope you will too. Here is her answer to the question of why there are so many antidepressants with basically the same mechanism of action. She calls these "me too" drugs which means they are in essence money-making incentivized copies of already successful drugs, "minor variations of drugs already on the market." Let's look at how that applies to the serotonin antidepressants.

We need to start with a little bit of neurophysiology. I've told you that the chemical messengers (neurotransmitters) that communicate messages between cells are typically released in tiny amounts when sending their "fire/don't fire" messages. Now we need to look at what happens to these neurotransmitters after they send their message. They need to be somehow removed from the scene so that they don't interfere with the next message coming down the pike. They are removed by either being deactivated by a nearby enzyme or being recycled. Most of the neurotransmitter is recycled as this is the most energy efficient process. On the surface of the sending cells are tiny pumps that return the neurotransmitter to inside the sending cell, ready to be used again. When a drug blocks the pump then the neurotransmitter is not taken up into the sending cell and therefore spends more time exposing the receiving cell to its message. That is it, the proposed mechanism of action of most of the antidepressants that you might have heard referred to as SSRI's. What that acronym stands for is **S**elective **S**erotonin **R**euptake **I**nhibitors.

(*Here is an amusing story that I once heard. The word that accurately describes the way the neurotransmitter is returned to the cell is by uptake. It's not specifically a reuptake because that implies that it was already taken up and is being taken up again. I know this is splitting hairs but just stick with me. If we use the word uptake to create the acronym for this class of drugs then they would be **S**erotonin **U**ptake **I**nhibitors or **SUI's.** Someone noticed that this also happened to be the first three letters in the word **SUI**cide. Whoops! Bad choice. So they rethought the problem and decided to call the action of the pumps that these drugs block as "reuptake" instead of uptake. Now the acronym could be **S**erotonin **R**euptake **I**nhibitor or **SRI.** Safe! The label you are used to hearing is SSRI which adds the word **S**elective, hence **S**elective **S**erotonin **R**euptake **I**nhibitor: **SSRI.** I don't know if this little historical tidbit is true or not but it easily could be. Compared to the marketing tactics by drug companies we will discuss in detail in chapter eight, this little name change is quite tame).

The difference then between serotonin antidepressants and the more powerful illegal serotonin drugs we mentioned is that the SSRI's do not promote a *release* of serotonin, they merely interfere with its removal so that there is a longer serotonin exposure to the receiving cell. But how did we figure this out? And how did we discover that serotonin cells are the culprits in depression? I can assure you one thing: not scientifically!

Turning back to Dr. Angell's book; she discusses the process by which new drugs are developed to treat diseases. It's called research and development (R&D) and she explains:

> You can't just randomly test chemicals to see if one will turn up

> that might be helpful in treating a disease. That would take an infinitely long time and be dangerous as well. Instead, most of the time you first have to understand the nature of the disease you want to treat—what has gone wrong in the body to cause it. That understanding needs to be fairly detailed, usually at the molecular level, if there is to be any hope of finding a drug that will safely and effectively interfere with the chain of events responsible for the disease. What researchers hope to find is some specific link in the chain that the drug will target (Angell 2004, p.22).

As an example of R&D, Dr. Angell traces the history of the development of drugs to treat AIDS. All there was at first (noticed in the 1980's) was this bizarre wasting condition and the presence of infections that most people don't get. That focused attention on the immune system which eventually, through *painstaking* work, resulted in the isolation of the HIV virus, the cause of AIDS. Then came the development of drugs to treat AIDS, but only after the cause had been clearly identified. That is traditional R&D. What I want to say about psychiatry is:

Psychiatry, you are so NOT a science!

So, how *were* antidepressants discovered? Dr. Angell said that you can't just randomly test chemicals to see if it would cure a disease because it would be an infinitely long and dangerous process. Well how about if you are testing a drug for one reason and, just by sheer luck, you notice that it helps a condition you weren't even testing it for? (Like the antihypertensive minoxidil, brand name Rogaine, unexpectedly leading to hair growth). That does happen, as it did in the 1950's when they were testing a drug for tuberculosis called iproniazid. It was noticed that some people taking iproniazid also seemed to experience mood elevation. When studied it was found that iproniazid inhibited the activity of the enzyme that removed dopamine, serotonin and epinephrine after it gave its message to the receiving cell. The iproniazid class of drugs is called MAO inhibitors or MAOI's but we are not going to really get into them in this book. Suffice it to say that side effect problems (some fatal) pretty much knocked the MAOI's out of the ballgame although they are still available today (as Nardil and Parnate) and used for some patients. Back to the history: Later in the 1950's another drug called imipramine was being tested for psychotic illnesses such as schizophrenia. Again, mood improvement was noticed as an unexpected effect. This drug was the first in a class that would be called tricyclic antidepressants which were found to inhibit the reuptake of serotonin and epinephrine into the nerve cells. Serotonin, epinephrine and dopamine are also called cathecholamines. Since both iproniazid and imipramine increased cathecholamine activity it was theorized that depression was *caused* by decreased cathecholamine activity. So doesn't this mean that like it was for AIDS, a cause for the illness was found?…well, not quite!

The virus that causes AIDS is a visible identifiable physical thing that can be isolated, cultured, implanted in animals for drug studies etc. Sorry, no such luck for cathecholamine depletion. It cannot be seen, cannot be isolated, cannot be tested for and cannot be confirmed as the cause of depression. In R&D it is best to isolate the cause of an illness and then develop treatments. The theory of the imbalance of the neurotransmitters serotonin and epinephrine causing depression (and many other psychiatric disorders) was arrived at in what I like to call a bass-ackwards sequence, i.e. find a drug that (?seemingly) helps the condition and then study what that drug does and hypothesize the cause of the disease based on the action of the drug. The argument against this type of logic is simple and compelling: *A headache is not the result of an aspirin deficiency.* Okay, so this is clearly not ideal R&D but it can still lead to the total package medical science shoots for: cause>treatment>cure. But this isn't quite how it has worked out in psychiatry.

The effects and purported mechanism of action of the "accidentally discovered" antidepressants were pretty well understood by, let's generously say, at the latest, around 1960, some fifty years ago. In referring to the medical model concept of depression as a biologically based mental disorder I will now make the following factual statements:

IN 50 YEARS WE HAVE NOT GAINED ANY GREATER UNDERSTANDING OF A DEFINITIVE AND DEMONSTRABLE BIOLOGICAL BASIS OF DEPRESSION

WE HAVE NOT DEVELOPED ANY DEFINITIVE MEDICAL TESTS FOR "BIOLOGICAL" DEPRESSION!

WE HAVE NOT DEVELOPED ANY PROCEDURE OR MECHANISM TO CLEARLY DISTINGUISH A "BIOLOGICAL" DEPRESSION FROM ALL THE OTHER VARIETIES OF EXPRESSIONS OF HUMAN UNHAPPINESS!

AND FINALLY: WE HAVE NOT DEVELOPED ANY MEDICAL TREATMENT THAT IS SUPERIOR TO IMIPRAMINE FOR THE TREATMENT OF DEPRESSION!

Just for fun let's take a time machine back to 1960 and imagine we are eavesdropping on a doctor and his patient:

Doctor: "What's wrong, you look terrible?"

Patient: "I don't know. I can't stop crying and I feel hopeless."

Doctor: "That sounds like depression to me. But don't fret, we have a new drug called imipramine that should help. If not, there are some other drugs called MAOI's we can try."

Patient: "Drugs?? I'm not physically sick. I'm depressed."

Doctor: "I understand. But we are learning that depression is a physical illness, only it's in the brain."

Patient: "Wait a second Doc, are you saying I'm nuts??"

Doctor: "No, no, not at all. You are perfectly sane, just depressed. And it is not your fault at all. The fact that I can give you medication is GOOD news. A lot better than my sending you to Dr. Gross for two years of psychoanalysis."

Patient: "You sure this is gonna work doc?"

Doctor: "Nothings for sure but I've heard some real promising stuff."

Patient: "So what labs and X-Rays do you need to see if I have this brain disease?"

Doctor: "Well that's the great thing. I can figure out whether you have depression by just asking you questions."

Patient: "Wow that's terrific. I hate getting blood taken. But listen, I think my wife is gonna want some proof before she goes along with me taking pills. So if it's just the same to you Doc, I think I better go get those lab tests."

Doctor: "Sorry. I guess I didn't make myself clear. There aren't any lab tests or X-Rays or anything else for depression right now but I hear they are working on them and there will be some tests for depression real soon."

Patient: "OK Doc this is a little scary but I guess if it's guaranteed to work I'll take the drug."

Doctor: (Starting to get a little peeved). "Look, let's be clear. I can't guarantee it's going to work. Nothing works 100% of the time"

Patient: "OK, OK, don't get angry. Hey, I'm the one who's depressed here. Just give me a percentage, 70, 80, 90 percent chance?"

Doctor: "I'm not angry. This is just kinda new to me too. I'm not sure about percentages. The studies are a bit confusing."

Patient: "Man this decision is getting harder the more we talk. I know I gotta make up my mind. Just one last question. These pills aren't dangerous are they?"

Doctor: "Well we will have to get an EKG before we start because there have been some reports of cardiac toxicity. You might feel tired or more nervous. You can gain weight, get blurry vision, get constipated and/or not be able to pee. You might sweat more and not be able to perform sexually."

Patient: (On his way out the door now). "Hey you know Doc, thanks but I think my depression is starting to go away…"

Doctor: "Wait I didn't get a chance to tell you about how overdoses can kill you, or the withdrawal effects when you stop."

I'm really not trying to just be funny here. (But I must admit I am kind of amusing myself). This is a completely legitimate possible conversation in the early days of antidepressant treatment. And, aside from the cardiovascular side effects of the antidepressant, it is just as legitimately possible as a doctor patient conversation today (although I expect the marketing phrase "chemical imbalance" might be tossed around a bit more). Actually, I think the care offered by biologically oriented psychiatrists was much better 30 years ago in 1980 than it is today. Why did I pick that date? I'll tell you: Sitting in front of me is a book published in 1980 entitled *Diagnosis and Drug Treatment of Psychiatric Disorders: Adults and Children.* It was edited by Donald F. Klein, Rachel Gittelman, Frederick Quitkin and Arthur Rifkin and published by Williams and Wilkens. It's the source I quoted earlier when I mentioned demoralization as a diagnosis I like to use. This book is a true "state of the art" compilation of medical model psychiatry just before DSM III was released. It focuses primarily on drug treatment. It was written before Prozac was even developed. There are seven tricyclic antidepressants listed in the book but with nineteen different brand names (hey, business is business). There are also four MAOI's. In the section that reviews the effectiveness of treatment there are so many rejoinders that it's just about impossible to pick out a meaningful number. They go to great lengths to make the case that tricyclics are "superior" to placebo even though a few studies showed the opposite. Among the confounding variables mentioned that made an accurate estimate difficult were the uncertainty of diagnosis and the possibility of spontaneous recovery. "Clearly superior", they say, over and over estimating a 2/3 response rate to drug versus 1/3 response rate to placebos. As you will shortly see, a 2/3 response rate would look pretty good today. But I need to point out that the studies are very different today for two related reasons. The first is that there is LESS discrimination in selecting study subjects today than there was in 1980. The second is that since Prozac hit the scene the world itself has changed pretty dramatically, not just around Prozac but, in part, because if it! (This is a complex sociological and cultural issue we will be covering in detail in later chapters).

I am glad that writing this book forced me to get Klein's book off the shelf and revisit it because I remember how much I liked it in 1980 when I was still just a resident in psychiatry. I was very enthusiastic at that time about our efforts to distinguish biological depressions from non-biological depressions because then the decision of when and how vigorously to use medication would make more sense and the psychiatrist would play an important role by being the person who made the discriminatory judgments necessary to formulate a rational treatment plan for each individual patient. None of us in 1980 could possibly have anticipated that our then, still relatively noble profession, would ultimately be reduced to the level of being a pitchman for pharmaceutical companies.

Sometimes when I am trying to explain this to my patients I use the analogy of being the owner of a store that sells tires. I ask them to imagine what happens when a customer drives up in their car and asks; "Do you think I need new tires or are these still OK?" It's pretty clear that if the tire store owner was assiduously honest he might end up sending away more customers than he could afford. So he bends the truth a little and recommends new tires to just about everyone who asks the question. Then the only issue is which brand of tire to "suggest", Goodyear, Firestone, Michelin? That decision might rely on factors regarding quality but might also rely on economic incentives and the marketing by the tire companies. Of course a lot of the customers might express their own preference or be influenced by some recent ad or TV commercial.

That's my analogy for today's psychiatric practice. If the psychiatrist sets too high a threshold for diagnosing a presenting patient as having a mental disorder (even if that threshold is still pure medical model, diagnosing a mental disorder *only* in those who clearly meet strictly applied DSM diagnostic criteria) then there might not be enough billings generated in follow-up "med checks" to keep the lights on and pay the staff. And this isn't just the psychiatrist's fault. The entire healthcare delivery system is set up in such a way that an initial intake and then med checks are the only services reimbursed to a psychiatrist. I'm a pretty radical critic of today's psychiatry but if you looked at my private practice appointment book you would have seen one hour intakes and 15 minute med checks there too. But it's interesting to look back at Dr. Klein's book published in 1980 because it reflects a medical psychiatry *centrally* focused on discriminating biological from non-biological conditions. There isn't much life left today in the type of discriminatory thinking that Dr. Klein recorded in his book. Let me give you some examples of what I am talking about.

In the chapter titled *Clinical Management of Affective Disorders* Klein discusses sub-types of depression each with their own specific treatment plans. The first type he distinguishes (that I believe still accounts for the majority of cases we see today) he calls "the dysphorias." Dysphoria is probably better defined by the word unhappiness than by the word depression. He then separates out the chronic dysphorias. Chronic dysphoria encompasses people with personality disorders, recurrent traumas and what used to be called neuroses. Here is a truer than true statement, at least to me. Dr. Klein says: "They are often refractory to the major antidepressants and to many years of psychotherapy as well" (Klein et al. 1980, p.438). Not a very optimistic appraisal, just honest and realistic. These types of patients fill mental healthcare and primary care physician's offices. So should these people be tried on medication? Today that is no longer a question. The chronically anxious/depressed patients are like lab rats to PCP's and psychiatrists. They end up on constantly "adjusted" multiple medication regimens. They often get re-diagnosed as bipolar or labeled as treatment resistant and, wait until I tell you what biopsychiatry has in store for "treatment resistant" depression now. (Here's a hint. It requires a scalpel). But I want to tell you what Dr. Klein recommended 30 years ago. He said: "…in the treatment of the chronic dysphoric, a 5-week trial of imipramine, reaching a minimum dosage of 300 mg daily during the 5th week, followed by a 1-week drying out period and then by a 5-week trial of phenylzine at a dose of at least 75mg per day, is probably an adequate test of clinical responsiveness of such patients to the major antidepressants" (Klein et al. 1980 pp.438-49). So five weeks of a tricyclic, then five weeks of an MAOI (phenylzine) and that's it. If it doesn't work, it doesn't work. What happened to this common sense biological psychiatric thinking? You'll see. But here's a hint. It has to do with the local tire store owner who had already partly compromised his integrity (selling new tires to people that didn't really need them) but going out of business *anyhow* because a Sears and Wal-Mart opened down the street and he just couldn't compete with their corporate muscle.

In this chapter Dr. Klein also describes a presentation of depression he calls Disappointment Reaction (*Reactive "Depression"*). He actually puts the quote marks around the word *Depression* to show that this isn't really depression. I love the term disappointment reaction, it so accurately describes and de-medicalizes this very common problem. Clinically Klein suggests a "wait and see" approach because this distress should clear up in about 2 months or the stressor might precipitate a real biological depression which he describes by the word endogenomorphic, meaning arising from within. Klein's specific recommendations for the treatment of a disappointment reaction is to just be supportive and monitor the patient for signs of whether or not the stressor sets off a biological depression. Knowing that patients in emotional pain want symptom relief the use of a Valium type drug might be warranted. But, he states in no uncertain terms: "Major antidepressants of the imipramine-like or MAOI class are not a wise choice for reactive depression and often have therapeutically adverse effects" (Klein et al. 1980 p.442). So don't just "jump in" with antidepressants. I haven't seen a recommendation like that in a proverbial month of Sundays.

To be fair there is a group of diagnoses in DSM IV called adjustment disorders that are similar to what Klein is calling a reactive depression. But notice, it's called a disorder, implying somehow that this is an abnormal or pathological response to stress. But it does distinguish these conditions from depressive illness, *at least on paper!* In the doctor's office it makes no difference. Antidepressants will enter the picture at some point. And once they do…there is no turning back. As psychiatrist David Kaiser puts it: "Unfortunately what I also see today are the casualties of this new biological psychiatry, as patients often come to me with many years of past treatment. Patients having been diagnosed with 'chemical imbalances' despite the fact that no test exists to support such a claim, and that there is no real conception of what a correct chemical balance would look like. Patients with years of medication trials which have done nothing except reify in them an identity as a chronic patient with a bad brain. This identification as a biologically-impaired patient is one of the most destructive effects of biologic psychiatry." (Kaiser 1996)

Thank you Dr. Kaiser, I couldn't have said it better.

So how did psychiatry, even medical model psychiatry as represented in 1980 by Dr. Klein, evolve (although the correct term is probably devolve) into what it is today, recently ironically "critiqued" by the new president of the American Psychiatric Association, Steven S. Sharfstein M.D., as a devolution from a "bio-psycho-social model" to a "bio-bio-bio model" where a "pill and a med check" have come to dominate treatment (Sharfstein 2005). The answer to that question is the overall topic of this and the next two chapters. Let's return to an examination of an essential factor in the progression from bio-psycho-social to bio-bio-bio psychiatry, the antidepressants from Prozac and beyond.

I recently visited Amazon.com and counted the number of books that they have for sale with the word Prozac in the title. I counted at least 35. I guess Prozac is a good word to have in the title when you are trying to get a book published. The point here is that what Prozac has come to represent in our culture is far, far more than merely an improved version of imipramine (one with less troublesome side effects) but a whole new vision of being human and our relationship to technology. When the book *Listening to Prozac* was published in 1993 (Kramer 1993) the incredible attention it garnered (especially for such a technical book) was because it introduced the notion of "cosmetic psychopharmacology", using these marvelous new SSRI antidepressants to *improve* the lives of humans, not just return them to normal from a state of illness. "Better than well" they called it. What a product for a sensation crazed culture, kind of like ecstasy and coke but less dangerous and ENDORSED BY DOCTORS. In the seventeen years that have passed since Dr. Kramer published his book this hype and hyperbole has died down considerably. Reality has a way of throwing water on the "medical miracle" fires, every time. Just a brief historical tidbit here: When heroin was first brought to the United States it was embraced by the medical establishment as a miracle cure for...wait...can you guess?...that's right—opium addiction. Silly doctors.

Clinical experience and the arrival of a number of "me too" drugs has shifted the emphasis away from Prozac as *the* miracle drug onto the class of drugs Prozac belongs to as being the curative treatment for a wide range of emotional problems. I believe this shift occurred, in part, due to the changes in our day to day life in America, where being "better than well" is no longer a driving force for us. We just want to feel less depressed, anxious and hopeless in a world increasingly driven by fear, uncertainty, epidemic insecurity, violence, greed and hate. (Gee Doc, aren't you just Mr. Sunshine?) That is one of the reasons why there is a whole new category of disorders being treated with the serotonin effect. These are the anxiety disorders which include generalized anxiety disorder, panic disorder, obsessive compulsive disorder, social phobia, and post traumatic stress disorder, all now with more than one SSRI and/or SNRI FDA approved for treatment.

Once there was competition for Prozac, first Paxil and then Zoloft, the drug companies (as I explained previously) started to use DSM IV as a marketing tool. After all, you can only get so far with trying to promote the idea that Paxil is a *better* drug than Prozac with all the research showing that no antidepressant is superior to any other antidepressant...period! That was one of my shocking tidbits mentioned above; officially no antidepressant is superior to the first one, imipramine developed in 1957. That's not my personal opinion; it is the official position of the American Psychiatric Association.

So we have these new antidepressants, the SSRI's, the SNRI's and Wellbutrin that I listed above. They have a wide range of indications from the FDA but I am going to save the details about this for chapter eight where we will look at how getting FDA indications became a sales and marketing battleground with DSM IV conveniently supplying the ammunition. What I want to do now is an appraisal of the price paid for choosing to take an antidepressant in terms of the possible negative consequences. We've covered two already: The "what the hell effect" and the identification of yourself as having a "broken brain." We'll look at the rest of the side effects shortly. First, we need to examine what was so "new" about the second generation antidepressants and why they have replaced tricycilcs as the medication of choice. Since I was in active practice through the tricyclic and SSRI era I can tell you the clinical advantages because they were quite welcome. There was ease of dosing, often just once a day. The first dosage strength was often the desired dosage. Tricyclics almost always had to be "titrated" which means raised in small increments to achieve the final dose. When this was done in the hospital, titration was no big deal. You could just rewrite the orders every day and get just the right dose and speed of titration. When the emphasis switched to outpatient this became a major pain for the doctor and patient. An initial Imipramine prescription would be something like Rx: "Take one 50 mg pill at night for three nights, then, if tolerated, one 50 mg pill morning and night for three days, then one 50 mg pill in the morning and two at night" and so on and so on, shooting for a final dose of 250 to 300 mg. The starting orders for Prozac Rx: "Prozac 20 mg, one every day". That's it! First dose equals final dose. Maybe this more than anything else resulted in clinicians embracing Prozac and sparked its spread from the psychiatrist's office to the family practice and primary care offices. (This plus the promotion of the *disease* along with the promotion of the drug…see chapter eight).

Another incalculably important advantage to Prozac is that overdoses wouldn't kill you. As you recall from my hypothetical conversation between doctor and patient in 1960 there is a cardiac risk with tricyclics. Overdoses had a good chance of killing you. If you took an overdose you needed to be on a cardiac monitor for at least three days before being released as no longer in danger. So think about it; psychiatrists treating depression, the emotional condition most closely associated with suicide, were forced to hand their patients a loaded gun by giving them pills that could kill in overdose. And if there is any "suicidal" act that someone does impulsively, even with no true intention of dying, it's swallowing a mouthful of pills. Sometimes patients had to be prescribed only one week's worth at a time, an incredible hassle for all involved. Weight gain, constipation and sleepiness, terribly bothersome side effects of tricyclics, were not initially reported as side effects of Prozac. In fact, when it first came out, Prozac was touted as a possible weight loss drug. I think the ease of use on both sides of the equation, doctor and patient, had a lot to do with the growing acceptance of a depressed mood being a medical condition responsive to medication.

Ah, but the bloom does come off the rose doesn't it? It's just a matter of how long it takes. After getting the cover of Newsweek as a miracle drug Prozac started getting some front page coverage as a drug that could cause suicide and violence. I am not going to cover this ongoing controversy (now encompassing all antidepressants) in any great detail here. It's a contentious issue that has recently resulted in a strong FDA warning of the potential for an increased risk of suicide from antidepressants in anyone under 24 years old. On top of this, more and more central nervous system drugs that are used to treat things other than psychiatric disorders are now receiving FDA warnings about suicide potential. Recent examples include Chantix (for smoking cessation) and Lyrica (for fibromyalgia). Neither of these drugs carried a suicide warning when first approved, this suicide "side effect" only emerged after the drugs were in wide use. What is Mother Nature trying to tell us here? That it's dangerous to blindly muck around with the biochemistry of the brain? Gee, you think so?

Let's turn to less life threatening concerns about Prozac and its SSRI and SNRI followers: Paxil, Zoloft, Celexa, Lexapro, Effexor, Cymbalta and Prestiq. The three major concerns about the SSRI's I want to discuss are the sexual side effects, the "Prozac poop out" syndrome and withdrawal symptoms.

There are doctors and clinics that specialize in treating sexual problems as I'm sure that anyone who listens to the radio knows. There are also widely advertised drugs for male erectile problems that anyone who watches TV knows about. (PLEASE: *GET OUT OF THOSE BATHTUBS!)* But there is also a less talked about problem that plagues some men that has nothing to do with the capacity for and desire to have sex, it has to do with things ending before they have barely started. It's called premature ejaculation and can be ruinous to a couple's sex life. Fortunately it has been discovered that this condition can often be treated (by making it take longer to achieve orgasm) by giving the man SSRI antidepressants. This successful treatment has nothing to do with depression; it works by taking advantage of a certain side effect of these drugs officially called delayed ejaculation.

The frequency, incidence and severity of sexual side effects from serotonin antidepressants has been a contentious subject with the drug companies quoting some pretty low figures around the 10% to 20% range but with independent studies citing a 60% to 70% incidence. I'm going to get deeply into the "tricks of the trade" by pharmaceutical companies in chapter eight but I do want to offer an explanation for how such a major discrepancy in the incidence of sexual side effects reported by drug company vs. independent research might easily occur. In drug trials by pharmaceutical companies they assess the type and incidence of side effects based on open ended questions to study participants; questions like "Are you having any problems with the medication?" and see what the patients report. Ask yourself, how likely you would be to report to this stranger in a white coat sitting across from you: "Oh, yes, I can't orgasm anymore, even by masturbating?" Or, "Why yes, I noticed that I have absolutely no sexual feeling towards my husband anymore and when he demands sex I just use a lubricant and go along with him until he's done." I'm talking here about people with normal sex lives before the drug study. All I can say is that in my clinical experience and that of the colleagues I have questioned, the higher figures are much more realistic and accurate. So what do you do about *this* problem? Well, don't ask me, ask Newsweek!

I'm not picking on Newsweek but do you remember that when I "deconstructed" the article in Time magazine about bipolar disorder in children and said that I was *not* suggesting that Time was bribed or pressured to run this highly prejudicial, one-sided story. As you recall I blamed the bipolar disorder in children article in Time magazine on discourse control. It's harder for me to be as "generous" in my lack of suspicion about a story in Newsweek run in November 2006. The title of the article is *"Depression Drugs: How to Avoid Sex Problems"* with the subtitle *"SSRI's are a potent weapon against depression, but sexual side effects scare off patients. Now there's help."* Well that's good news! When I picked up the article I thought there actually might be something in there about some new research on an antidote for sexual side effects of antidepressants that I had not yet heard or read about. That wouldn't be the first time I heard about something important in a newspaper or magazine. But that was not the case. This one page article was literally an advertisement for the pharmaceutical industry that straight out LIED to the reader about solutions to the problems of overcoming the sexual side effects of SSRI's. Every reassuring recommendation and strategy mentioned in the article has been discussed and tried for years but not a single published study has ever supported any of the mentioned strategies or antidotes as legitimate or effective. The article starts by accurately reporting the incidence of sexual side effects at around 60%. Hooray for that. But then it goes on to positively spin ways to deal with the side effects that are not effective. The first suggestion is to simply be patient. Over time the sexual side effects will just wear off. Huh?? Try telling that to my patients. Then they suggest adding Wellbutrin, the one antidepressant without sexual side effects. Let me assure you, we have all tried it. And let me assure you, in the vast majority of cases, it doesn't work. If it did the Wellbutrin people would have published studies that it works and have been hawking it to doctors for years. (Remember, drug companies have NO obligation to publish negative studies). The only viable option with Wellbutrin (and this is legitimate) is to use it to replace the SSRI. The next (and I will tell you very old) recommendation is to take a "drug holiday". Basically that entails skipping the Friday and Saturday dose of your antidepressant and having a pre-scheduled sex session Saturday PM. (Hey, no performance pressure there). But make sure your drug isn't Paxil or Effexor because the withdrawal syndrome (discussed below) comes on very rapidly with these drugs. Oh, and it can't be Prozac because it stays in the body too long and will not be out of your system for weeks.

None of my patients has EVER reported that the drug holiday strategy worked out for them. Then the article suggests Viagra. Of course that is only for men and will not help if their problem is lack of libido or difficulty having an orgasm, the latter being by far the most common complaint. How are we doing so far? So, what about the ladies? Newsweek's suggestion is so insensitive and sexist I don't want there to be any mistake about who made it so I will quote directly from the article. "To improve lubrication for women, [Dr. Michelle] Riba suggests either a lubricant or more foreplay before sex." Let's do a little mini-deconstruction on that sentence. The woman's sexual problem, like the man's, can be either a loss of desire, a loss of ability (here the female equivalent of an erect penis is a lubricated vagina) and/or difficulty or inability to orgasm. Often, there is a bit of all three in SSRI treated patients. So the solution recommended for women has nothing to do with increasing sexual desire or the capacity to orgasm, just to make the vagina moist so the man can enjoy himself. Hey, I have an idea. Why not suggest **not starting the drug** in the first place and try out other strategies for dealing with unhappiness before you just jump right in to taking drugs that will more likely than not impair your sex life for as long as you take it? Or...just read the fairy tale in Newsweek and figure hey, it will be okay. The doctor can fix it, and if he can't then "what the hell". (psst. This strategy works best if already on antidepressants).

What's Prozac poop out? Maybe you've heard the term, maybe not. It refers to the all too frequent phenomenon of the felt positive impact of antidepressants (not just Prozac) fading over time. To staunch biopsychiatrists this decrement in effectiveness of antidepressants is a fascinating phenomenon that they can add to their list of things to wildly speculate about. You recall that I mentioned the large number of serotonin receptors that have been discovered? Maybe the receptors have been over-sensitized, or maybe under-sensitized; or maybe the number of receptors has gone up...or down.

Suggestions for dealing with this problem have included raising the dose of the current drug or lowering the dose of the current drug. Or add another drug… or switch drugs. Or redo the history and find some evidence of "mood swings" and re-diagnose the patient as bipolar and start some mood stabilizers. Have you begun to notice that the suggestions for dealing with ANY CLINICAL PROBLEM in psychiatry are basically the same Chinese Menu choices I just listed? Does that scare you? It should.

I too have a speculative explanation for the Prozac poop out problem but it has nothing to do with brain chemistry; it has to do with human nature. Ever watch the show *House Hunters* where a family has outgrown its current house and wants a bigger one? They always tell the real estate agent the minimum requirements for the new home, two bathrooms, room for a home office, a garage…whatever. Once they find a new house that meets their requirements and that they can afford, they get ecstatic. "Oh, it's everything we ever wanted; now the kids can each have their own room and I finally have a bathtub." You know the scenario. But what do you think might be heard if you dropped in on this family three years after they got the new house. C'mon…you know. The ecstasy would clearly be gone and a new list of "must-haves" has emerged as they begin fantasizing about the next house. Its human nature, wait, check that; it's American human nature! We are consumers through and through and as such are programmed to never be fully satisfied with what we've got. Is it possible that this same aspect of our nature influences our relationship with our antidepressants as well? When the serotonin stimulation impact first hit it was novel, new, thrilling ("I've never felt this good in my whole life!"), but then as the novelty wears off, and life with all of its tedium and stresses continues unabated, the antidepressant no longer *seems* to be working so good even though in terms of its chemical impact on brain tissue, there has really been no change. Shouldn't this possible explanation also be in the mix when discussing Prozac poop out? Of course it should. But it isn't because that would violate the bio-bio-bio model of psychiatry that Dr. Sharfstein (?) criticized. (Not really *criticized* by the way, like he was intending to do something about it. More on that later).

I want to highlight one last side effect of the antidepressants before we look at the recent $35 million study on how well antidepressants work. I am purposely leaving out a list of other side effects like weight gain, nausea, anxiety and the like for brevity sake because this chapter is itself starting to spin out of control. You can find a list of common side effects any number of places. I want to wrap up this portion of the chapter by briefly mentioning the withdrawal issue. As it has for many classes of drugs certain problems do not really show themselves until the drugs are in wide use over a longer period of time. Antidepressant withdrawal is just such a problem. Only in the last 10 years have psychiatrists recognized the severity of this problem. Next, of course, you will expect me to list the symptoms of withdrawal. I would, except the list is so long it would almost look like I am saying that just about anything can result from antidepressant withdrawal. (psst. I am). Let me just list a few: profound dizziness, electric like shocks in your arms or head, nausea, vomiting, fatigue, muscle pain, insomnia, vivid dreams, crying spells, anxiety, agitation and irritability. (Antidepressant withdrawal, fortunately, does not appear to be life threatening). The likelihood of having withdrawal symptoms is not the same for all the drugs. The ones most rapidly eliminated that have no active metabolites (Paxil and Effexor) are much more likely to cause withdrawal than slowly eliminated drugs or those with active metabolites (Prozac and Zoloft) but there are no hard and fast rules. It seems that Wellbutrin does not have a withdrawal risk although all drugs suggest tapering off slowly. There are growing indications, including lawsuits, that some people have had a very, very difficult time coming off of antidepressants. How long does withdrawal last? When does it start? Sorry, don't know. Hey I know what; I've been waiting to say this so now I will: **Ask your doctor**. Hah!

My interest in withdrawal is more about the paradoxical and confusing factor that it introduces into the medication issue. How do you figure out when someone doesn't "need" antidepressants anymore? Are there guidelines? Maybe you've heard that you should be on for six months or a year. Perhaps you've heard that after one episode of major depression you have a 50% chance of another, after two episodes you have a 70% chance of a third and should therefore stay on meds to prevent future episodes. Depression can come in episodes?? Do you mean that you can get suicidal and depressed and not want to get out of bed and that if you don't kill yourself, the depression will eventually go away without any treatment? How long will that take? And what if I go off of antidepressants and I have anxiety and insomnia and crying spells; does that mean I am still mentally ill and need to go back on the medication or is it withdrawal? How long should I wait? What am I supposed to do? I feel awful. Do I just wait it out?

"I have something to confess doctor. I went back on my Paxil and felt better right away. (psst., she was in withdrawal).Let's you and I make a little agreement doc. Don't EVER suggest I try going off my antidepressants again. I'm staying on them, and that's that!"

I've warned you that the closer we inspect medical psychiatry, the more detailed the interrogation, the worse it is going to look. There are no right (or wrong) answers to all of these questions because there is no basis in a legitimate science to the whole bloody endeavor. That has a way of catching up with you over and over again. But I can report some things that are observable:

1. More people than ever take antidepressants.
2. Most people probably stay on them chronically or go back on them after they quit.
3. There is very little to no dialogue in psychiatry about distinguishing depressive or anxious states that don't require medicine from those that do.
4. It looks as if the profit hungry drug companies are totally running the show and getting exactly what they want from the power elite, a.k.a. "thought leaders" in psychiatry, period.
5. End of story:

(Regime of truth in control: check.
Discourse control: double check.
Foucault proven right? Must I even answer?)

So am I saying this is a total scam? Not at all. I think I have made it very clear that there is a contribution that medical model psychiatry can and should make to mental healthcare. That the *dominance* and *exclusivity* that characterizes medical model psychiatry is doing more harm than good is the concern of this book. And I can't think of a better way to prove that than by deconstructing the most up to date and largest study of the effectiveness (and lack thereof) of antidepressants, the recently completed STAR D* NIMH sponsored multi-center research project.

When I discussed Dr. Klein's 1980 book above I mentioned that it was very hard to establish based on the studies at that time what the response rate to antidepressant treatment was but he (very biased towards the medical model) surmised a rate of about 2/3 on medication vs. 1/3 on placebo. But (deconstructively speaking) what does it mean to say *response?* How is that determined? I'm not 100% certain how that was dealt with in 1980 but I do know how it is done now. So I will explain it to you. As I do you will once again be uncomfortably reminded how unscientific and uncertain (and simplistic, reductionistic and dehumanizing) this medical model that rules psychiatry truly is.

The STAR*D (Sequenced Treatment Alternatives to Relieve Depression) study is the most up to date major study on the clinical effectiveness of antidepressants for the treatment of major depressive illness. Its four stages were completed by the end of 2006. The study was sponsored and paid for by the National Institute of Mental Health (NIMH), which means of course, paid for by taxpayers. (References for the STAR*D study are NIMH press releases and the Medical News Today article, all listed in the bibliography). The idea was to not have drug companies sponsor the research to hopefully remove any concern that the study design would favor any particular drug. (Gee, I wonder why such a concern would even exist). The study would involve multiple thousands of patients with depression and be run at mental health clinics, regular health clinics and doctors offices so that the study would not be biased by the factors that can bias studies where most are conducted, university clinics and free standing clinical research centers (you've heard the ads). Again, we sense a concern about the possibility of prejudicial results emerging from the "normal science" conducted by big pharmaceutical firms (big Pharma). Hey, is this like an admission of something? (See chapter eight). So now we just need to identify study subjects. No problem; psychiatric researchers have been doing it for years. How? By evaluating prospective patients with a twenty one item questionnaire and then adding up the score on the first seventeen items. And then...what else? Nothing. That's it; a onetime twenty one item multiple choice quiz. No further assessment, no independent evaluations and, as we know so very well, no lab, X-Ray or any other kind of biological test. Score above the pre-selected threshold for the diagnosis of depression and you are in! There is a question that needs to be asked here. With so much on the line and results that could potentially affect millions of people why isn't the diagnostic assessment done more thoroughly and carefully? That is a very good question.

Let's imagine that this study was being done in 2006 but with a 1980 mindset. You could use your quiz to screen for the *symptoms* that are seen in depression and *then* get to work on diagnosis. In 1980 we might want to do some interviewing to screen out the "unlikely to respond" chronic dysphorias. Then we could screen out the disappointment reactions and the demoralization patients as either not qualified or put them into a separate arm of the study. What happened to this type of discriminatory and very reasonable thinking in medical psychiatry? DSM happened! The domination of biopsychiatry happened. And the voice of the practicing clinician grew fainter and fainter as the voice of research and administrative psychiatrists (funded by big Pharma) grew louder and louder. Biopsychiatry, as defined by the dominant voices, needs one and only one thing: numbers; because studies in science must have numbers. Otherwise there would be no way to come up with those most manipulative words in science: "statistically significant." So people need to have depression "scores" so that there can be post-medication depression "scores" to numerically compare. And if all you need for the research study are some pre and post treatment numerical scores to compare then why go through all the time and expense of discriminating demoralized people and personality disorders from the depression study group? It would screw up the numbers because the most important thing in statistical analysis is having a large "n" or number of experimental subjects. Remember the foundational factors in Heidegger's concept of "Gestell"? Utility, efficiency, ordering and control (and then I added the late 20th Century factor of profitability). The STAR*D study certainly meets (and even exceeds) Heidegger's description of the priorities of Gestell. (For example, some of the follow-up interviews to assess the study subject's emotional status were done by an automated telephone program).

Okay, so what exactly is this multiple choice questionnaire used to make diagnoses and to numerically assess treatment response? It is called The Hamilton Rating Scale for Depression (HAM-D). It has twenty one questions but usually only the first seventeen are counted because the last four questions are related to the "type" of major depression (i.e. with delusions, with melancholia and/or with severe anxiety symptoms). So what are the questions on which hangs the entire drug industry's case for efficacy of antidepressants? The test is administered and scored by the clinician. Each item (or question) is labeled with the symptom it is exploring. So here are the seventeen symptoms the HAM-D asks about:

1. Depressed Mood.
2. Feelings of Guilt.
3. Suicide.
4. Insomnia- Early.
5. Insomnia- Middle
6. Insomnia- Late
7. Work and Activities
8. Psychomotor Retardation (body motor activity slowed)
9. Psychomotor Agitation (body motor activity increased)
10. Anxiety- Psychic
11. Anxiety- Somatic
12. Somatic Symptoms- Gastrointestinal
13. Somatic Symptoms- General
14. Genital Symptoms
15. Hypochondriasis
16. Weight Loss
17. Insight

THIS IS A VERY STRANGE LIST. It doesn't really conform precisely to DSM criteria and seems to be really over weighted in the insomnia and anxiety areas versus depression. Nevertheless this has been the standard for nearly all research studies in depression. (Other rating scales do exist and are used in some studies). Each of the seventeen items on the HAM-D has three to five choices for the examining clinician; the higher the score on each item, the more serious the symptom. For example the choices under suicide are:

1. 0=absent
2. 1=Feels life is not worth living
3. 2=Wishes he/she were dead or has any thoughts of possible death to self
4. 3=Suicidal ideas or gestures
5. 4=Attempts at suicide

So zero to four points for the suicide symptom of depression. Are the distinctions between the choices a little fuzzy or is it just me? Here are the choices for the Agitation symptom of depression:

1. 0=none
2. 1=Fidgetiness
3. 2= "Playing with" hands, hair, etc.
4. 3=Moving about, can't sit still
5. 4=Hand wringing, nail biting, hair pulling, lip biting

Again, not real clear distinctions. And notice how hand wringing can earn you just as many depression points as a suicide attempt? And wouldn't just about any calming agent from a drink to a tranquilizer calm you and reduce your agitation score without really having any antidepressant properties. Oh, I'd love to tear this test apart for a couple more pages but let's move on but there is still a lot to cover in this chapter.

So the $35 million STAR*D study signs up around 4,041 potential candidates whose only entrance qualification for having depression was a HAM D score of fourteen or higher. 1,165 of these Level 1 subjects were excluded from the final data analysis for various and sundry reasons. That left 2,876 Level 1 subjects. All of them were treated with Citalopram, an SSRI antidepressant, for twelve weeks. Dosage adjustments were left to the discretion of the doctor. At the end of the twelve weeks the subjects were once again evaluated by the HAM D. A successful response to medication was defined as a remission of depression which numerically meant a HAM D score of less than or equal to seven. The choice of remission is important here because there is a different endpoint criteria used in all of the studies used to gain FDA approval for antidepressant effectiveness. That other endpoint is called response. A response to an antidepressant is defined as a 50% reduction in HAM D scores. So for example, a subject with an initial HAM D of twenty six would be considered to have had a positive response to medication with a final HAM D score of thirteen, far from the remission score of less than or equal to seven.

Okay, I can imagine everyone waiting with baited breath. How did the Level 1 STAR*D patients do? In the three month period on Citalopram, around 30% of the subjects achieved remission. Stated another way, seven out of ten *did not* achieve remission. (This is called spin. 30% sounds pretty good, seven out of ten sounds lousy. Would you like to guess how the STAR*D data was reported?).

On to Level 2: Non-responders were then moved on to Level 2 where perhaps the most important research relevant to practicing clinicians was set up. But I need to mention that 1,127 non-responders DROPPED OUT at that point so only 1,475 of the total of 2,602 non-responders went on to stage two. That's a heck of a lot of dropouts. I wonder what effect something like that that has on the validity of the data. Anyhow Level two is what all the clinicians were waiting for. In both primary care and psychiatry offices we are all dealing everyday with patients who don't respond to their first antidepressant. This would rarely be after three months however because neither the patients nor the doctors (especially PCP's) can handle waiting three months without improvement before trying a second drug. Even if they do the question remains the same: Which drug should be second? Is there a logical choice to guide this decision? On the surface there would appear to be. Since in this study (and most often in the real world) the first drug tried is an SSRI which theoretically works almost exclusively on serotonin, then it seems logical that the second drug should have a different mechanism of action. Why would another serotonin-only drug work? So the Level two choices included:

1. A second SSRI (Zoloft),
2. An SNRI (Effexor) and
3. Wellbutrin (thought to work primarily on dopamine).

In addition there was the option of staying on Citalopram but adding a second drug to "augment" or strengthen the effect of the Citalopram. This second stage of the study was also run for twelve weeks. So, what happened? Around 25% of the patients who switched and around 30% of the patients who chose augmentation experienced remission of symptoms. However, much to the chagrin of the clinicians and, even more so to the makers of Effexor and Wellbutrin I would imagine, there was no best second choice. Statistically all of the options performed about the same. The study was now six months long and well below 50% of the original enrollees were better (or had already dropped out). Well, fear not; on to Level three.

There were 1,062 subjects left to try the third treatment option. Not surprisingly, about 40% (432) dropped out. The remaining 630 depressed subjects were either switched to less often used antidepressants (Remeron or the tricyclic nortryptiline) or had their current drug augmented. Here only 10% to 20% achieved remission. Notice the percentages dropping at each level. Finally, nine months into the study there were 268 non-responders left. Two thirds (169) dropped out. The remaining 99 subjects were switched to either an MAOI or the rather exotic combination of Remeron and Effexor. Only about 10% achieved remission. The study, mercifully, was over.

There are a few more facts to add before I comment on the results of this study. The first is that there was no placebo utilized. That means that if anyone got "better" the drug would be credited because there was no comparison group of people on fake pills who also got better. This effectively hid the fact that there is often very little separation of drugs from placebos in psychiatric studies. Of course it doesn't take much to make a "statistically significant" difference. I told you those are scary words. They allow barely different data be used to make black and white statements: "Scientifically proven effective in the treatment of…" even if the statistics barely achieve significance. (Using the HAM-D it takes only a two point difference to achieve a statistically significant result).

Okay, so what is the typical placebo response rate in double blind antidepressant studies in which remission is the outcome measure? Generally around 20% to 30% (Fink, 2006). WHOA!! That's pretty close to the outcome in the first arm of this study. In chapter eight we are going to look more closely at exactly how psychiatric research studies are conducted, how statistics are manipulated, and how and why the only rich psychiatrists are research and administrative academic psychiatrists while the clinical psychiatrists are making less and less money every year.

But before we leave STAR*D I have two more points to make. The first is that Heidegger is spooky. His predictions about "Gestell" are being lived out in the real world right in front of our eyes. These research subjects are *exactly* what Heidegger called "standing reserve." Major, extremely important research studies on *relieving human emotional suffering* (what should matter more, higher resolution video games?) are being rendered ever more efficient and cost effective by utilizing things like automated phone interviews to assess a subject's emotional status. I've got to share a quote I found made by the research director of the STAR*D study, Dr. A. John Rush. He was quoted as saying that patient self reports on their response to antidepressants cannot be trusted because "they are not going to be accurate" and that patients "cannot be precise." I hope you remember my characterizing medical psychiatry as dehumanizing and reductionistic. Dr. Rush's statement reminds me of the story of the harried hospital administrator bemoaning that they could really turn the hospital into an efficient, orderly and profitable business if it weren't for those damn doctors and patients. Why is it that the sloppy edges of humanness are such a hindrance in today's corporate climate?

I will come back to STAR*D in chapter eight. But I do want to leave you with some food for thought, one last tidbit to chew on from this study. It was reported that at Level 1 a response to medication was positively correlated with the following psychosocial variables: Those most likely to get better on antidepressant medication were:

1. White
2. Well educated
3. Employed
4. Married
5. Had fewer complicating problems

So this purely biological illness that MUST be treated medically just happens to separate out along racial and economic lines. What an incredible coincidence. Well I'm convinced. I guess this rock solid data rules out any other approach to the epidemic of depression in this country.

Okay. This has been going on long enough. We have reached the final topic of this very long chapter, what to do when antidepressants just plain do not work. Switching, augmenting, and combining…nothing. The patient is still depressed. Remember the non-negotiable rules of the medical psychiatry game: No reformulating of the case along psychosocial, psychoanalytic, existential, spiritual, philosophical or any other dimension. It is still a chemical imbalance. So how do we affect brain chemicals when swallowing psychoactive drugs just doesn't work? I know. Let's go to the brain itself. Let's just mess with the brain directly. How about giving it a big electric shock, cause a seizure, scramble up all the brain chemicals and see if that works. This reminds me of the recommendation you get when you call a help line about a computer problem: "Just unplug it and then plug it back in." And you know, sometimes it works. So too, claim its proponents, does what I just described above: Electroconvulsive Therapy (ECT). I am going to skip commenting on ECT because I have had such limited clinical experience with it. I have met some pretty bitter patients who feel that their memory was ruined by the procedure. But ECT has been around a long time, longer than the antidepressants, and is still endorsed by a lot of psychiatrists. I'll put some references in the back of the book for you if interested. But I will say one thing, it is a hell of a radical decision to undergo this procedure ten or twelve times for an "illness" as poorly understood and defined as depression.

A new acronym has started to pop up in my daily dose of psychiatric "literature" I get in the mail. The acronym is **TRD** which stands for **T**reatment **R**esistant **D**epression. What an amazing coincidence that this "topic" starts filling my mailbox and conference invitations so soon after the FDA issued their approval for a radically new treatment for TRD. It's called (acronym time again) **VNS** which stands for **V**agal **N**erve **S**timulation. This is the "treatment" I was alluding to as "starting with a scalpel". Yes, it is an *invasive surgical procedure* for depression. Here is what is done. A pacemaker is implanted under the skin of your chest. A wire from the pacemaker is run into your neck and wrapped around a very large nerve next to your carotid artery called the vagus nerve. The pacemaker sends electrical signals directly to the brain through the vagus nerve. The psychiatrist's job (if its correct to still call the doctor a psychiatrist) is to make adjustments to the signal being sent to the brain by using a magnetic device to adjust the signal strength and frequency of the pacemaker. Hey…and that's it. Now just sit back and wait a year or two to see if it helps. I know you think I'm kidding. I wish I were. When I said be afraid, I meant it and when I said psychiatry is spinning out of control, I meant it too. (I recently saw a segment on 60 Minutes where the doctor decided to just stop fooling around and stuck electrodes *directly into* a woman's brain to electrically stimulate the alleged mood center. The doctor doing the procedure had an economic stake in the company making the device and tried his best to put a positive spin on the very ambiguous results he achieved. That was when I decided: I love Leslie Stahl. SHE NAILED HIM!)

I first heard about VNS from a salesperson who visited me in the office. I learned it was a procedure used in the treatment of medication non-responsive epilepsy (seizures). Of course in that application you had some pretty good evidence if it was working or not because you can see, measure and record seizures. Now here it was being applied to a condition that we can't even prove is a physical illness. Apparently someone "noticed" that some of the patients receiving VNS for epilepsy reported an improvement in mood. (Aha! Depression is an implant deficiency disease!) I knew this couldn't possibly be related to cashing in on the depression treatment craze because the device only cost $16,000, less than most decent cars. Of course the salesperson did mention that the often frequent pacemaker adjustments are a "reimbursable" procedure and did mention a procedure code I could use to get about $100 per adjustment. My interest sparked, I just had to know more. (Let's see $100 for a ten minute visit times we'll say 10 patients a week times 50 weeks. That's

$50,000 a year for 100 minutes of work a week. Yeah, sounds good. Oh, by the way…does it work?)

We have entered a new and even more perilous phase in biopsychiatry. I'm starting to get the distinct feeling that the pharmaceutical industry has finally caught on to the 21st Century "hypereality" game. THE PRODUCT DOESN'T MATTER ANYMORE, JUST THE PROMOTION. I'm seeing these incredibly slick, polished, multimedia marketing campaigns for the most questionable new "treatments". A new sleeping pill is running a massive advertising campaign to doctors and the general public. They have set up websites galore and have established a network of sleep disorder faculty to give lectures, attend meetings and participate in online training and communication. Every trapping of an ultra successful business (like Disney) has been put into place. The only thing bugging me is the product. Again, I'll turn to the PDR. **"INDICATIONS: Rozerem is indicated for the treatment of insomnia characterized by difficulty with sleep onset."** Two studies showed that Rozerem reduced the amount of time to fall asleep by enough minutes to meet the threshold for statistical significance. It did not increase total sleep time or decrease the number of awakenings during the night, generally the most problematic aspects of insomnia in terms of next day impairment; so, a very modest product at best. Not being scheduled as a Class IV abusable drug does set it apart from the other new sleeping pills. But the launch and marketing of this drug was massive; you'd think it was a cure for cancer or something. And I ought to know. I was one of their paid speakers. (More on this later)

A sleeping pill with modest effect is one thing. A dangerous and costly surgical procedure for TRD is quite another. There had better be some pretty robust data supporting this treatment option! (Shouldn't there be?) The following statistics were provided by Dr. Charles R. Conway, a "practicing psychiatrist and assistant professor in the department of psychiatry at the Saint Louis University School of Medicine" as reported in the Orlando Medical News, 12 September 2006. The first rather striking bit of information about VNS is that response time is no longer measured in the nearly unbearable weeks to months we ask medicated depressed patients to wait for; now the time to response is reported in years. Here are the statistics as reported in the article. "In clinical trials, about half the patients had at least a partial response as defined by symptom improvement of 25% or more. At the one year mark, 27% of patients in the clinical trial were identified as responders, as defined by 50% or more improvement in their symptoms, and one in six of the total population (16%) were remitters with few or no symptoms of depression. Only 7% of non VNS patients remitted in the same time frame. In the one case where there was a placebo group, (people actually getting the surgery but not having the device turned on), showed nearly identical response to the active group, varying on only one of four measures used in the study. Only when both groups had the machine turned on so it could be compared in efficacy to what Dr. Angell calls "nothing" could the statistics be "interpreted" in favor of this extremely questionable procedure. It should also be noted that we "standing reserve" humans remain a major pain in the butt to companies developing products to make us feel better. Like it was for choice of antidepressants and dosages, no characteristic voltage or frequency emerged as best. "...in the clinical trials some patients responded with tiny doses of currents while others received much higher currents to no avail, leading investigators to believe there is some individual variability in optimal dosing." Oh, and yes I should mention that messing with the vagus nerve can also have some side effects like chronic hoarseness and a significant change in your voice (and God knows what else; this is a major cranial nerve!).

Well there you have it dear reader: The current *state of the art* of the treatment of depression and anxiety disorders by medical model DSM driven psychiatry. Enough said. I think so. Let's move on to an examination of the other drugs you will be offered to treat you and your family and loved ones as soon as you set foot in the psychiatrist's office or complain to your family doctor.

Chapter Seven:
PSYCHOPHARMACOLGY
It Aint Rocket Science

In this chapter we will examine the other four classes of psychiatric meds: Sedative/hypnotics, antipsychotics, mood stabilizers and stimulants. I will show you how the lack of rigorous testing and the ambiguous (at best) FDA indications for many of these drugs has resulted in a clinical situation where the choice of medicines and the dosing strategies are so arbitrary and capricious that you don't know (and the clinician has apparently lost sight of the fact that) we are dealing with some potentially very dangerous medicines here. I say "it aint rocket science" because logical guidelines based on clear-cut clinical results do not form the basis for medication choices. That opens the door to everyone from the family doctor's physician assistant to mental health counselors sending their clients to the local "doc-in-the-box" with a medication "suggestion" feeling a comfortable level of "expertise" in utilizing these limited number of often quite similar medications. No, its not rocket science or brain surgery or even regular medicine; it's the unique and stunning world of psychopharmacology. We've covered the all-purpose drugs called antidepressants; let's peek at what else is in the medicine cabinet.

SEDATIVE/HYPNOTICS

These are familiar medications like Valium and Ambien and Ativan that work primarily by an overall calming effect on the central nervous system (CNS). The mechanism of action of most of these drugs is better understood than antidepressants and may surprise you. To explain this I need to take another brief foray into neurophysiology and look at some additional information about how nerve cells in the brain send signals and communicate with each other.

The action of nerve cells in the brain (neurons) is amazingly simple. The cell bodies send tiny electrical signals down long narrow channels called axons. At the end of the axon the electrical signal causes the release of chemicals into the space between the axon and the cell it is communicating with. That space is called the synapse and the signaling chemicals include the familiar ones we are talking about in this book such as serotonin, epinephrine and dopamine as well as probably hundreds of others, many as yet undiscovered. As mentioned in the discussion on serotonin, the cell that receives the chemical message deciphers that message at special places on its membrane called receptors. So receptors receive messages. These receptors then "interpret" the message from the sending cells because some messages say "fire" while some say "don't fire." Affecting these chemical messengers is how most CNS drugs and goodies like alcohol and cocaine work. Occasionally, however, we come across drugs that don't work by affecting the chemical message sent between cells but actually bind directly to receptors on the receiving cell; in other words they are "recognized" (in a sense mistakenly) by nerve cells as being a chemical that naturally occurs in the body. If that sounds confusing just let me mention a familiar word: endorphins. Endorphins are called the body's natural opiates because after we found out that opiates like morphine and heroin bind directly to nerve cells in the CNS, we went looking for opiate like compounds in the body and, by gosh, there they were. Well the same is true for Valium, Xanax and all the rest of the benzodiazepines (let's call them benzos for short). They bind to nerve cell receptors called, quite naturally, benzodiazepine receptors. So they too act directly on brain cells, causing them to be more resistant to firing. That is why, like in the case of opiates, we can say with certainty that *no one feels nothing* when they take a benzo. Some people may not like what they feel but there will always be a felt effect from a drug that mimics a natural chemical in the body and directly acts on neurons. And it is why it is also true that there is no delay in the onset of action of these drugs. No waiting 3 or 4 weeks for them to work like we are told to do for antidepressants (without any, as yet, plausible explanation for this delayed action, by the way). This is why the use of benzo's, like opiates, is such a confusing mess for doctors and patients. Opiates relieve pain better than anything else but they can also deliver a "buzz"; a sense of euphoria and wellbeing that can be so attractive to people that they begin to chase that high on a full-time basis. The most potent opiates, like oxycodone (in long-acting form the "hillbilly heroin" Oxycontin), are therefore tightly regulated as Class II substances. (Of course that does little to prevent them from getting onto the streets). Benzos, on the other hand, have a mechanism of action that is different from opiates and are thus much less likely to deliver a true euphoric "buzz." The Drug Enforcement Agency (DEA) ranks the benzo's as Class IV drugs, the least addictive of all the scheduled compounds. But that doesn't stop the *idea* of being "addicted" to Valium, Xanax, even sleeping pills like Ambien from exerting a powerful effect on doctors and patients.

Clearly, these minor tranquilizers (benzos) have street value and are abused by some people. Most often (in the vast majority of cases) this abuse is by people who also use other drugs and alcohol to get high. A few years ago the daughter of the then Governor of Florida, Jeb Bush, was arrested for trying to falsely obtain Xanax without a prescription. This brought legal attention, unwelcome publicity and forced drug treatment to this very prominent family. But according to what I read, Xanax was not the Governor's daughter's drug of choice, it was cocaine. Xanax was just something she was trying to get to calm her nerves while trying to live a drug-free life. Benzo's are good drugs to have on hand to help ease the withdrawal from binges on cocaine or to enhance the effect of downers like alcohol or just to help ease the anxiety of living the life of an addict.

What about the legitimate use of this class of drugs? For some reason, I'm not sure why, the temperature is rising on this issue. There seems to be a growing pressure not to use these drugs, especially chronically. Apparently Medicaid and other insurances have expressed their stand on this by no longer being willing to pay for prescriptions, even though these mediations are generally quite inexpensive. One day, in the town where I was in private practice, most of the family doctors started refusing to continue to prescribe benzos; even to the patients they have had on them for years. So I got a lot of "new" patients coming to me expressly to obtain their benzos *while continuing to receive all of their other psychiatric medications from the family doctor.* When these patients presented to me I had two choices: continue the benzos (only now with my name on the prescription) or assist them in detoxing off of them, a very difficult thing to do. Either way I kept adding to the large number of patients who, despite my background in substance abuse treatment, or, correct that, *because* of my background in substance abuse, I was already comfortable with giving this class of drugs. (It's because in working for years with serious addictions to cocaine, alcohol and heroin I can put the benzo "addiction" issue into perspective. I never have and suspect I never will see a patient hooked "exclusively" on benzo's looking or acting anything like people addicted to those other drugs. It simply doesn't happen!)

So let me spell out *my* position on this class of medications without arguing right/wrong. There is one fact about benzos that is clearly true. If you stop them suddenly you are risking a severe withdrawal syndrome, one that could kill you. So there is a physical dependency that occurs if these drugs are used for more than a month or so. Beyond that, however, is the question of the medically appropriate usefulness of these drugs. Obviously, like in the case for opiates, if there is another, non-addictive alternative available, you would prefer to use that. Think about all of the prescription and over-the-counter non-opiate pain medications out there. If any were as effective as opiates we wouldn't be talking about opiates at all here because they would have disappeared. Well, they haven't. Is the same true for benzodiazepines? Are there non-addictive alternatives that are just as effective for anxiety, tension and insomnia? See answer for opiates.

What are the alternatives to benzos for anxiety? Two non-controlled medications are sometimes utilized for anxiety. The first is buspirone (brand name Buspar), an unusual drug with some impact on serotonin that was marketed exclusively for the treatment of anxiety. The problem is that because it works by a mechanism of action similar to antidepressants it takes three to four weeks to have an effect (if it does work at all). It has not been all that reliable for me although other doctors have more favorable opinions. Sometimes the antihistamine Vistaril is used but it's not really very potent. When you have serious anxiety or serious insomnia you want relief. A growing trend is to use small non-therapeutic dosages of the antipsychotic Seroquel (discussed below) in what I see as a kind of "anything but benzo" mentality in treating anxiety. Seroquel is in a class of drugs called major tranquilizers and clearly does help calm anxiety. But it is very sedating and so is generally given in multiple very small doses throughout the day. Psychiatric hospitals have apparently embraced this strategy and it works well for them. No problem: that is until the patient is discharged. They naively head down to the pharmacy to fill their discharge prescriptions and are shocked by the price tag for their four Seroquel pills a day. What, it's not covered by my insurance? $550? I can't afford that. Bye-bye Seroquel.

The other mainstay of treatment for anxiety problems should come as no big surprise—the serotonin antidepressants. I already mentioned what a good business move it was by Paxil to "get the indication" for social anxiety disorder. Among the antidepressants you will see FDA approval for every type of anxiety problem from generalized anxiety to panic disorder to obsessive compulsive disorder to post traumatic stress disorder. So why would I ever need to use benzo's? Is it because having an FDA indication doesn't insure a positive treatment outcome? If you guessed that, give yourself a pat on the back. You are learning! And remember where the bulk of my patients came from, family doctors who had already tried the patients on multiple antidepressants, sometimes to their detriment. Every clinician knows that antidepressants can also *mobilize* anxiety, i.e. make it worse. And this happens a lot, especially if you dose too aggressively at first. Many of the patients I've seen who have severe anxiety *refuse* antidepressants due to bad past experiences with them. Some of my patients had such a worsening of anxiety on a single dose of an SSRI that they report having contemplated suicide. (I believe that some suicides are the result of unbearable anxiety with or without depression. Severe anxiety is probably the most noxious emotion we experience). Bottom line, I used a lot of benzodiazepines in my practice because they worked, rapidly and reliably. There is something about drugs that bind directly to brain cells that is different from drugs that have a secondary effect. Plus, the fact that our brain cells have benzodiazepine receptors points to the fact that there is something our body produces that is a natural tranquilizer just like endorphins are natural painkillers. Researchers have named these natural tranquilizers enzopines. To me that opens the door to the possibility of a lot of ways things can go wrong biologically and cause dysregulation of anxiety and result in what I also believe are among the biologically influenced psychiatric illnesses: Panic Disorder, Obsessive Compulsive Disorder (one you would not wish on your worst enemy) and Generalized Anxiety Disorder (which manifests as *constant* worrying).

That doesn't mean that my patients always accept my advice to take benzos. Many of them are more worried about taking them than I am about prescribing them. "I don't want to get addicted", they say. I understand. It's a complicated decision. But one massive advantage that benzos have over those other drugs with a bad reputation, opiates, is that there is very little risk for the development of tolerance, meaning that once an effective dose is established it tends to remain effective for a very long time. Some of my patients had been on the same dose of Valium or Ativan for decades. Their only problem was when a doctor came along telling them that they were addicted and tried to take them off. I want you to understand that these were people with no other history of addiction or destructive behavior related to alcohol or drugs. It was just plain cruel to force them off their tranquilizers after all those years.

Poor Suzy; she was such a mess, chasing help for her personality disorder and severe anxiety over so many years with so many doctors. On top of that she had some legitimate physical problems but her anxiety and behaviors made it very difficult for doctors to evaluate if she was having serious symptoms or was just being hysterical. The paradigmatic story about Suzy was this: At times she would get so desperate for help that she would literally crawl on her hands and knees into the local Emergency Room (where she was well known). Eventually, it got to the point that when she crawled in the desk person would not even get up from her chair. "Hi Suzy, what's wrong today dear?" she would ask.

No psychiatric care or psychotherapy had ever penetrated Suzy's defenses and lack of capacity for insight. Notice I say lack of capacity for insight. That is just how it is for some people, they simply cannot see themselves as others see them or be taught to do so. So everything was an emergency with Suzy. She would leave rambling messages on my answering machine that would cut off in mid sentence because she exceeded the storage capacity of the tape. Needless to say, Suzy was a challenge. She had been on all classes of psychiatric medications and, she reported, they were all ineffective or made her condition worse…all except one: Xanax.

Suzy's daily dose of Xanax was one mg. five times a day. Xanax is a potent, short-acting benzodiazepine, so potent in fact that it comes in a 0.25mg dosage strength. For an elderly woman this 5 mg per day was a hefty dose. But it was the only thing that would keep her reasonably calm and out of hospital emergency rooms. The only time I had any real trouble with Suzy was when she would encounter a new doctor who insisted that she was addicted to Xanax and start to detoxify her. I'd get a nice long emergency phone message every time that happened.

The antianxiety drugs are all generics now and some have very familiar names. To review: the general class these drugs belong to is called benzodiazepines and they are Class IV controlled substances.

Benzodiazepines used primarily for anxiety:

1. Diazepam (Valium)
2. Chlorodiazepoxide (Librium)
3. Clonazepam (Klonopin)
4. Clorazepate (Tranxene)
5. Lorazepam (Ativan)
6. Oxazepam (Serax)
7. Alprazolam (Xanax)

Benzodiazepines used primarily for sleep:

1. Estazolam (ProSom)
2. Quazepam (Doral)
3. Temazepam (Restoril)
4. Triazolam (Halcion)

Non-benzodiazepine antianxiety drug (not a controlled substance)

1. Buspirone (Buspar)

Non-benzodiazepine sleeping medications (Class IV)

1. Ambien (Available as generic Zolpidem)
2. Ambien CR
3. Lunesta
4. Sonata

Non-benzodiazepine sleep medication (not a controlled substance).

1. Rozerem

Again, this looks more complicated than it is. All of the benzodiazepines work by precisely the same mechanism of action and differ only in speed of onset and duration of effect. The familiar drugs Ambien, Sonata, and Lunesta work a little differently and are used only for sleep, not anxiety. They are generally very effective (but far from trouble-free).

Let's talk a little about sleep before I move onto the next class of drugs. Many, many, many people have trouble sleeping. Sleep represents an extremely complex neurophysiological process, so complex it's a wonder any of us get a good night's sleep (after childhood). There is initial insomnia (difficulty falling asleep), middle insomnia (waking up during the night), and terminal insomnia (waking up and not being able to go back to sleep). Whatever the presenting complaint of a new patient, I always ask about sleep. Because sleep problems don't just accompany other emotional and cognitive problems; sleep problems can be the cause of the other difficulties. I've been sleep deprived as an intern and resident in medicine. It stinks. I could barely function after 20 hours with no sleep. What do we do with prisoners of war to break down their defenses and get them to talk? Sleep deprivation. So I always ask about sleep quality and duration and do not hesitate to use the new and very effective sleep aids Ambien, Sonata and Lunesta. But what about dependence on these drugs? Don't people get "hooked" on them? Isn't that a bad thing? Of course that is a concern. You want people to regain their ability to get a natural night's sleep. Many do but some don't. I have found the best way to handle the sticky issue of duration of drug use was the advice I got from a respected colleague whose entire practice is devoted to insomnia. He tells his patients that he is going to give them pills to help them sleep and that he will prescribe them for as long as needed and never cut them off. That takes care of about 90% of the worries patients express about using sleeping pills because he did not make an issue out of duration of treatment or drug dependency. So there is no "elephant in the room" that everyone ignores. The fact is that nearly all patients auto-regulate their intake of sleeping pills, most choosing on their own not to take them every night and eventually simply stopping them on their own or using one or two a week. It feels nice as a psychiatric clinician to do something of immediate value and clear-cut benefit to these people who are suffering. The same is true for the benzodiazepines, immediate and lasting benefit. I truly believe that some of my patients with clear-cut anxiety disorders, especially Panic Disorder and Generalized Anxiety Disorder would be non-functioning hermits, barely leaving their homes, if it wasn't for the benzodiazepines I give them. They are at times truly miracle drugs. (More about anxiety disorders and their treatment in chapter ten).

ANTIPSYCHOTICS

The next class of drugs is a large one. In part this represents the fact that what these drugs were designed to treat is a condition that few disagree is a biological dysfunction of the brain. The condition is psychosis and the drug class is antipsychotics. (Of interest here is that antipsychotics, especially the older first generation drugs are also sometimes called Major Tranquilizers, distinguishing them from the antianxiety benzodiazepines, also called Minor Tranquilizers. I wonder why they are called "Major"?

Zzzzz...)

Despite this being a large class of psychiatric drugs I will not be dealing with them in any great detail. I will, however, more closely examine the so-called "second generation" antipsychotics, a group of very expensive drugs that are desperately trying to expand their market in two ways. The first is to get an indication from the FDA for something (*anything!*) having to do with bipolar disorder. The second is to work behind the scenes in psychiatry fueling the rapid expansion of what medical model psychiatrists diagnose as variants of bipolar disorder, the Bipolar Spectrum Disorders we covered in detail in the chapter five.

The following is a partial listing of some of the better known *first* generation antipsychotic drugs:

Thorazine, Haldol, Mellaril, Navane, Stelazine, Prolixin...

Here is a complete list of the second generation antipsychotic medications; all are brand names as none of these medications has as yet gone generic (except Risperdal):

1. Zyprexa
2. Risperdal (generic: Risperdone)
3. Seroquel
4. Geodon

5. Abilify

I want to give you a brief education about the difference between first and second generation antipsychotics. The first generation drugs had some *serious* side-effect and tolerability problems. But in that they helped alleviate the symptoms of psychosis, many cases unremitting, these drugs were seen as a miracle. (There is still a strong controversy about this class of drugs that is beyond the scope and purpose of this book. I would once again recommend the book *Mad in America* for a much more detailed analysis of this controversy). These "first generation" antipsychotic drugs come with a price. They have a high number of side effects including excessive fatigue, dizziness, weight gain, blunted affect, growth of breasts in males, urinary retention, blurred vision and more. But the worst side effects, relatively unique to this class of medication, are called extra-pyramidal side effects (EPS). These drugs cause EPS because the brain chemical they affect, dopamine, is involved not only in the sensory and cognitive processes that have gone haywire in psychosis, but is also an essential brain chemical in the control of our muscle movements. By blocking the activity of dopamine in the part of the brain responsible for muscle control, these drugs led to conditions such as pseudo-parkinsonism (characterized by the same slowing of muscular movements and loss of control we witnessed from true Parkinson's Disease in Pope John Paul II) to dystonic symptoms caused by the uncontrollable contraction of muscle groups. Dystonic reactions can range from awful symptoms like torticollis, a contraction of neck muscles resulting in the head twisted horribly to one side, to oculogyric crisis where the eyes roll up into the head and cannot be brought down. Dystonias are both terrifying and very painful. Between the sedation and parkinsonian symptoms, (often resulting in the slow, small step gait and lack of upper body movement sometimes called the "Thorazine Shuffle"), and the dystonias (causing abnormally twisted bodies) chronic psychotic patients who were freed of their psychotic mental states often still looked quite bizarre and abnormal. But we have not as yet gotten to the worst side effect of all. That is a condition called tardive dyskinesia. All of the side effects mentioned thus far are theoretically reversible by discontinuing the drug or using other medicines to lessen the side effects. Tardive dyskinesia (TD) is an irreversible side effect where the patient tragically develops permanent movement abnormalities usually involving a darting tongue, facial grimaces and abnormal jerky and spasmodic movements of the upper body. Stopping the medication or using side effect medications does not reverse this permanent condition. (I will bet you that if you think back you can probably recall seeing people with TD but didn't understand what was wrong until now). So antipsychotic medications might have been a "miracle" but they came with a very big price tag; that was until the development of the second generation drugs.

The major initial selling point of the second generation (sometimes called atypical) antipsychotics was a reported very low risk for EPS and TD. All of these drugs were initially approved for schizophrenia and seemed to represent a welcome advance in the treatment of this horrendous disease. However, it seems that the bloom is starting to come off the rose. These drugs are far from side effect free and still carry warnings of the possibility of causing EPS and TD. Since I am not personally aware of any patients developing TD on these new medications I will not say in print whether any cases have developed or not. The bigger problem with these drugs (some clearly worse than others) is their predilection to cause weight gain and Type II diabetes as well as increased blood fats (sometimes called the metabolic syndrome). When the second generation antipsychotics hit the market most schizophrenic patients were (rightfully) converted to them despite the high cost. (Ballpark figure of about $8 to $15 a pill). Of course since schizophrenia is such a disabling illness most of the time Medicaid foots the bill. Or should I say taxpayers. These new drugs were also highly touted as more tolerable.

There were even studies showing that these drugs reduced not only the so-called "positive" symptoms of schizophrenia (delusions, hallucinations) but the "negative" symptoms (apathy, lack of emotions) as well, a response allegedly not seen in first generation drugs. Predictions were made that the outpatient treatment of schizophrenia would be much more successful with these new more effective and tolerable drugs because one of the chief reasons for failed outpatient treatment in this disorder was non-compliance with medication.

Well, here are the sobering results of a recently completed government sponsored study on medication compliance in schizophrenic patients, the Clinical Antipsychotic Trials of Intervention Effectiveness (CATIE) study. The only question asked in this study was what percentage of schizophrenic patients stabilized on one of the new antipsychotics (and in a control group of patients on one of the first generation drugs, Trilafon) would still be taking their medications as prescribed (compliant) eighteen months later. The results were abysmal. Only around 25% remained on their meds, 75% stopped taking them. It was exactly the same percentage in the control group on the older (and incredibly less expensive) drug Trilafon. Ah, the best laid plans... That is all I want to say about antipsychotics in the treatment of schizophrenia right now. I will have a lot more to say about some of the second generation antipsychotics in the next section where I will, in detail, discuss the class of drugs used in the treatment of bipolar disorder the

MOOD STABILIZERS

Here is a list of the currently available FDA approved mood stabilizers used in the treatment of bipolar disorder (many other drugs are used but this is the FDA approved list). After the listing I will explain the *specific* indications for each drug because there are some important differences you need to know about:

1. Lithium (Lithobid, Eskalith and other brands as well as generic)
2. Valproate (Depakote, Depekene as well as generic Valproic Acid)
3. Lamictal
4. Zyprexa
5. Risperdal
6. Seroquel
7. Geodon
8. Abilify
9. Symbyax

That's it. The whole list of FDA approved medications for the treatment of bipolar disorder. Recall, however, that in DSM IV there is more than one type of Bipolar Disorder. In fact there are four diagnostic choices: Bipolar I Disorder, Bipolar II Disorder, Cyclothymic Disorder and Bipolar Disorder NOS. In addition there are also different pathological mood states in a bipolar patient having an active episode. The patient's mood can be depressed, hypomanic, manic or "mixed". There is also the possibility of periods of normal mood (technically called euthymia) between active episodes. These periods of normal mood may last for weeks, months, years or even decades. Finally, we need to recall that psychiatric clinicians are diagnosing patients as bipolar spectrum disorders whenever there is any evidence of mood cycling, no matter how rapid the "cycling". You will also recall how the widely respected psychiatrist Dr. Hagop Akiskal is proposing six diagnostic categories for bipolar disorder with subtypes in each category. Have the above named medications been studied and approved for the treatment of all these types of bipolar "disorders" and if not, what have they been specifically approved for?

PREPARED TO BE SHOCKED (but not awed).

The goal in treating bipolar disorder is *prevention*. As I've explained previously, true (Type I) mania is a disabling, destructive, and dangerous condition. It is important that we have identified appropriate treatments for acute attacks of mania but to truly reduce the negative impact of this disease and allow the sufferer to have a fighting chance at a normal life, the primary goal is to *prevent* manic and depressive episodes from occurring. Of the list of 9 drugs above **ONLY ONE** has a clear-cut and unambiguous FDA indication for prevention of manic and depressive episodes (also called maintenance therapy) and a sufficient track record to back up that indication. It is the medication first approved for bipolar disorder in 1970. It is not a complex molecule developed after years of expensive research by a pharmaceutical company or university. In fact, it is not really a molecule at all; it is element #3 on the periodic table, Lithium. It was in 1949 when lithium was in a sense rediscovered as a possible treatment for bipolar disorder. Due to the fact that it was merely an element (and because years before it had been found to be toxic in high dosages) it took a long time for doctors to accept Lithium as a bona fide psychiatric medication. But it is and has been the mainstay of maintenance treatment of bipolar disorder now for decades. It is not free of side effects and risks. I told you before that bipolar medicines are not something to be taken lightly. But despite all the hoopla and advertising onslaught about other options in bipolar disorder it remains (in my mind at least) the most trustworthy and reliable bipolar medication and, unless there is a specific reason not to, is my mainstay of treatment for my bipolar I patients. Okay, now you are asking, "well what about all those other medications on the list? Why are they also called mood stabilizers?" I will tell you. I am going to pull out my trusty "little" 3500 page 2006 PDR and directly quote actual the bipolar "indications" for the other 8 drugs on the list.

1. Depakote: This is an anticonvulsant (epilepsy) drug which is also indicated for "the treatment of manic episodes associated with bipolar disorder...The efficacy of DEPAKOTE was established in 3 week trials with patients meeting DSM III-R criteria for bipolar disorder *who were hospitalized for acute mania." (Italics mine).*

2. Lamictal: This is also an anticonvulsant. The exact bipolar indication for this drug is so ambiguous and abstruse I decided to just quote it for you directly from the PDR and let you see if you can figure it out:

"LAMICTAL is indicated for the maintenance treatment of Bipolar I Disorder to delay the time to occurrence of mood episodes (depression, mania, hypomania, mixed episodes) in patients treated for acute mood episodes with standard therapy. The effectiveness of LAMICTAL in the acute treatment of mood episodes has not been established."

I invite you to chew on that one for awhile......

Here are the questions I need to ask the Lamictal folks:

1. When exactly do you start Lamictal in a bipolar patient?

2. Why would you put a "stabilized with standard therapy" patient on a second drug?
3. Do you stop the standard therapy or keep it going and for how long?
4. How do you know if Lamictal is working? If its effect is to delay the time to onset of a new episode then wouldn't you need to know if a mood episode *would have occurred* absent the Lamictal? How would you ever know that? In fact, how did you figure out you were lengthening cycles and get the FDA indication in the first place?

I really could go on and on here. The bipolar indication for Lamictal just doesn't make much sense to me. Maybe I'm just dense or something because from what I'm seeing a lot of psychiatrists are real comfortable with Lamictal and are prescribing it to a lot of patients. (Pssst...I'll explain the real reasons later)

Let's go on. Next come all of the second generation antipsychotics that have only rather recently gotten the bipolar indication. Their indications are essentially the same. They are all indicated for the treatment of acute manic or mixed episodes in patients with Bipolar I Disorder. Let me repeat the salient words "acute" "manic" "Bipolar I". Okay great. That takes care of treatment for, what did Dr. Lieber tell us, the 1% of the population with bipolar I disorder (three million people). But what about the other twelve to twenty one million people with Bipolar II, Cyclothymia and Bipolar Spectrum disorders? Whatever shall we use to treat this massive patient population who are bipolar but don't happen to be hospitalized type I patients in acute manic or mixed states like all of these drugs were tested on? Whatever shall we do?

"Wait a second Batman, I got it!"

"What is it Boy Wonder?"

"I know the FDA didn't approve or test these drugs for all of the types of bipolar and bipolar spectrum disorders but isn't it true that doctors can use drugs for whatever they want? I know the pharmaceutical companies are strictly forbidden by the FDA to promote the use of drugs for anything other than the indications approved by the FDA but if you can get doctors to associate the concept of bipolarity with a specific drug, don't you think they will use it on patients who have any evidence of bipolar type symptoms like mood swings and impulsivity and temper tantrums and stuff?"

"Boy Wonder, no wonder they call you Boy Wonder!"

"Aw, gee whiz Batman, even a dummy could figure that out."

We have two more items to explore on these mood stabilizers. The first are the indications that Zyprexa and Abilify have gotten for maintenance treatment. Zyprexa has received FDA approval for maintenance treatment in Bipolar Disorder. They did this by running a single long term trial of patients who were initially in a Bipolar I mixed or manic state and responded to Zyprexa for two weeks. These Zyprexa responders were then divided into two groups. One group continued to receive Zyprexa while the other group got placebo. There were a high number of drop-outs on both sides. The PDR does not report the length of the study but does say "patients receiving continued Zyprexa experienced a significantly longer time to relapse." Similarly Abilify's indication for maintenance treatment was established in a single study in which Bipolar I patients stabilized on Abilify for 6 weeks were then randomly assigned to Abilify or placebo and followed. The PDR says: "During the randomization phase, Abilify was superior to placebo on time to the number of combined affective relapses (manic plus depressive), the primary outcome measure for this study. A bit "jargony" I'd say but basically the same as the Zyprexa justification for its usefulness in maintenance. Like in the Zyprexa study, the PDR summary of the Abilify study does not report the duration. That is actually kind of a big deal. Remember when I said that medical model psychiatrists will often tell their patients that bipolar disorder is like diabetes and that they will need therefore to stay on treatment for life? I have to say that a single placebo controlled trial of what I would guess is of a relatively short duration hardly puts these drugs into the same ballpark as Lithium which has undergone hundreds of clinical trials and has proven its clinical efficacy over the last 36 years. I don't think I'm ready just yet to switch my Bipolar I patients over to these new options based on the data presented in the PDR. There is something else about these studies you may have picked up on so I think it is as good a time as any to deal with the issue of placebos.

What you may have picked up on in the Zyprexa and Abilify maintenance studies is that the study groups were derived from patients who were already on the active medication and were having a positive response to it. Do you think that maybe, just maybe, the subjects switched to placebo might have noticed the difference? Do you think they might have been, therefore, more psychologically prone to feeling depressed or manicky? Why are all these FDA studies always an active drug versus placebo? Why not against another active drug or some sort of placebo that at least mimics some of the felt effects of the study medication? And while we are at it, how come the casinos in Vegas are allowed to create games in which the house always has a statistical advantage? Why don't they run true games of chance with equal odds for both sides?

In her book *The Truth About the Drug Companies,* Dr. Angell deconstructs the placebo issue. As you recall Dr. Angell expresses concern in her book about the "me too" drugs that represent the major proportion by far of new drugs brought to the market every year (She puts the figure at 77%). She labels this a "travesty". She says: "This travesty is made possible by one crucial weakness in the law—namely, drug companies have to show the FDA only that new drugs are 'effective'. They do not have to show that they are *more effective than* (or even as effective as) what is already being used for the same condition. They just have to show they are better than nothing. And that is exactly what the companies do. In clinical trials, they compare their new drugs with placebos (sugar pills) instead of with the best current treatment. That is a very low hurdle indeed. In fact, on the basis of placebo-controlled trials, drugs can be approved that are actually *worse* than drugs already on the market. The last thing drug companies want is a head-to-head comparison" (Angell 2005 pp.75-6).

Okay, let's go back to the title of this book and recap where we are at in our fear of pill-pushing psychiatrists and look at how what we are learning about the whole "bipolar" disorder deal, from soup to nuts, might be causing you to seriously consider cancelling your trip to Psychiatryland.

Diagnosis:

Questionable and dangerous as soon as you get past the classic symptomatology of the lasting and severe manic and depressive episodes seen in Bipolar I disorder. When you start to speculate that the bipolar pathology can be expressed in less serious and obvious symptoms you run the risk of the inclusion of larger and larger numbers of distressed or misbehaving adults AND CHILDREN into what is turning into a catch-all psychiatric diagnosis.

Treatment:

Recall the statement from the Time magazine article that claimed that "Pharmacologists are perfecting combinations of new drugs that are increasingly capable of leveling the manic peaks and lifting the disabling lows." How does that match up with what we see in our survey of FDA indications in the 2006 PDR? All we have seen in terms of anything new is a parade of drugs that are better than doing nothing at all in the very small number of obviously ill hospitalized patients with Bipolar I manic or mixed episodes on which they were tested. I don't want to sound too irreverent here but I've seen Bipolar I manics in the hospital and I would argue that just about anything with sedating or calming properties would outperform sugar pills in calming the mania. We use injections of sedatives like Valium or Ativan all the time on them. The few new drugs approved for long term treatment aimed at preventing manic and depressed episodes have either very ambiguous indications or only one or two studies supporting the idea that they might be effective in the long run.

So we started with classic bipolar type I disorder and the fortunate discovery that an unlikely drug, the element lithium, actually helped. We knew that in 1970. What has happened since? In 1980 DSM III was published and the dominance of medical model psychiatry began. As a result of that we now have a rapidly growing number of ill defined bipolar disorders being diagnosed in family practice, psychiatric and primary care offices and, perhaps most disconcerting, in child psychiatrist and pediatric offices as well. So be afraid!

Okay Dr. Phill, hold on a second. I can see the problem but c'mon, be afraid? So the diagnosis of bipolar disorder has gotten a little sloppy and loose. So some kids and adults are being treated with "mood stabilizers" that they might not really need. I agree, maybe psychiatry is spinning out of control, but why the fear? Isn't that a little over the top?

You know, perhaps it is. But I'll let you decide after we cover this next topic, the side effects and dangers of "mood stabilizers." We'll start with lithium. I will get my information here directly from the 2006 PDR. So I need to explain to you exactly what the Physician's Desk Reference contains. Number one: over 3500 pages of very small print. Most of those pages are taken up by the "package inserts" that are produced by the pharmaceutical companies. The package inserts are EXTREMELY detailed accounts of just about everything known about a particular drug. They are therefore chock full of information but are so detailed and complex you really need to know how to separate the relevant from irrelevant information. These package inserts are also quasi legal documents by which the drug companies protect themselves from liability by listing any and every possible side effect associated with the drug and any reported untoward reactions, any possible drug-drug interactions. That is why I always find it amusing when a patient calls asking if some problem could "possibly" be a side effect of a medication. I can almost always answer yes because nearly everything is a "possible" side effect of any medication. For example, I counted the list of possible side effects listed for Zyprexa in the PDR. The package insert (PI) in the PDR for Zyprexa is eight pages of triple column tiny print. One section is labeled "Other Adverse Events Observed During the Clinical Trial Evaluation of Zyprexa": Divided into frequent, infrequent and rare the number of adverse events listed in this section is around 224. Obviously no doctor could keep that list in his or her head. But we don't need to. The more worrisome side effects and dangers that are more clearly caused by the drug are listed under "Contraindications", "Warnings" and "Precautions". There are still other lists of side effects reported in tables comparing the incidence in the active drug versus the placebo groups in clinical trials. (Placebo patients report a surprising number of side effects from just taking sugar pills). This is a lot of information. And the FDA knows it. So they developed a way to list certain warnings in the PDR that would insure that the doctor notices. It's called the "Black Box Warning." Black box warnings are not buried in the package insert and are not hard to find. They are located right after the name of the drug, before any other information, and are in larger and bolder type than the rest of the package insert. Plus they are set off by a black line surrounding the warning. It is literally a black box. You can't miss it!

Okay, back to Lithium. Since the PDR only has full package inserts for brand name drugs we will use the information from the brand of lithium called Eskalith . The information in the insert would apply to any form of lithium taken for bipolar disorder. There is a black box warning for Lithium. It says: **WARNING:** Lithium toxicity is closely related to serum lithium levels, and can occur at doses close to therapeutic levels. Facilities for prompt and accurate serum lithium determinations should be available before initiating therapy." Yes, you are getting it right; lithium can kill you. Of course so can many other medications if you take enough of it. Even water can kill you if you drink too much. The reason this problem with lithium earned a black box warning is that the dose needed to kill you is not a whole lot larger than the dose needed to treat you! That's what it means when it says that toxicity can occur at doses close to therapeutic doses (evaluated by "serum levels", the amount of lithium in the blood). So initiation and ongoing treatment with lithium requires monitoring of serum lithium levels by blood tests. You also have to look at other blood tests before you even start lithium because any problems with the kidneys or thyroid glands might rule out using lithium before you even start. Lithium is "cleared" by the kidneys so any kidney dysfunction can result in inadequate clearance, raising serum lithium levels to the toxic range. Concerns have been expressed about lithium possibly leading to permanent kidney damage although this remains controversial. No doubt, you have to keep an eye on the kidneys during treatment with lithium. Lithium also clearly affects the function of the thyroid gland in a number of ways. Frank thyroid failure has been associated with the chronic use of lithium. Finally, under the heading of terrifying side effects is this: Lithium is teratogenic. I threw in this big word because even the word looks scary, as it should, because it refers to the fact that lithium is known to produce birth defects. In particular, a heart defect in the fetus called Ebstein's anomaly. The rate of occurrence of Ebstein's anomaly in the babies of women treated with lithium during the first trimester has been reported as anywhere from one hundred twenty to four hundred times that of the general population. Okay, that takes care of the really scary stuff. Now let's look at common side effects of lithium treatment that often the patients are asked simply to put up with:

1. Constant hand tremor
2. Weight Gain
3. Acne
4. Hair Loss
5. Nausea
6. Excessive thirst
7. Frequent urination
8. Mental cloudiness and forgetfulness

I told you that it stinks to be bipolar. This mainstay of treatment which, due to its unquestioned effectiveness, is the one I try to use on all my bipolar patients. But it is also clearly a drug that exacts a big price, just not as big as the cost of unchecked manic episodes and painful bipolar depressions. So it's a trade off, pure and simple. Obviously both the patient and doctor would like some other choices when it comes to treating bipolar disorder. Since lithium was so incredibly unique there was not a spate of "me-too" lithium like drugs developed by the pharmaceutical industry. They simply manufactured lithium in different forms and delivery systems. The next class of drugs that showed promise in bipolar disorder were the types of drugs use to calm excessive nerve cell firing in the brain, the anticonvulsants. As I said in an earlier chapter, a desperate psychiatry, stuck with the singular option of lithium, enthusiastically embraced every anticonvulsant, looking for anti-bipolar properties. Only two are listed in the 2006 PDR as FDA approved for an indication related to bipolar disorder. Of course as the Boy Wonder pointed out, doctors are free to use drugs for any purpose, so in clinical practice a number of anticonvulsants are used even though they don't have a bipolar indication. These include Carbamazepine (brand name Tegretol), Oxcarbazepine (brand name Trileptal), Gabapentin (brand name Neurontin) as well as the non-generic Topomax. But as listed above the only two anticonvulsants with FDA bipolar indications are Valproic acid (brand name Depakote) and the non-generic Lamictal.

I have to admit that your old friend Dr. Phill was himself surprised when researching Depakote. (I'll use the brand name here for easier reader recognition). I have seen so many patients over the years on Depakote and have treated more than a few bipolar patients with it myself, that I was really shocked to see that Depakote does not (in the 2006 PDR) have the maintenance indication. But it does have the Bipolar I indication (reported as effective against mania in hospitalized bipolars) so it is at least in the ballpark. Now the question is; does it offer a clear advantage over lithium in having less toxicity and less terrible side effects? Let me list them and then you can decide for yourself. But I'll give you a hint: NO!

Does Depakote have a black box warning? No, it doesn't have *a* black box warning. It has THREE black box warnings. Let's go to the PDR. Actually, its three warnings are contained in one big black box taking up over half a column. (If you want to see it for yourself look on page 427 of the 2006 PDR). The lettering is different from that in lithium's black box. The text is in all capital letters, with the headings highlighted in bold. It clearly grabs your attention more than the black box on Eskalith does but I'm not sure that has any significance. Here are the black box warnings for Depakote:

1. **HEPATOTOXITY:** This means toxicity to the liver which can, in the worse case scenario result in liver failure and death. The black box warning then goes on to be more specific in saying that the risk is greatest in patients under two years of age, especially if on additional anticonvulsants. But the possibility of liver failure is not ruled out at any age and remains a potentially fatal side effect of the use of this drug. (Hmm, excuse me a second, a memory is trying to come forward in my mind. Something about Depakote and children. Oh yeah, I remember! It was in the Time magazine article about bipolar children. It was that 9 year old Brandon Kent. He was put on Depakote and Risperdal and his body began to swell. So they switched him to Topomax but he got sleepy so then they ended up putting him on Tegretol and Risperdal. This might be a good time to ponder the implication of diagnosing bipolar disorder in children. They get put on the same medications that, as we are seeing, are no picnic for adults. And those kids, their brains and organs are still growing.)

2. **TERATOGENICITY:** Uh Oh. Birth defects again. Isn't it usually true that the greatest risk to the fetus is in the first trimester? Isn't that the time when you are least likely to know you are pregnant even when you are? I hate the birth defect warning because it's always dumped back on the doctor to "weigh the risks" of birth defects against the risks of not treating the underlying condition. As Borat would say: "Niiice". Great choice, especially in psychiatry where you can never be certain that

anybody has anything. For example, in discussing lithium and birth defects, the biological psychiatrists who wrote *The Concise Guide To Psychopharmacology,* (published by the American Psychiatric Association Press in 2002), say: "The increased risk of malformations must be weighed against the risk of harm to both mother and fetus if lithium discontinuation results in manic relapse." In other words the doctor either makes or heavily influences the decision. But here is what I think. It's not the doctor; it's the mother and child who will live with the results of a "wrong" decision for the rest of their lives. For God's sake, if at all possible don't take ANYTHING if you are pregnant; that's my advice. By the way, the birth defect associated with Depakote is spina bifida.

Now we get to black box warning number three. This warning is of a danger of a higher order of magnitude than any previously mentioned. Leaving aside the birth defect issue, the warnings of the dangers on lithium had to do with a higher than required blood level of the drug, a situation that can generally be avoided by careful dose and serum level monitoring. But this next type of warning is of a potentially fatal side effect that cannot be anticipated, avoided or reversed. I'm going to quote the PDR warning word for word.

3. **PANCREATITIS:** CASES OF LIFE-THREATENING PANCREATITIS HAVE BEEN REPORTED IN BOTH CHILDREN AND ADULTS RECEIVING VALPROATE. SOME OF THE CASES HAVE BEEN DESCRIBED AS HEMORRHAGIC WITH A RAPID PROGRESSION FROM INITIAL SYMPTOMS TO DEATH. CASES HAVE BEEN REPORTED SHORTLY AFTER INITIAL USE AS WELL AS AFTER SEVERAL YEARS OF USE. PATIENTS AND GUARDIANS SHOULD BE WARNED THAT ABDOMINAL PAIN, NAUSEA, VOMITING AND/OR ANOREXIA CAN BE SYMPTOMS OF PANCREATITIS THAT REQUIRE PROMPT MEDICAL EVALUATION. IF PANCREATITIS IS DIAGNOSED VALPROATE SHOULD BE DISCONTINUED. ALTERNATIVE TREATMENT FOR THE UNDERLYING MEDICAL CONDITION SHOULD BE INITIATED AS CLINICALLY INDICATED.

If any of my readers are currently taking Depakote they are probably saying to themselves right now, "HOLY CRAP!!" Chances are your doctor did not mention this side effect when you agreed to take Depakote. It's what they call a deal buster! We see that no incidence figures are given here and I would guess the risk of this horrendous side effect is extremely low; but it is not zero. This is a very, very alarming type of drug side effect because there is no way to monitor anything that would allow you to stop the Depakote in time to prevent progression of pancreatitis. Serum amylase is a blood test that can be used to monitor pancreas function but my neurologist friends who use a lot of Depakote tell me that by the time serum amylase is abnormal, it is too late. Obviously doctors who don't fully inform patients about this particular side effect before initiating therapy with Depakote are making a judgment that the risk is so low that the benefits clearly outweigh the risks and that there is no need to unnecessarily terrify the patient. In principle I agree that the doctor should exercise clinically experienced judgment when confronted with the informed consent issue. I had a couple of patients in my private practice on Depakote (they came to me on it and if they are indeed Bipolar I and are stable, I will choose to sometimes leave well enough alone). I had one patient who had severe and dangerous prolonged manic episodes in the past. He came to me on both lithium and Depakote (this is not an unusual or rare situation). Once I got to know him better and had reviewed his past records I decided to simplify the case and get him down to one medication. Faced with the choice of stopping either lithium or Depakote I saw it as a no brainer; stop the Depakote. Not just because of the pancreatitis issue, but because of lithium's proven track record as a maintenance drug in Bipolar I Disorder.

There are *no drugs* FDA approved for Bipolar II, Cyclothymia, and Bipolar NOS (Bipolar Spectrum).

So what exactly do you think psychiatrists and other doctors are using when they diagnose Bipolar II disorder, Cyclothymia, Bipolar NOS and Bipolar Spectrum (and any other condition where a "mood stabilizer" is deemed clinically appropriate such as patients presenting with complaints of impulsivity or anger outbursts)? Is this psychiatry spinning out of control? You tell me! If it isn't what is it…science? C'mon. Our next "mood stabilizer", one that is rapidly growing in popularity is Lamictal. Guess what? It can kill you too but in a way that if I had my choice I'd go for the acute hemorrhagic pancreatitis. At least it's a pretty quick death. But before we turn to that lovely topic, I do need to mention a few common side effects of Depakote reported at therapeutic doses (this list might sound familiar): Weight gain, tremor, indigestion, nausea, drowsiness and both transient and persistent *hair loss.* (For real. Your hair falls out. We just ask our patients to "tolerate" these non-fatal side effects)

Okay, it's Lamictal's turn. As mentioned above the exact indication for Lamictal is simply not very clear. I remember when the "buzz" was that Lamictal would be indicated for the treatment of bipolar depression, a particularly nasty swing of the mood in Bipolar I disorder, often difficult to treat. Some help in that department would have been most welcome. Instead Lamictal was released with the bipolar indications detailed earlier. Also an anticonvulsant, Lamictal had an advantage in clinical use that was very attractive: No blood tests required. Unlike Lithium and Depakote, Lamictal posed no risks of organ damage and no risks of toxicity. Well that isn't quite true. Anybody ever ask you: "What is the largest organ in the human body?" In case you are ever on Jeopardy, here is the answer: the skin is the largest organ in the human body. And Lamictal does pose a threat to that organ, so much so that it as earned itself a black box warning. From the PDR here are some excerpts from that warning: (As I said before I don't know if it means anything but this black box warning is in both caps and bold type. You really can't miss this one):

SERIOUS RASHES REQUIRING HOSPITALIZATION AND DISCONTINUATION OF TREATMENT HAVE BEEN REPORTED IN ASSOCIATION WITH THE USE OF LAMICTAL...IN CLINICAL TRIALS OF BIPOLAR AND OTHER MOOD DISORDERS, THE RATE OF SERIOUS RASH WAS 0.08% (0.8 PER 1000) IN ADULT PATIENTS RECEIVING LAMICTAL AS INITIAL MONOTHERAPY AND 0.13% (1.3 PER 1000) IN ADULTS RECEIVING LAMICTAL AS ADJUNCTIVE THERAPY.

Let's take a break and "unpack" here. What are they talking about, serious rashes requiring hospitalization? A rash can kill you? How? Well I'm no dermatologist but what I have been able to find out is that what we are talking about here is called Stevens-Johnson Syndrome and/or Toxic Epidermal Necrolysis. The description of this condition is not pretty. It is said that the skin can peel off in sheets. Blisters form in the mucous membranes such as the eyes, mouth and vaginal area. You lose your top layer of skin as well as your hair and nails. Like in burn victims you are in unbearable pain and can die from infections that easily gain entrance through your unprotected flesh. (Sometimes it's better to just not know all the horrible things that can happen to the human body. I like to watch the educational channels on cable TV but sometimes I see things on Discovery Health and similar channels that I wish I had never seen). But here is this terrifying fatal skin rash in a black box warning about a drug being used in psychiatry to treat all the variants of bipolar disorder. I need to make clear that in the medical articles I accessed it is stated that the most frequently cited cause of this skin condition is as a reaction to drugs and actually lists quite a few drugs thought to be causative. I don't know what the FDA and PDR rules are that advance a regular warning to a black box warning although I assume it has something to do with degree of risk. For example the anticonvulsant Carbamazepine is mentioned in the article on Stevens-Johnson syndrome but when I looked it up in the PDR this complication was listed in the WARNINGS section, but not as a black box warning. (Don't feel sorry for Carbamazepine, it does have a black box warning too, only its for Aplastic Anemia and Agranulocytosis, which is when your body stops producing red and white blood cells which can lead to death from infection too. Sheeesh!). Back to Lamictal because there are more details regarding risk factors in the black box:

NEARLY ALL CASES OF LIFE-THREATENING RASHES ASSOCIATED WITH LAMICTAL HAVE OCCURRED WITHIN 2 TO 8 WEEKS OF TREATMENT INITIATION. HOWEVER, ISOLATED CASES HAVE BEEN REPORTED AFTER PROLONGED TREATMENT (E.G. 6 MONTHS). ACCORDINGLY, DURATION OF THERAPY CANNOT BE RELIED UPON AS A MEANS TO PREDICT THE POTENTIAL RISK HERALDED BY THE FIRST APPEARANCE OF A RASH.

ALTHOUGH BENIGN RASHES ALSO OCCUR WITH LAMICTAL, IT IS NOT POSSIBLE TO PREDICT RELIABLY WHICH RASHES WILL PROVE TO BE SERIOUS OR LIFE THREATENING. ACCORDINGLY, LAMICTAL SHOULD ORDINARILY BE DISCONTINUED AT THE FIRST SIGN OF A RASH, UNLESS THE RASH IS CLEARLY NOT DRUG RELATED. DISCONTINUATION OF TREATMENT MAY NOT PREVENT A RASH FROM BECOMING LIFE-THEATENING OR PERMANENTLY DISABLING OR DISFIGURING.

Reading this, you might think I have some personal grudge against Lamictal but I don't, I really don't! My grudge is against a psychiatry spinning out of control in both diagnosis AND treatment. I'm pulling my information right out of the PDR. I am not exaggerating or making anything up. You may also be asking who in their right mind would take a risk and go on a drug like this or any of the other mood stabilizers we've discussed. Patients, that's who. They go to the doctor for help and they more often than not do what the doctor recommends. I must admit that I've seen my fair share of patients who were on Lamictal from other doctors who did not exactly share this *precise* warning with them. They were told things like: "If you get a rash, give me a call." Invariably when I open the PDR to page 1449 and let them read the warning they choose to go off the drug. But my question is this: Why is psychiatry so hell bent on expanding and loosening the diagnostic criteria for bipolar disorder when the direct implication of that diagnosis is the necessity of utilizing mood stabilizer medications for life? It would just seem to me that we should be doing all we can to search for alternative conceptualizations and treatment plans for moody, impulsive and needy patients, reserving the bipolar diagnosis for only the most serious and undeniable cases. The PDR warning on Lamictal is not just a hollow warning. Some people *have to die* before the FDA forces a warning such as this. Here is a case from one of my many "throw away" journals I get every week. It's from *Current Psychiatry,* vol. 5, no. 2 / February 2006. It's in a section called "Malpractice Verdicts". Here is the case.

> *"A 43-year-old woman sought treatment for emotional difficulties. The psychiatrist diagnosed her with bipolar type II disorder and prescribed Lamictal. Within 5 weeks, the patient developed Stevens-Johnson syndrome and died from its complications."*
> *The patient's estate claimed*
>
> *a. That the psychiatrist misdiagnosed the patient, who the estate alleged, had posttraumatic stress disorder (PTSD).*
> *b. That prescribing Lamictal was inappropriate because the patient didn't have bipolar disorder and the drug is not first-line treatment for bipolar II disorder. (*Note, there is no first line treatment for bipolar II disorder)*
> *c. The psychiatrist failed to inform the patient that Lamictal may cause hypersensitivity reactions and neglected to obtain informed consent to use the drug.*

To satisfy your curiosity, the jury awarded the estate $3 million, reduced by capitation to $1.65 million. But I am hardly advocating that this problem with speculative, unprovable diagnosis and overzealous prescribing of CNS active medications be halted by court actions and malpractice awards. I want it to stop because psychiatrists come to their senses! I'm writing this book because I don't expect that to happen any time soon so I'm trying to get the consumers of psychiatry to be the ones who come to their senses first.

Okay, Lamictal is scary. What about the other new drugs for bipolar disorder. I've been seeing a lot of ads in Newsweek, Time and other magazines for Abilify as a treatment for bipolar disorder.

That is correct; you have been seeing A LOT of ads for Abilify. We'll look at why that is in chapter eight. For now, let's just go over all the antipsychotic drugs that have recently (and will most likely in the future) get FDA approval for bipolar disorder. Recall, first of all that most of these approvals were given for acute mania or mixed states in hospitalized Bipolar Type I patients. Only in the flawed logic of medical psychiatry would this then automatically imply effectiveness in all the other hypothesized forms of bipolarity. But recall that antipsychotics are also called Major Tranquilizers and I will guarantee you that any one who takes them will definitely feel *something*. And if you, your family and your doctor interpret this slowing and sedation as "improvement", then you will most likely experience what you are feeling as just that. The trouble is, you're probably going to have to buy new clothes...bigger clothes. Even though I disagree with what they did I am going to go along with the FDA on this and let you know that they issued a class warning about weight gain and diabetes on all members of the second generation atypical antipsychotic class. That includes, therefore, Zyprexa, Seroquel, Abilify, Risperdal and Geodon. The reason I disagree with the FDA deciding to issue a class warning is because an independent panel of endocrinologists, internists and psychiatrists reviewed the data and assigned variable numbers of pluses (meaning increased risk) to the individual drugs. Under weight gain Zyprexa got three pluses (+++), Risperdal and Seroquel two (++) and Abilify and Geodon uncertain (+/-). Under risk for diabetes and worsening lipid profile only Zyprexa got a plus (+). It seems clear that this panel saw Zyprexa as the worst offender; the FDA class warning did not back this up. (American Diabetes Association 2004)

Speaking of Zyprexa, its maker Eli Lilly did something very interesting a few years ago. I think it's fair to say that they took advantage of a bit of a loophole in FDA regulations. They came out with a new drug called Symbyax, only it wasn't anything new at all. Symbyax was a combination medication, putting together in one capsule two Eli Lilly drugs, Prozac and Zyprexa. No new ingredients, just varied numbers of milligrams of Zyprexa and Prozac. The loophole was that this could be patented as a new drug. Now, why would they do this? Well it turns out that the most common way to treat episodes of depression in patients with bipolar disorder is to utilize *both* a mood stabilizer and an antidepressant together. This is because an antidepressant alone can cause a depressed bipolar to overshoot and go manic. That is not a good thing. But you can't patent two drugs for one illness if the two drugs must be used at the same time. In terms of clinical care by the psychiatrist, that is no big deal. Choose a mood stabilizer, lithium, Depakote etc., and choose an antidepressant, any one you like. But, by putting Prozac (the antidepressant) and Zyprexa (the mood stabilizer) into the same capsule, Eli Lilly could now advertise Symbyax at the time (IF I'M LYING I'M DYING) as "the FIRST and ONLY FDA-approved treatment for bipolar depression." Enough said? (More in chapter eight).

Sometimes we physicians get warnings from the FDA that take us totally by surprise. Such was the case in 2005 when out of nowhere we received an FDA warning that the use of atypical antipsychotics (any of them) in the treatment of behavioral and cognitive disturbances in elderly patients with dementia was associated with an increased all-cause risk of mortality. At that time nearly all confused, psychotic and aggressive Alzheimer's patients WERE being treated with atypical antipsychotics precisely because they were viewed as LESS risky and more tolerable to the elderly than the first-generation typical antipsychotics. Now what are these psychiatrists who "specialize" in nursing home psychiatry going to do? These FDA warnings come at you anytime and without warning. On December 8, 2005 we all received an FDA warning "Advising of Risk of Birth Defects with Paxil"! This was in 2005. Paxil was approved by the FDA for the treatment of depression in 1992!! "Whoops, sorry ladies and infants; our bad." Speaking of risks, let's go on to our fourth class of psychiatric medications, the stimulants. Unlike the more obscure problems like Stevens-Johnson syndrome and tardive dyskinesia, the risks attendant to the use of amphetamine-type stimulants are, unfortunately, very well-known.

STIMULANTS

This time let's go right to the PDR. I am looking at page 3168 of the 2006 PDR. This is where the package insert for a drug named Adderall is located. A lot of people are on Adderall or its timed release formulation Adderall XR. Most people on Adderall are children and teens being treated for ADD but as we discussed in chapter five, a growing number of adults are being treated for ADD as well. I am not picking on Adderall here but I do find that most people on this medication (or in the case of children, their parents) are shocked when I read the two main ingredients of Adderall to them from the PDR. These two main active ingredients are dextroamphetamine and amphetamine. Wow, that sounds a lot like methamphetamine, the main ingredient in crystal meth, a drug of abuse ravaging this country. Are they alike? Well..yes they are. When a chemical name contains the word amphetamine that means it is a member of a class of CNS stimulants also known commonly as speed. I want to quote something for you from the book we previously discussed *Driven to Distraction*. It's from a section of the book where the author, psychiatrist Edward M. Hallowell, M.D., is discussing the choice of medication for treating ADD. He says: "The main reason we usually start with Ritalin, as opposed to another stimulant such as Dexedrine, is that decades ago, when stimulants were first used to treat ADD, many people thought of Dexedrine as a street drug, a drug of abuse. Although when Dexedrine is used properly it is not a drug of abuse, it had a major public image problem. Therefore, most physicians prescribed Ritalin, which had no such image problem. The trend continues to this day" (Hallowell and Ratey 1994 p.239). I know that this is ludicrous but what if someone snorted two lines of cocaine or crystal meth, 8AM and 1PM to help cope with the demands and rigors of the multitasking fast-paced world of work (and play) in America. Then the poor guy gets busted and faces years in prison. Would the "Adult ADD defense" work? I think I'll send this idea to the writers at the TV show Law and Order. I bet that they would take this on.

ADD. What a diagnosis.
Diagnosed at 10 times the rate in the U.S. versus Great Britain.
80% of the world's Ritalin supply used by the United States.

A widely diagnosed illness not demonstrable by any solid physical evidence but as real as real can get in our culture (reified) for children and teens. And pretty soon for adults. Because I'll guarantee you "they" are working on it. And who are "they"? C'mon already! Business people looking to make money. That is what it is all about and you know it! I am going to go into the whole dirty business of creating and selling disease in the next chapter but I just can't resist sharing with you something I once got in the mail. It arrived packaged in an oversized box. It was a little booklet advertising Adderall XR, the amphetamine mentioned above. The little booklet was wrapped in plastic and had a button showing through. The button said to "learn more, push here." The following is the honest to God exact transcription of the message (minus the sound effects and trained voices). I'll try to write it like a script.

Opening: A police siren is sounded and then a walky-talky with official sounding "chatter" is heard indistinctly (lending an air of authenticity).

Deep male voice, irritated: "Do you have any idea how fast you were going? Please step out of the vehicle".

Immediate segue to irritated high pitched female voice: "Can you believe he wants a divorce??"

Immediate segue to irritated male voice: "This is the third meeting you missed! You need to start getting to work on time!!"

Immediate segue to concerned female voice: "Sarah, your unemployment benefits run out next week! What are you going to do?"

Immediate segue to reassuring and comforting voice of narrator saying: "The stakes are high. These are some of the potential consequences of Adult ADHD. Your ADHD patients need effective symptom control that lasts all day. Find out why Adderall XR is the number one prescribed brand of Adult ADHD medication and how it can help."

I'm just kind of amazed. I finally decided to write this book that has been percolating in my mind for years. But as I am writing this chapter in real time in early 2007 unsolicited evidence keeps arriving to convince me that spinning out of control may be too tame a term to describe what is going on in my chosen medical profession. I mean seriously, what has to be going on in a society to allow for the emergence of this insultingly childish ad that I just got in the mail? I hope I don't need to explain to you why I find this insulting. I suspect that if you are still reading then you know. But here is a question worth asking; why would they send this advertisement to doctors? Why is this ad targeted at MD's? I've worked with drug companies. I've worked on TV. I worked for a while for the company that makes and sells Ultra Slim Fast. This much I can tell you for sure. Major advertising campaigns are launched by big corporations because they work! What do you think it cost Shire US Inc. to produce and mail this ad to doctors? More than most of us will make in a lifetime, that's how much. This wasn't produced by a couple of first year MBA graduates. It was produced by highly paid professionals who are playing more and more of a central role in our lives, advertisers. But how do they expect this moronic, simplistic script to sell Adderall? If someone gets a speeding ticket, gets divorced, is late for work…these are the secret markers of otherwise unrecognized Adult ADD? According to whom? Based on what? Science? These ads are designed the same way all ads are designed…to leave a residual trace in the mind of the doctor so that the idea that a patient in life crisis just might have ADD comes to mind. Then, if all goes well for the drug company, the doctor will pull out a handy little checklist that, interestingly enough, also comes from the drug company, and, by jove, there it is, Adult ADD. Who would have thunk it? THAT is worth millions of dollars to the drug company

Okay, back to stimulant medications. How about starting with the black box warning, shall we? Here it is:

> AMPHETAMINES HAVE A HIGH POTENTIAL FOR ABUSE. ADMINISTRATION OF AMPHETAMINES FOR PROLONGED PERIODS OF TIME MAY LEAD TO DRUG DEPENDENCE AND MUST BE AVOIDED.
> PARTICULAR ATTENTION SHOULD BE PAID TO THE POSSIBILITY OF SUBJECTS OBTAINING AMPHETAMINES FOR NON-THERAPEUTIC USE OR DISTRIBUTION TO OTHERS, AND THE DRUGS SHOULD BE PRESCRIBED OR DISPENSED SPARINGLY.
> MISUSE OF AMPHETAMINE MAY CAUSE SUDDEN DEATH AND SERIOUS CARDIOVASCULAR AD-VERSE EVENTS.

Let us pause for a moment to ponder a contrast. Let us contrast this official warning above from the FDA with the cutesy little advertising gimmick I received from the makers of Adderall designed solely to increase the number of customers by cherry picking from the extremely speculative and questionable potential manifestations of Adult ADD a few common negative aspects of the human condition…EVERY HUMAN! If this doesn't astound you; if this doesn't literally blow you away then we are all lost. I mean that sincerely. We are allowing our profit-hungry corporations to totally and completely run the show. The American adult has existed and thrived for over two centuries without anyone even considering that there was a hidden epidemic of Adult ADD lurking just beneath the surface responsible for the ruination of millions of lives and lost potential for vast numbers of citizens. What does that mean? The American adult has not accomplished enough? We are a bunch of addled, distractible and unfocused brain damaged people that, thank the Lord, the new science of psychiatry has finally unmasked? Or is it possible..just possible…that like the oil industry, like Halliburton, like nearly every moment of American life it has become…Rick?

***Another Roderickism:**
"All about that s..t called money!"

Are the FDA's concerns legitimate? Is there evidence that Ritalin, Adderall and the other stimulants are being abused? PLENTY! Here are a few quotes from the **DEA's official website** about methylphenidate (Ritalin)

> "[Ritalin]...has a high potential for abuse and produces many of the same effects as cocaine or the amphetamines."
>
> "The abuse of this substance has been documented among narcotic addicts who dissolve the tablets in water and inject the mixture."
>
> "The *increased use of this substance for the treatment of ADHD* has paralleled an increase in its abuse among adolescents and young adults who crush these tablets and snort the powder to get high."

Sounds like Dr. Hallowell's statement about Dexedrine being a minor abuse problem decades ago might have been a bit of a soft sell. In May 2000 DEA Deputy Director Terrance Woodworth said: "continued increases in the medical prescription of these drugs without the appropriate safeguards... can only lead to increased stimulant abuse among U.S. children." Safeguards, I wonder what those might be. Here are the recommendations in *The Concise Guide to Psychopharmacology* published by the American Psychiatric Association in 2002.

> The potential for stimulant abuse is a controversial topic. In general, clinicians should closely monitor the use of stimulants and be aware of the risks of potential abuse by patients and those around them, including family members, friends, and school personnel responsible for dispensing medications. One should exercise great caution when considering treatment with stimulants in any patient with a history of substance abuse or dependence (APA 2002, p.157).

That is actually all it says on the topic. Exactly how the doctor should "closely monitor" the use of stimulants is not spelled out in detail. Actually, that is for a very simple reason...YOU CAN'T! The only way to exercise any control over the growing abuse of pharmaceutical stimulants is to stop prescribing them. I still remember a patient I saw for the first time from a local college. She had been on stimulants for years but somehow I got her to spill the beans. She told me the college students abuse Ritalin all the time. She said you could stay up and drink longer and party harder if there was some Ritalin available. She said Ritalin abuse was rampant on campus and that the ADD students were highly valued by their classmates. And, oh yes, she also told me that these bright and sophisticated young men and women thought that the psychiatrists were a bunch of naive morons. They knew exactly what to say to get their Ritalin from them. "Doctor, I think the medication is helping but around 4PM I start to get drowsy and lose focus. Do you think we could add another pill at 4PM?" "Duh, sure!"

When I worked at a substance abuse hospital early in my career the director of the program (a world famous addiction specialist) called me into his office to share some words of wisdom before my first day on the drug treatment unit. Here is what he said: "There are three things you must always remember when treating drug addicts; you can never go wrong if you just remember these three things. Here they are: They lie, and they lie, and they lie." Honest that is what he said. It stood me in good stead for the next five years of my career.

One of the incredible theories floating around psychiatry today is that there is a high prevalence of substance abuse in patients *with* ADD. Well that doesn't sound too complex to manage. Just..uh. Just..uh. Just give them the stimulants and make them promise not to abuse the pills. Yeah, that ought to work.

Well, this chapter is starting to spin out of control, just like chapter six. So I think I'd better wrap it up. Yes there is a non-addictive treatment for ADD called Straterra. I haven't used it for any patients so I can't comment on its effectiveness or side effects from personal experience. I do see a lot of patients that other doctors have on amphetamine stimulants. A new, and I think very crazy trend, is diagnosing bipolar disorder *and* ADD in the same patient. It's not from the diagnosis side that this seems particularly nutty compared to other "co-morbid" diagnoses; it's the treatment implications. The bipolar part is treated with a mood stabilizer to prevent the patient from getting manic (hyper energetic, wired, euphoric, sleepless, crazy) but then treated for the ADD part with a stimulant, a class of drugs well known to cause hyper energetic, wired, euphoric, sleepless and crazy states. I just don't get it. I really don't. It's as if reason and common sense have been abandoned by psychiatry and some other force is painting this once eclectic and fascinating specialty deeper and deeper into a theoretical corner from which there will be no escape. For a full accounting of this "other force", see chapter eight, coming right up!

Chapter Eight:
"PSYCHIATRY, MEET BIG BUSINESS"
"I'm sure this is going to be the beginning of a beautiful relationship!"

"If there is anything resembling geist left in the world today, it is advertising."

Rick Roderick

I will get to explaining Rick's comment in just a moment. It took us a while to get here (there was a lot you needed to learn before we could deconstruct this) but we have finally arrived at chapter eight where all (that I know) will be revealed about the unholy alliance between the big pharmaceutical companies (Big Pharma) and the leaders and promoters of medical model psychiatry. As you will see, this alliance has successfully invaded every aspect and moment of your daily life and has radically and fundamentally altered your innermost understanding of yourself and the world around you. Just business as usual? As you'll see; sadly, yes.

Am I exaggerating, overstating the case? Well let's just go through this together and then you can decide. As always I am going to do my best to present to you *easily verified* factual material without knowingly attempting to slant or distort it. My primary source of critical commentary and opinion will once again be Marcia Angell's book *The Truth About Drug Companies.* I previously explained why I consider her an unimpeachable source for this information. There are numerous other credible sources of critique of the pharmaceutical industry and its relationship to psychiatry which I will provide in a list at the end of the book. When something is my own personal opinion I will clearly let you know. Before we get to the main meal however I want to start you off with a little appetizer because as I am working on this chapter in the winter of 2007 it is so "in your face" right now that I think you will find that it amuses and teases your palette. So our first course from the menu today will be Cymbalta.

In 2007 Cymbalta was the newest antidepressant; it is produced by Eli Lilly. At the core it is clearly just another "me-too" antidepressant drug with no new or radical mechanism of action deriving from newly discovered or hypothesized causes of "depression." It is just another drug that blocks the reuptake of serotonin and epinephrine, two of the catecholamines implicated in the fifty year old theory of the biological basis of depression. (You remember; the theory that yields a 30% drug versus 20% placebo rate of remission.) But……BUT…BUT…THERE'S MORE!

If you don't know what the "more" is I'm giving you a D-minus in TV watching. The rest of us, the normal TV watchers, know there is a very special additional action to Cymbalta. It treats PAIN! And not just any pain, the pain ASSOCIATED WITH DEPRESSION. Now how does that TV commercial go? *Where does depression hurt? Everywhere! (Have miserable looking woman rubbing her shoulder while grimacing from pain). Who does depression hurt? Everyone! (Have miserable looking man staring down at his needy and concerned looking dog).* And so on. It is a very good commercial. Nearly every patient to whom I quote the above lines recognizes that it is from the commercial for Cymbalta. THAT is what a good advertisement is supposed to do! (In contrast there is a very clever and entertaining set of ads running right now that features Abe Lincoln, a beaver, a chess set, a deep sea diver and a sleepy guy. The theme of the commercial is that "your dreams miss you", with Abe Lincoln, the beaver etc. being the players in the sleepy guy's dreams that he is not having because he is not sleeping. Not one of my patients knew that this entertaining and clever commercial was for the new sleeping pill Rozerem or why they might ask their doctor for this particular drug. I'm not sure Rozerem is getting what they want out of this commercial. As we've all learned in recent elections, getting the message across in expensive TV ads is in many ways the ESSENTIAL element in any business or political venture. Isn't that right "Swift Boat Veterans for Truth"?)

Back to Cymbalta. This is an incredible marketing scheme that represents a number of elements of the games drug companies play (and play very well). The first is the hiding of the "me too" status of the drug that we will talk about in detail when we discuss medical research. The second is making a "me-too" drug appear unique by testing it for effects other than those traditionally tested for by previous similar drugs. The most stellar example of this is the Prilosec/

Nexium "shuffle" that we will discuss later also. (Remember, this is just an appetizer). What I want to do now is simply blow your mind by showing you how a drug company can operate. From day one the makers of Cymbalta, Eli Lilly, have been intensively promoting the pain relieving properties of this antidepressant. This is what distinguishes Cymbalta from all of the other antidepressants. None of them have an FDA indication (remember you cannot promote anything but FDA approved indications) for pain except Cymbalta. And what depressed person doesn't have pain? And who wouldn't welcome some pain relief along with relief from depression? Seriously, who wouldn't? There is, however, a little technical problem here. Pain IS NOT a recognized symptom of depression AND CYMBALTA DOES NOT RELIEVE PAIN!! Now wait a second Dr. Phill. Didn't you just say that a drug company cannot promote a drug except for approved indications? And didn't you also say (more than once) that you don't want to get sued? Didn't you just slander the drug company that makes Cymbalta?

I'll tell you what...Let's go to the PDR and you decide.

On page 1730 of the 2006 PDR is a section in the Cymbalta package insert labeled: **INDICATIONS AND USAGE.** There are two sections under this heading. The first confirms Cymbalta as indicated for major depressive disorder. Okay, granted; it's an SNRI antidepressant. No big surprise there. The second section covers Cymbalta's pain indication. It says: "Cymbalta is indicated for the management of neuropathic pain associated with diabetic peripheral neuropathy." Is that it, the pain indication? Uh, what's that mean? Well, take it one word at a time. Diabetic means it is a complication of the *disease diabetes.* Peripheral means farthest from the center (hands, legs and feet). Neuropathy is pain and discomfort originating in nerve tissue (caused in this case by damage to the nerves by diabetes). Putting it all together diabetic peripheral neuropathy is pain in the hands, legs and/or feet caused by diabetes. Now why is that lady in the commercial rubbing her shoulder? Why indeed.

Remember when I told you that the atypical antipsychotics have been desperately trying to increase their market by getting in on bipolar disorder because the market for schizophrenia is so limited? Then I showed you how they did "better than placebo" studies on hospitalized manic or mixed Bipolar I disorder patients and were therefore able (with FDA approval) to put the name of their drug and the word bipolar in the same sentence. Apparently after meeting that "name association" minimal requirement all bets are off and the drug companies can go to town with their new "indication." Cymbalta's entire advertising campaign to the general public AND doctors has been based on the idea that physical pain in general (not just diabetic peripheral neuropathy) is an integral and characteristic SYMPTOM of depression. But look in the DSM IV. (Not my favorite document, as you know, but the source of official diagnostic information in all drug trials). If you recall Major Depression is diagnosed when at least five out of the nine listed symptoms is present for a period of greater than two weeks. That's nine choices and NOT ONE mentions the word pain, not one. Physical pain IS NOT a diagnostic symptom of depression. Period. It just isn't. That is why I said that the advertising campaign for Cymbalta is strongly implying that there is another type of depressive disorder, one that DOES have pain as a primary symptom. That is what I mean by "inventing" a disease to fit the drug. If you look at the Cymbalta ads you'd think that the creators of DSM, all psychiatrists and all doctors have been cruelly IGNORING the physical pain in their depressed patients because the entire print ad campaign for Cymbalta has revolved around the idea that if we doctors are "merely" treating the *emotional* symptoms of depression, we are only doing half the job. This is graphically illustrated by images such a bicycles missing one wheel or a dumbbell with weights on only one end. I have no doubt that Eli Lilly has paid big bucks for this ad campaign. Cymbalta is statistically significantly better than placebo in relieving the pain in diabetic peripheral neuropathy, only. Even by the incredibly liberal standards set by the FDA to prove efficacy, this is all they have shown. So unless your depressed patient happens to ALSO have diabetic peripheral neuropathy, Eli Lilly can make NO CLAIMS that physical pain in your depressed patient will be relieved by Cymbalta.

This obvious lack of checks and balances regarding how the drug industry presents their products (how did this commercial get on the air??) is kind of terrifying. But, from everything I've seen, it works. I've had other doctors switch my patients from the antidepressants I had them on to Cymbalta because, the doctor would tell them, it helps relieve pain. True chronic pain is awful, a tortuous experience. Many of my patients have pain complaints: fibromyalgia, rheumatoid and osteoarthritis, failed back syndrome and post traumatic (e.g. automobile or motorcycle accident) chronic pain. If Cymbalta could prove efficacy in any of those conditions I might sit up and take notice. But to imply efficacy based on one very tangentially related indication…that bugs me. One of my sour grapes is that I'm tired of being in the profession that presents itself as so formulaic and simplistic that no one, PCP's, physician assistants, nurse practitioners, or even mental health counselors feel the slightest hesitation in making or suggesting alterations to my treatment plan. By the time they get to me many of my chronic pain patients have tried everything including strong opiates, injections, implants and surgery and have still not gotten lasting relief. My treatment "plan" with these individuals is to try to help them accept and adjust to pain as a part of their existence so they can make the most of what they've got by moving on from a daily preoccupation with their pain. So it really irritates me when another doctor undermines my plan by giving into the advertising and switching my patient from their current antidepressant to Cymbalta; one more "miracle" drug to try. Sometimes I try to imagine what would happen if I, a clinical psychiatrist, changed one of my patient's cardiac or cancer meds based on an ad I saw on TV and a visit by a drug rep; something would hit the fan, that's for sure.

ADDENDUM: February 2010:

It turns out that Cymbalta did eventually get approval for the treatment of fibromyalgia. But this was well after they initiated the ad campaign and marketing strategy I outlined above. So this new approved indication does not change the point of my "deconstruction."

So there you have it, a little appetizer. I know you are wondering why doctors don't carefully read the package insert before they prescribe a new drug. Clearly that would have brought a halt to Cymbalta's early "pain of depression" campaign. That is the level of expectation any patient should have. But something has happened in the last twenty or so years in this country that seems to render the above mentioned practice by a physician somehow superfluous and meaningless. I know this is hard to believe but in a very real way it *doesn't matter* anymore whether the physician reads the package insert (except for the technical stuff about how a drug can harm you or interact with other drugs) because trying to use "facts" to counter a well conceived and mounted marketing campaign is generally an exercise in futility. Remember, we are in Psychiatryland and what matters now is not reality in the traditional sense of the word (with its rational arguments and proofs), but "hypereality" the "more real than real" world of images and beliefs grounded in marketing and advertising. To expand on this, it's time to get back to some philosophy.

In the opening quotation in this chapter I used the word geist. This is a word used by the 19th Century German philosopher Hegel. You know Hegel's work, we all do. In fact, the vast majority of us in America are staunch Hegelians, even if we don't realize it. We are Hegelians because we believe in ***progress.*** Hegel strongly believed in the idea of progress. He was the philosopher who is famous for the concept of the dialectic, something some of you might remember as thesis-antithesis-synthesis. This dialectic represents Hegel's analysis of history when it is looked at in retrospect. Basically, he proposed that in each era in history there are predominant ideas and beliefs but there are also often very strong counter-beliefs that are active as well. Eventually, these battles of beliefs end by some sort of synthesis of the opposing beliefs. This then is the source of progress in humankind as a whole. But, progress towards what?

Pause and ask yourself where you think we humans are heading. What drives us and keeps hope and motivation alive in the human race? Is the endpoint in your mind some time in the future when there will actually be a full and total scientific understanding of the nature of reality, an unimaginable technology that will allow all humans to truly live in peace and harmony? A utopia? That would not be uncommon because the idea of an eventual utopia drives many civilizations. This may surprise you but we are clearly living in a utopia right now…at least as it was envisioned 100 years ago when people were giving up their lives while blasting tunnels for the first transcontinental railroad. Perhaps you are not sure, in fact maybe have no idea, how the current "dialectics" of Western democracy versus Islamic theocracy or the even more fundamental dialectic of religion versus atheism will work themselves out, but at some level you just know they will. Humankind is progressing; it is a slow and often painful process, but there is progress. And just *where* is this progress located? Where can it be *seen?* It's kind of just there, in the *shared consciousness* of the human race, in what humans learn and pass onto each successive generation, in the collective human *spirit.* This is what Hegel called geist. Hegel himself was very hopeful and optimistic about where geist was headed—God-consciousness. Humans would eventually become one with the mind of God. That is the ultimate trajectory of history. Does that "feel" right to you? I'll venture a guess that it does. So where is Rick Roderick coming from with his *deflationary* comment that the only thing left in the world that resembles geist is advertising? Well, Roderick is not a Hegelian. He is a postmodernist. So am I. Here is why I agree with Rick. I'll bring it closer to home.

As tempting as it might be to want to believe that there is a productive dialectic process going on in the mental health field, my lived experience as a psychiatrist argues otherwise. I can say with a high degree of personal conviction that the complex dialectic I've watched play out in psychiatry between the conceptualization of normal and abnormal mental functioning and emotion as a broad humanistic concern (sharing fuzzy boundaries with psychology, philosophy, sociology, art, literature, religion and spirituality) and biopsychiatry, a narrow, hard core pseudo-scientific field of inquiry (with its clearly demarcated boundaries of wellness and illness) has not and will not result in a welcome synthesis of these opposing points of view. Rather it has already yielded a clear WINNER (scientism) and a clear LOSER (humanism). So it hasn't acted like a Hegelian dialectic at all. It has acted like exactly what it is: a power struggle.

There is a very different sense of geist in a power struggle, one that you don't have to look hard to find because it is all around you every moment of your life. In a power struggle someone (or thing or idea) has to "win the hearts and minds" (the spirit) of the masses. That is how you get a winner and a loser. That is how you got the Nazi party mobilizing the German people to attempt world conquest a mere half century ago. That is how you get power, money, wealth, fame and the presidency. That is how you get people to buy Toyotas or Harleys. Persuasion: Winning the hearts and minds of the masses. And where is that "persuasion battle" played out in today's world, in the early 21st Century? Why in the media of course. That is the basis for hypereality; creating a persuasive *image* is the name of the game, not a persuasive argument. An argument is too rational, too long and drawn out.

Nobody wants to choose a brand of car or TV or computer or lifestyle by undertaking a rational and detailed investigation of every choice. Its way too complicated. It would take a month just to research what they are talking about when they tell you that you should buy this truck because of its "unibody" construction. Nobody can do that. So they show the car in a "lifestyle" commercial. Is it a slick "hot" car for single people on the prowl? Is it a status car just oozing messages about your wealth? Is it a safe car for a suburban family? Or is it (why this motif keeps running I cannot understand) a kick-ass car with 350 horsepower that can accelerate from 0 to 60 in 4 seconds and then is shown driving down a country road or around a test track at 140 mph.? We don't want facts and technical details. We want images to teach us what to think and believe. We *want* to be persuaded. We watch and are entertained by the battle of persuaders. The race for the Democratic presidential nomination in 2008 started 18 months before the election, more than enough time to dig up some really good dirt or watch a candidate go down in flames after a "Howard Dean moment." Or perhaps we will get to enjoy yet another tear-filled "apology" that we will then be told how to interpret, (sincere or insincere?), by our media pundits. Maybe we will even get to vote on the sincerity of the apology by text messaging or using our remote controls.

(As I am editing this today the entire nation is waiting with baited breath for Tiger Woods' "apology" to be televised nationally on TV. Just a single camera and no questions from reporters are the rules. I sure hope Tiger has some highly paid writers and coaches to help him look genuinely remorseful. A lot of money is riding on this).

Some presidential "candidates" dropped out as soon as they realized they had no chance of raising the $100 million or more needed for the nomination campaign. Why so much money before you can even start thinking about being a serious candidate? Advertising is expensive! The media and advertising have spun totally out of control and biopsychiatry has come along for the ride.

There really is no choice. Join the crowd or toil away in obscurity. You have no idea how many excellent books, papers, lectures and elegantly detailed arguments against the domination of medical model psychiatry ALREADY EXIST and have gotten less than one hundredth of the attention of a single television commercial for Cymbalta (and not a snowball's chance in hell of "winning the minds and hearts of the people"). That is why it doesn't matter if your doctor reads the Cymbalta package insert or not. The carefully crafted "truth" is already out there. Cymbalta relieves the pain associated with depression. That is the image Cymbalta wanted and that is the image they got. The game is over. It was over before your doctor wrote his first Cymbalta prescription.

Let's examine what has happened in the psychiatric field and the pharmaceutical industry in the past 20 years to bring this about, because achieving this level of discourse control and the establishment of such a powerful "regime of truth" is no easy task. There are a lot of steps involved and some key figures need to join the "right" side early on. (I will not possibly be able to cover all the critical events that have lead to the current biopsychiatry regime of truth in psychiatry but I will list some interesting books on the subject in the back). Right now, let's look at a key figure in medical psychiatry and examine how he came over to the "dark side." It's time to revisit the father of medical model psychiatric diagnosis, Robert Spitzer.

As you recall I have characterized the framers of the DSM model of diagnosis as good intentioned (see title of chapter three). We have gone over a statement of those intentions as included in the introduction to DSM IV where, to remind you, it says on page xxiii: "The specific diagnostic criteria included in DSM IV are meant to serve as guidelines to be informed by clinical judgment and are not meant to be used in a cookbook fashion." Okay, fade out sentence from DSM IV and fade into a large ballroom of an obviously lush resort hotel. The year is 1993. The room is lined with neat rows of cloth covered tables facing a stage with large screens at the front of the room. Gentle music plays in the background. At each seat are water pitchers, glasses, pens, bowls of hard candy and a largish shiny blue box with lettering on the side. Pan in for a close up: The lettering reads ***PRIME MD*** brought to you by Pfizer Pharmaceuticals, makers of Zoloft. In the distance we hear a murmur and clinking of glass that sounds like a lot of people eating in another room. They are; an elegant breakfast buffet starts the day. A chime sounds. The eaters start filtering in, coffee cups in hand. The seats fill up. Soon there are over 350 people in their seats, men and women, dressed casually, many looking like they are dressed to play golf. The lights go down. The show begins; its time to find out what is in those shiny blue boxes...

I'm not making this scene up. I'm running it over in my memory. Because along with Dr. Spitzer I was a speaker at that meeting, in fact I was the only other speaker aside from the special guest who would "entertain" during lunch, Cyril Wecht, MD the pathologist famous for refuting the single bullet theory in the JFK assassination. After lunch...golf. That is how we used to do it; free trips to resorts, speakers, activities, entertainment, all in all a very nice perk, and a welcome break from the demands of medical practice...but no more. (See below). Right now though we need to peek inside the blue box and see what all the fuss is about.

The box was labeled PRIME MD. Inside the blue box were multiple copies of two items. First there was a tablet of one page tear-off 26-item yes/no questionnaires, the PQ or Patient Questionnaire. Then there were multiple copies of the CEG or Clinician Evaluation Guide, an algorithmic guide to allow the clinician to firm up any mental disorder diagnoses suggested by the answers on the PQ. You know what I'm talking about...if "yes" skip to item 3, if "no" go to next question, that sort of thing. I was glad to find that I happen to have a copy of a video tape promotion for Prime MD made in 1995 because I want to share it with you.

The tape is obviously professionally produced with both a narrator, two "case examples" and guest appearances by Robert Spitzer himself and his wife and co-worker Janet Williams DSW. The tape starts with a brief narrator introduction defining the problem that PRIME MD was designed to address, which is how the vast number of people with psychiatric disorders "present first to their primary care physician." Then Robert Spitzer himself appears. He says: "PRIME MD will make it easier to make early, accurate diagnoses of depression and other mental disorders in an area that has been largely neglected, the primary care setting." His wife, Janet Williams adds (I suppose to allay the concerns of already overburdened PCP's) that after about five patients' worth of experience "the average time to administer is about 10 minutes." A mere ten minutes to make a diagnosis that could change someone's life forever. Not bad huh? Let's look at one of their case examples.

She is a forty six year-old woman whose divorce became final six months ago. She has been forced to take a low level job due to financial pressures. She is raising two teenage boys on her own and they are still struggling with the impact of the divorce. Her chief complaint to the doctor is "fatigue." Since that is way too non-specific; let's get out the PRIME MD and see what is *really* wrong with this lady's brain. She fills out her PQ and then the doctor comes in with his CEG in hand to assist him in finding which mental disorder(s) this middle aged divorcee is suffering from. He goes through the depression "module" which is basically the diagnostic criteria from DSM put into question form: "For most days over the past two weeks have you...?" Occasionally the patient tries to expand or qualify her answer; sometimes she tries to talk about the divorce (especially when asked about the depression symptom of guilt) but the doctor cuts her off to get back to the yes/no questions he is instructed to ask. Not surprisingly she turns out to "suffer" from major depression but "not dysthymia" because she has not "felt down" for two years. For some strange reason the onset of her depressive feelings just happened to coincide with her divorce. (Remember readers, it was Dr. Klein in 1980 who was talking about "reactive" depression, something he would not treat with medication. In our more modern and up to date psychiatric thinking we put the divorce down on Axis IV as a stressor labeled: "Interpersonal Problem"). Okay, we are clear that our patient has "clinical depression" caused by a chemical imbalance, a problem that will resolve once she is put on the right medication. Did she answer yes to any other screening questions? As a matter of fact she did.

Our patient checked off yes in response to a question about anxiety. Our diligent doctor turns to the anxiety module. In the course of answering more stilted questions about anxiety symptoms the patient actually appears to get a little annoyed. She says: "Maybe I'm missing the point here somewhere; I came here because I'm tired all the time." Her annoyance seems to annoy the doctor who gives her a brief lecture about how underlying psychiatric disorders *cause* symptoms like tiredness (in other words, back to the biopsychiatric model) and then gets back on task. He rules out an anxiety disorder and then goes on to the alcoholism module because our patient answered yes to the following yes/no question: "Have you ever thought you should cut down on your drinking?" The doctor probes further and she reports: "I'm embarrassed to admit this. A couple of times I've been out with some of my friends and I drank too much and I drove myself home and almost had an accident. I have teenagers; I'm not setting a very good example am I?" After stiffly responding "Yeah, I understand", the doctor got her back on task, asking four more questions about alcoholism that she responded to with four no answers. End of exam. No more modules to go through. So the doctor invites the patient to sit down in his office and go over the various treatment options (medications) available.

Back to the narrator who summarizes the findings. We get major depression of course (not a word about the divorce) and then a little surprise tack-on diagnosis. The narrator says "Because the patient answered yes to one of the questions on the alcohol module this indicates a diagnosis of probable alcohol abuse or dependence." I know, I know…man!! The speculation that she may be an alcoholic is now in a doctor's official medical record. This might come in real handy for the ex-husband if he decides to sue for custody. (Once again, as Borat would say…Niiice!) I feel I must remind you again. I am not making this stuff up. I am not distorting or exaggerating. I took the quotes directly from the videotape, verbatim. Now we need to examine the significance of PRIME MD in terms of the big picture.

PRIME MD was not a huge hit in and of itself. I remember that when I was touring with this Pfizer lecture series how odd it was that when the doctors left the ballroom to go have lunch and then play golf, a lot of them left the PRIME MD kits behind. I don't have any statistics but I assume that few PCP's really use PRIME MD. It is kind of stiff and formal. I think another problem is that, despite Janet William's enthusiastic endorsement of it taking a mere ten minutes to administer PRIME MD, ten minutes is *way too long* for a PCP to spend on a psychiatric screening exam. Ten minutes is what the clearly overburdened PCP's allot for the entire head to toe office visits of their regular patients; that's all the time they've got. So I don't ever hear about PRIME MD anymore, a complex and expensive project funded by an "unrestricted grant" from Pfizer (more about unrestricted grants and other sources of financial support by drug companies later). Well you win some and lose some. Don't worry; I think Zoloft did pretty well anyhow. As have all of the other antidepressants once things like PRIME MD opened the floodgates to rapid, simple and uncomplicated psychiatric diagnosis and treatment plans that could be done by anyone. Highly trained psychiatrists no longer needed. Even a PCP's physician assistant or nurse could handle this with ease.

I like and respect Robert Spitzer. But he just had to be aware that the vocational dignity and necessity of clinical wisdom that he and his followers argued for in demanding that DSM not be used like a cookbook would be utterly invalidated by things like this questionnaire. Who needs clinical wisdom and experience? PRIME MD said to the world loud and clear: "Psychiatric diagnosis and the recognition of biologically based mental disorders is a snap, as easy as pie." Now the drug companies had it all; the products, the money to push them and the official endorsement of the chief honchos in psychiatry. The few voices of protest (e.g. David Kaiser MD, David Healy MD, Peter Breggins MD, the AAPP, the ICSPP and the rest) would have their voices DROWNED by the tsunami of carefully coordinated promotions of the biopsychiatric perspective in medical journals, the popular press, print ads, news releases, television commercials and talk shows. Discourse control, remember? This multilevel coordinated onslaught is so impressive that it rivals, gee I don't know, Disney?

PRIME MD might be gone now but questionnaires still abound in the business of psychiatry. They are online, they are in magazines, and they are in doctor's waiting rooms in the brochures placed there by drug reps; they are simple and easy to take. Some of the new questionnaires make PRIME MD look like an S.A.T. by comparison. Here is one of my all-time favorites. I used to see it every week because it was attached to the front cover of the magazine

Entertainment Weekly that mysteriously started to appear in my mail at the office. (I'm grateful; I like the magazine). The questionnaire was attached to a six page glossy color brochure that enclosed the magazine (I actually threw out a couple of copies of the magazine before I realized that the ad wasn't a cover for one of the many pseudo-journals I get every week). The predominant color of the brochure was blue with bold yellow lettering. A drawing of a sad looking but very attractive woman was accompanied by the question "are you taking antidepressants and still **FEEL** depressed? Below the picture: "If so, you may have a different medical condition. **Find out more inside.** Turning the page we are asked:

> Did you know...In a study of patients with depression, nearly **1** in **5** people who had been on more than one medicine for depression and still experienced symptoms screened positive for a different medical condition that included depression as a main symptom. You may be experiencing the same thing.
> For more information visit www.sayhowyoufeel.com.

Ever wonder what the really bright college graduates are doing for a living nowadays? I think some of them are paid big bucks to make up clever names for websites. What do you think? Anyhow, you don't need to go to the website because the question of what mysterious medical condition you have is answered right on the same page. Set off by a black border and on a white background is the following:

> **say something**
> to your healthcare provider
>
> If you've been on more than one antidepressant and still feel depressed, it's possible you may have a different medical condition called **bipolar depression.** Talk to your healthcare provider about how you feel. The following questions may help you start a conversation with your healthcare provider about symptoms you may be experiencing. He or she will have additional questions about your symptoms and medical history to make an accurate diagnosis.
>
> Have you ever been told by your
> healthcare provider that you have anxiety?
> __Yes __No

Do you sometimes feel that people
are acting unfriendly towards you?
__Yes __No

Have you been diagnosed with
depression within the past 5 years?
__Yes __No

Has anyone in your family ever been diagnosed
with manic depression (bipolar disorder)?
__Yes __No

Have you ever had any legal
problems (minor or major)?
__Yes __No

Talk to your healthcare provider and explain that you still feel depressed. Be sure to ask if you could have **bipolar depression.** He or she may reconsider your treatment options.

Note to Healthcare Provider:

These questions are not designed to be a stand-alone diagnostic tool.

They are intended to serve as one of several factors you consider in assessing your patient's condition.

This is an honest-to-God verbatim copy of this ad put out by Glaxo SmithKline, another one of the pharmaceutical giants, to advertise their bipolar product Lamictal although no medication is mentioned in the ad. I have to tell you that this ad and quiz took even my cynical breath away, it is so embarrassingly bad. Its obvious goal is amazing (and amazingly successful): **GET THE PATIENT TO MARKET TO THE DOCTOR! INCREDIBLE!!** You can't imagine how much this hurts. The profession that gave us Sigmund Freud, Carl Jung, Alfred Adler, Adolph Meyer, Karl Jaspers, Victor Frankl, Freida Fromm-Reichman, Ludwig Binswanger, Medard Boss, Harry Stack Sullivan, Elizabeth Kubler-Ross, Martin Buber, Hilda Bruch, Abraham Maslow, Jim Phillips, David Healy, John Sadler and so many more brilliant deep thinkers is now represented to the public by this blatant hucksterism? Aside from the one on genetics, the questions on the quiz don't even make any sense!! Thinking people are "acting unfriendly" towards you as a symptom suggesting bipolar disorder? Huh? Who made up this quiz? What psychiatrist passed on this and approved its publication? I will give you the word that accurately describes this kind of garbage: Propaganda. I get really angry about all of this sometimes. I worked so hard for my membership card to a profession that I am now often embarrassed and humiliated to be associated with.

"Suddenly, a voice from the audience cries out: HYPOCRITE!! How much money did you make lecturing for drug companies?" I cannot tell a lie. I made a lot of money. So let's talk about my days as a drug company hired "educator." It all started in Camp Iroquois when I was a young boy. I found out in camp that, unlike most people, I was not intimidated by speaking, telling jokes, even singing in front of an audience. I guess I just had a talent for an easygoing and confident manner in public speaking. Being in the right place (working at a prestigious psychiatric hospital near New York) at the right time (the mid 1980's) got me noticed. All of a sudden I am on one TV show after another and then, without any additional letters after my name or the words Harvard, Princeton or Yale in my resume, I'm touring with Robert Spitzer. Ah, but things were really different back then. Tucked away in some boxes in the back of my current office are thousands of 35mm slides I collected over the years to use in my lectures. I traveled all over the country and stayed at posh resorts and got paid well to do it. It was a terrific escape from the grind (and shrinking remuneration) from my office practice. So I would get a topic (always from a drug company although I limited my speaking engagements to drugs that I could honestly say I saw really help some of my patients) and I would get busy on my slide sorter putting together an entertaining and informative sixty minute lecture. There was zero control exercised by the drug company on the content of my talk. Of course it was understood that somewhere along the way I would mention their product in a positive way. But it wasn't hard sell. I spent the majority of my time in lectures in those days talking about diagnostic issues and the uncertainty of diagnosis. I even talked about alternative treatments and no one hassled me. But then that turn started...the infamous "last twenty years" I've previously mentioned. Following the government's successful investigations into overcharging and overutilization at psychiatric hospitals (an investigation of the NME run PIA hospitals was "settled" for a consent agreement of $750 million), attention, for reasons I'm not sure of, turned to how pharmaceutical companies market their products to doctors. Before I go on here I have to share a fact I just learned with you that I found utterly astounding.

THERE IS ONLY ONE COUNTRY IN THE WORLD THAT ALLOWS TELEVISION ADVERTISING FOR PRESCRIPTION MEDICATIONS: THE UNITED STATES.

I have gotten so used to TV ads for drugs that I just assumed this was some sort of international phenomenon. The reason I mention it here is because this liberal attitude about hawking drugs directly to the public stands in such marked contrast to the continually evolving tighter and tighter regulations about doctors "selling" drugs to doctors. There were some major scandals of course, usually involving marketing plans to sell drugs to doctors for indications other than those approved by the FDA. But some of the tightening up seemed just kind of mean spirited. For example, spouses were no longer allowed to attend dinner meetings with their wife or husband physician. That was too bad because in my lectures the spouses usually paid more attention and had the more interesting questions. Any gifts given to physicians by drug companies came under tight scrutiny. Soon all paid for activities such as golf or tickets to shows were gone. It started to get a lot tougher to get doctors to meetings. But for the speakers, the real bummer lay ahead.

All of the speakers were at first free to use whatever slides they wanted to give a lecture on the general topic they were selected for. For example, for the sleeping pill Ambien, most of us did a comprehensive lecture on insomnia, mentioning Ambien at the end as an effective treatment option. But the education for our fellow physicians was about insomnia, not a sales talk for Ambien. Many of the sleep disorder specialists who spoke for Ambien spent a good deal of time in their lectures on sleep apnea, a topic they believed their audience needed to learn more about. (In fact, sleep apnea is not really a traditional insomnia condition or target market for Ambien). We were also free to mention competing drugs and their effectiveness as well. They gave us a set of 35mm slides created by their company but their use was not mandatory. I would usually pick a couple of slides the drug company gave me to mix in with my slides, many of which I made myself. I could even use slides from rival companies if I wanted. Most of us had two or three New Yorker type cartoon slides mixed in as well. It was fun putting together these lectures. Now skip ahead to 2007. Although radically reduced in number (to free up money for TV and print ads?) doctor dinner lectures are still going on. The content of the lecture, however, is strictly controlled by the drug company. We receive slides as downloads on our computer. The slide sets are created by the drug company and microscopically scrutinized by their legal department to make sure nothing on the slide deviates from the officially approved package insert. At first we were sent slides on PowerPoint and could change the order and maybe delete a few excessively boring ones from the lecture. We could even "import" a few of our own slides but that was frowned upon. Next the slides started to come as "read only" files for PowerPoint which meant no deleting or changing the order and no importing of other slides. Although I never learned how, some speakers tell me there is a way around the "read only" restrictions that allows adjustments to the presentation. The current "slide decks" I receive, however, are in a pdf format to guard against any manipulation. I haven't discussed this with any fellow lecturers because most companies no longer have in-person speaker training sessions. The training is on-line now and boring beyond belief. I no longer do any lectures for drug companies.

I need to briefly touch on the incredible paradox at the core of this massive overhaul of how doctors are being marketed to by drug companies. As the companies officially present it, these new guidelines were voluntarily imposed by the conglomeration of pharmaceutical companies called Big Pharma. This was in response, in part, to the heightened government scrutiny of marketing to doctors but also, ostensibly, to insure that the doctors receiving the lectures would get a "fair and balanced" (uh-oh, scary words) presentation. The paradox is that experienced clinicians like me, employed to give the lectures, were now limited in what we were allowed to say by the scripted set of slides the company compels us to use. So now, rather than a doctor to doctor lecture sharing clinical experience and an introduction to a new medication, the doctors in attendance are getting a pre-packaged sales pitch with the only mention of competitors products or alternative treatment options being tightly controlled by the company's own slide kit. Fair and balanced???

One last memory. Back when we used to have in person speaker trainings a new specialist started showing up on the speaker program, the company attorney. He or she would make sure that we understood in no uncertain terms that if we ad-libbed at the lecture and presented any claims about the medication other than those approved in the package insert, that we, the lecturers, faced the possibility of both civil and CRIMINAL prosecution. And yet the print and TV ads…I just can't figure it out. All I know is that if the government would crack down on prejudicial and manipulative perk filled marketing practices in other industries, we could kiss our luxury hotels, fancy restaurants, convention centers and basketball arenas goodbye. (Maybe a lot of strip clubs and golf courses too). Isn't "manipulative" marketing how we do business in this country? It's called sales. But don't despair; this intense scrutiny of how drug companies market to physicians does not seem to be affecting the rules of how drug companies market to the public. One of the most interesting outgrowths of this is how doctors now get marketed to, no longer as doctors with technical and scientific expertise, but as if we too are part of the consuming public.

I have sitting in front of me the current copy of Psychiatric Times, a glossy newspaper distributed to about 50,000 psychiatrists monthly. It's a good publication that even offers a forum for some dissent (Dr. David Kaiser and I have both published articles in the Psychiatric Times) as well as the usual biopsychiatry biased articles. I just counted; forty-five of its total of seventy-one pages is either a full page drug ad or one with an ad or ads that dominate the page. It reminds me of Cosmo or Elle magazine, which appear to me to be almost all advertisements. It also reminds me of ads in those magazines in another way; nearly all of the ads in Cosmo, Elle and Psychiatric Times feature physically attractive people. I don't think the drug companies create separate ads for doctors except for the ones showing graphs and research results but why the beautiful people? They certainly don't resemble most of the people I see in my practice. A healthy percentage of my patients are morbidly obese. It makes you wonder how the drug companies view their physician customers. Apparently pretty generically, susceptible to the same sublimated sexual messages that are used to sell everything from Victoria Secret underwear to automobiles. Of course it doesn't have to be subliminal sexual messages to get our attention. In my eyes Eli Lilly chose a completely different theme to launch their ad campaign for their combo drug Symbyax. The theme they chose was fundamentalist Christianity.

When I got my very first ad for Symbyax I literally chuckled to myself because the symbolism was so subtle…NOT! A man is stranded on a cliff face, at risk for falling down into the abyss. With an expression of desperation on his face he lifts one arm skyward to the waiting hand of a figure atop the cliff. The rescuer wears a long white coat, is young and handsome and, for some strange reason, is holding an old-fashioned lantern emitting a brilliant light. There is something very odd about that lantern. Its light does not diffuse in all directions but instead forms a kind of coherent cone of light illuminating the man on the cliff. (I can't say for certain, not being an art historian, but isn't that kind of an iconic Christian symbol associated with Saints?) Anyhow, behind our (pardon the expression) Christ-like rescuer/doctor lies a blue sky with puffy clouds, green grass and lush trees. Could it perhaps be paradise? I've received and seen dozen of Symbyax ads from Lilly and although none quite matched the undisguised Christian symbolism of that first one, the lantern, and the Christ-like figure (in some ads a female) leading the patient from the darkness into the light is the theme of every ad. May I say:

WHEN IS THIS GOING TO STOP?
WHY IS THIS GOING ON?
WHERE IS THE RESPECT FOR THE PROFESSION OF MEDICINE?
IS IT REALLY ALL JUST DISNEYLAND?
……is it?

I see these ads as totally disrespectful but I have to believe that their market research supports it. Speaking of print ads I want to discuss one that is so ubiquitous that I'm sure most readers have seen it, the print ad for Abilify.

Obviously each drug company has their own marketing plan and a lavish but still limited budget. The company that makes Abilify has surprisingly decided to spend a good portion of their advertising budget on print ads in national and local publications. (Update: September 2007: I have just received in the mail a preview copy of Abilify's planned television commercial, so get ready). I have seen the same ad in Newsweek, Time, USA Today and as a full page color ad in my local newspaper. It is clear that they are trolling for bipolar business because schizophrenia (the initial indication for Abilify) is not mentioned in the ad. But why direct to consumer advertising for a drug for something as serious as bipolar disorder? At the time of this writing Abilify only has an indication for Bipolar I disorder and, as previously discussed, there might be at most 3 million Bipolar I patients in the US. Since it is such a serious illness, most are probably already under a doctor's care. So why are they taking out frequent very expensive ads in national publications?...Hmmm. Do they by any chance have in mind what that bipolar quiz we discussed above came out and said directly? Do they want the members of the general public to tell their doctors they are bipolar and perhaps ask to try Abilify?? Well duh... Perhaps to expand the market?? Well, double duh. So how do they communicate this message in a delicate fashion because it's not that far a stretch from the label bipolar to the label nuts!! Let's look at the ad.

The ad has the Andrew Wyeth-like picture of a young slender woman with her back turned to us gazing out over a field of grass and wildflowers. Why that particular image? I don't know but in me it invokes two feelings simultaneously, one of serenity but also one of searching, feeling lost and alone. So my question is did the ad designers want us to see this young woman as a treated and cured bipolar or someone with mood swings looking for answers? I really can't tell. But I can tell you one thing for sure. She doesn't look at all like many acutely manic bipolar I patients I've seen who are being strapped down with restraints by beefy security guards while screaming obscenities at the hospital staff. Now here is what the print ad says: Top line in large print: **TREATING BIPOLAR DISORDER TAKES UNDERSTANDING: You've been up and down with mood swings. You may want to move forward. Maybe ABILIFY can help.**

Can you pick out the key words here? Of course you can if you remember what you read in chapter five. The key words, the "marketing" words, are **mood swings.** That is what the consumer will see and remember because the rest of the ad doesn't make much sense as a marketing strategy in Newsweek, Time and my local newspaper. It says that Abilify can help

- Control your symptoms of bipolar mania
- Stabilize your mood
- Reduce your risk of manic relapse

Then the ad says that "ABILIFY is used to treat manic or mixed episodes in adults with Bipolar I disorder and maintain efficacy in patients whose symptoms have been controlled on ABILIFY for 6 weeks." This is, of course, merely a restating of the FDA approval for Abilify and Bipolar I disorder. But...do you see how this is an example of hiding in plain sight? Most doctors outside of psychiatry would not know what the diagnostic label Bipolar I disorder is particularly referring to (versus Bipolar II, Cyclothymia and Bipolar NOS), let alone the average Newsweek reader. This is technical stuff inside the field of psychiatry. Just "hide it" in plain sight. So it is not that the ad particularly distorts the truth although the use of the term mood swings is clearly manipulative (psst. They are looking for Dr. Lieber's bipolar spectrum patients here); it is the fact that this ad is run in major publications all over the country nearly every week that is the real focus of concern. We should all *be very afraid* of the existence of a cultural atmosphere that makes it worth the money to purchase these ads soliciting bipolar disorder "customers" in popular magazines. Recall the quote in the introduction to this book by the NY Times columnist Judith Warner:

> Rebecca Riley was not killed by biological psychiatry or Astra Zeneca or the Massachusetts Department of Social Services or parents like you or me who may or may not be medicating our children but are, indisputably, part of a culture in which doing so is the norm.

This is a deep insight into the real problem. But it also points to a possible solution (one which I have, by the way, been leading up to since page one). In simple terms: IF THE CULTURE WON'T CHANGE THEN THE ONLY WAY TO COPE IS TO RISE ABOVE THE CULTURE AND FIND A WAY TO CHANGE <u>YOU</u>! (This is what I advised at the end of chapter five; rising above the "herd" when it really counts). Of course the very first step in this is to come to both see and *believe* that you are completely immersed in and encompassed by your culture. You are part of the herd, the anonymous "they-self" that believes without question, for example, that science is truth and psychiatrists are scientists. Only when you CLEARLY SEE will you have a chance to transcend your immersion in the everyday world and be able to think and decide about crucial issues like you and your family's mental wellbeing for yourself. I want you to understand there is GREAT HOPE here. But you've got to believe. That is why I have been spending these first eight chapters deconstructing biopsychiatry. It isn't easy to swim against the tide or resist the pull of advertising driven popular culture. But like it was for the Tinman, the REAL problem was not his rusted joints; no, the REAL problem was a culture whose norms and beliefs empowered the Evil Witch of the East in the first place. So have HOPE. We are almost there and you are almost ready for some genuine personal empowerment. Just remember that knowledge is a big part of power so I want to ask for your patience and indulgence while I catalogue a few more dirty tricks of the trade by drug companies and their pals in psychiatric "research". To do this I will follow the outline of the problems as spelled out by Dr. Angell in her book *The Truth About Drug Companies*. Please be prepared for a little more shock and awe (or at least shock).

We will start with the "me-too" drug phenomenon since so many psychiatric drugs are of the "me-too" variety. In fact, Dr. Angell points out that between 1998 and 2002 77% of newly patented drugs were me-too's, defined as non-innovative drugs no better (or even worse) than those already on the market (Angell 2005, p. 75). Remember we discussed how no antidepressant has yet been developed that is superior to imipramine, released in 1957! So that powerful class of currently popular drugs, the SSRI's (patent names Prozac, Paxil, Zoloft, Celexa, Lexapro, and Luvox) are much more alike than different in hypothesized mechanism of action and efficacy. Effexor, Cymbalta and Prestiq as well as Serzone and Remeron are slight variations on the theme. Only Wellbutrin with its clearly different mechanism of action and very different side effect profile seems genuinely innovative and unique. So how does the FDA allow so much time, energy and money be devoted to me-too drugs? (By the way this occurs in many classes of drugs such as the highly profitable cholesterol lowering statins: Lipitor, Crestor, Zocor and the like). Dr. Angell points out a loophole in FDA regulations that allows new drugs to be patented and approved for a particular indication if they demonstrate statistically superior efficacy to placebo. In other words a new drug does not need to work better *or even as good* as an older drug; it only needs to work better than a sugar pill. This little "loophole" is especially beneficial for psychiatric medications whose only proof of efficacy is based on answers to standardized questionnaires.

Let's say you have a compound you want to test as an antidepressant. The FDA requirement is for two studies to show statistical superiority to treatment with a sugar pill. What numbers create the basis for the statistics? Nothing measured in a lab or counted on a microscope (like you might use in testing a new drug for leukemia). No, it is numbers created by the previously described questionnaires like the HAM-D. So arbitrariness and a lot of wiggle room are intrinsically built into the system from the beginning. Now add on top of this the FDA rule that you are only required to produce two positive tests. Tests in which the drug does not outperform the placebo (or does worse) are not counted. And there can be as many negative tests as you want. Amazing huh?

Let me describe a graph they use in some ads for Lexapro in the treatment of depression. (I am not picking on Lexapro. Remember the cardinal rule of the disappointing class of drugs we call antidepressants...all of them have equal "efficacy"). It is a line graph where the vertical height represents severity of depression and the horizontal axis is time. All subjects' lines start at the top and slope down over time as the subjects' HAM-D scores improve. The "improvement" line for Lexapro barely differs from the line tracing the improvement from placebo for the same eight week period. At certain points along the Lexapro line little asterisks appear. These are the points at which Lexapro demonstrates statistical superiority. But let me tell you, it aint much! I show this to my patients who are all gung-ho to get on a happy pill and they are shocked because to the untrained, common sense eye it looks like almost no difference at all. (Thank goodness our mathematicians are here to correct our common sense "errors"). What is particularly striking is how the down-slope of the placebo line so closely parallels the Lexapro line. Once again common sense would tend to argue that if an active drug is truly effectively "treating" a pathological cellular or biochemical abnormality, then at some point in time the placebo line should just level off (how many weeks can you be fooled?) while the drug line would continue to plummet and a visibly apparent large separation of the lines would occur. But it doesn't. This has caused some critics to reasonably ask whether in these very typical depression studies there is any drug effect at all. On the HAM-D there is a total possible "score" of around sixty points. As mentioned before, "statistical significance" (oh those scary, scary words) can be achieved by a difference of only two points between drug and placebo. And since the active drug, likely to have some clearly felt side effects, can often be distinguished by both the subject and the researcher there is plenty of room for "error" on both sides of the typical allegedly double blind study (Greenberg and Fisher 1997). Why might a study subject be inclined to positively bias the results? Hope, among other things. Many believe that the high placebo response rate seen in psychiatric studies is related to a very obvious variable that is not biological and is not related to medicine. Depressed and anxious people improve in these studies because they get attention, validation and caring (Fournier 2010). Someone gives a damn about how they are doing emotionally and, study or no study, that makes people feel better.

Next topic: Why would the *researcher* be inclined to bias the results? Well it could be because of a word starting with m and ending in y that seems to have a lot of influence and power. I told you that I've gotten paid a pretty good fee for my drug company lectures but it is like chump change in comparison to what you can get for doing drug company sponsored research. So the next major issue to address is whether pharmaceutical companies can influence "independent" research on their products. A similar question is: "Does a bear poop in the woods?"

In chapter two of her book *The Truth About Drug Companies* Dr. Angell describes the steps a drug company needs to take to get FDA approval to market and sell a new drug. Once some basic lab and animal research is done the drugs obviously have to be tested on humans. The human trials are done in three phases. As Dr. Angell points out, these three phases are usually done only AFTER the drug company has patented the drug so the profit clock is already running on the 20 year patent exclusivity the drug company gets. They therefore would like the phase one to three drug trials to go smoothly and be done efficiently. Since these trials can ultimately involve testing on thousands of people the drug company has to farm out the work to doctors at universities and, increasingly, to doctors and clinics devoted exclusively to clinical trials. Is a bell ringing? Have you heard or seen all the advertising on radio and in print asking if you are depressed, anxious…diabetic…impotent…dying from cancer…please call…free exam…free trial medications. "So that's what that business is." They are testing drugs for drug companies. YES! But why all the advertising? Can't doctors just test their own patients or patients at a clinic or something? I have to confess here that I do not have direct first person experience in the drug trial business. When I looked into it I was totally put off by the tedious record keeping required and by the need to SUPPLY THE PATIENTS. I take it back; I did participate in one kind of drug trial for schizophrenia but it was a phase four (post approval) trial, something we will discuss shortly. Anyhow, I haven't done big time drug trials but I've met some people that do. There is some major money in doing drug trials but there are major pressures also, the greatest of which is getting subjects. Ah, but here is where psychiatry is so special…it just might be a little "easier" to find people with let's say depression or adult ADD or even bipolar disorder than it is to find study subjects with real diseases diagnosed on the basis of lab tests and physical findings.

In her book Dr. Angell tells us:

> At one time, most trials were done at medical schools and teaching hospitals. Companies would give grants to faculty researchers to carry out clinical trials under institutional auspices. That is no longer the case. Because there are so many more trials

> nowadays, and because drug companies are so eager to get them done quickly they have shifted much of their business to new, for profit companies set up exclusively to organize and carry out trials for drug companies. These are called contract research organizations (CRO's). In 2001, there were about a thousand of them operating around the world, with revenues from their drug company clients of some $7 billion. They establish networks of physicians who, working under the organizations' supervision, are paid to administer the study drugs and collect information on their effects (Angell 2004, p.29).

So there really IS a lot of money floating around out there which means a lot of INCENTIVES to deliver the drug companies what they want. And, as always, it means there is a lot of competition for those dollars. In fact, Dr Angell reports that in 2001 there was an estimated 80,000 clinical trials going on in the USA. She mentions that the government (the National Institutes of Health or NIH) spends about as much as the drug companies on research but it is generally not about specific marketable commodities; it is what is called basic research. The biggest problem faced by the drug companies in running drug trials, Dr. Angell tells us, is "the scarcity of human subjects." Sometimes, maybe often, subjects are actually paid to participate in a research study, however "Whatever they are paid, it is dwarfed by payments to doctors." Here are the figures Dr. Angell dug up, and some consequences that might attach to such an incentive plan:

> To get human subjects, drug companies or contract research organizations routinely offer doctors large bounties (averaging about $7000 per patient in 2001) and sometimes bonuses for rapid enrollment. For example, according to a 2000 Department of Health and Human Services inspector general's report, physicians in one trial were paid $12,000 for each patient enrolled, plus another $30,000 on the enrollment of a sixth patient. One risk of this bounty and bonus system is that it can induce doctors to enroll patients who are not really eligible (Angell 2004, p.31).

From the point of view of the drug companies or CRO's running these studies, I can only imagine they want some bang for their buck. So if you are doing, oh let's say, a "study" on the effectiveness of ADD treatment in adults whose initial presentation is depression, (gee, where did I come up with that? And..gee...I wonder how many "depressed" adults might feel more energetic and focused with a daily dose of legal amphetamines?), I'm sure that among the physicians competing for these generous paychecks, the ones who can most rapidly deliver the largest number of study subjects might well be a "preferred" doctor by the drug companies and CRO's. Might there be some incentive to therefore perhaps loosen even further the already subjective diagnostic criteria employed by psychiatry? To answer this I will turn to a question I recently asked: Does a bear poop in the woods? Beyond that how do you think a drug company or CRO views a research group or physician if they return a lot of negative outcomes versus those who return the positive outcome results the drug company needs to get their drug approved? Is it possible that the doctor can influence the outcome of double blinded placebo controlled drug trials? Please, I don't want to mention the bear again. We previously discussed how both the patient and clinician are often able to judge from the side effects whether they are receiving active drug or placebo. Now listen to what Greenberg and Fisher (1997) tell us they found in reviewing numerous antidepressant drug trials:

> The source of outcome ratings is another possible distorting factor in determining the size of an antidepressant effect. In a meta-analysis of antidepressant studies that were presumably blinder because of greater design complexity, we found small but significant antidepressant effects when outcome was determined by clinician ratings but no advantage for antidepressants beyond the placebo effect when patients rated their own outcomes (Fisher 1997, p.137).

For some reason that quote from Dr. Rush, chief investigator in the STAR*D study, that I gave in chapter six comes to mind, the one about how you cannot trust patient reports because they cannot "be precise." Could it also be that study subjects don't tell you what you want to hear?

Dr. Angell also discusses the phase four study issue. These are studies done after the drug has already been approved and is being widely used. Phase four studies are done for a number of reasons. Sometimes it is to search for the incidence of known side effects and the emergence of new side effects once the use of a drug is expanded from thousands of people (pre-approval), to millions (post-approval). This is generally a good thing. Phase four studies (which are not as stringently controlled as phases one to three) can also be used to search for new "indications" for existing drugs. You had better believe that this is a big, big deal in psychiatric medications and their ever-expanding lists of "disorders" they treat. (See, for example the Prozac/Serafem maneuver discussed below). Finally, Dr. Angell tells us "And a great many—perhaps most—are really, in the view of many critics, just excuses to pay doctors to put patients on a company's already-approved drug." I know this is true because I have been solicited for precisely these types of "studies" although I never participated in one.

Enough dirty little tricks? Sorry...there are more you need to know about. One of particular interest in psychiatry is called patent extension which is increasing the number of years that the drug company holds exclusive rights to profit from a drug. Patent extending has been a great source of anguish to me in my personal practice. I like drug reps and I've enjoyed speaking for drug companies, but when they start pulling the patent extending tricks... it starts to turn my stomach. As an illustration of patent extending tricks I want to turn away temporarily from psychiatric drugs to tell you the purple pill story. Dr. Angell uses the example of the Prilosec to Nexium switcheroo in her book but I found a detailed accounting I want to share with you in a New Yorker article, October 25, 2004 called *High Prices* written by Malcolm Gladwell. First a little background. I'm sure everyone remembers the purple pill commercials for Prilosec. They saturated the airways for a long time, helping to launch the class of stomach acid treatment medications called proton pump inhibitors to the front of the line for the treatment of heartburn. Prilosec itself dominated the market, its closest proton pump rival being Prevacid. If you need any further proof of the power of saturation advertising or an answer to the question of why political candidates need so much money for TV ads then you need look no further than Prilosec. Doctors and patients alike totally embraced the purple pill and it earned its maker, AstraZeneca, nearly $6 billion over a five-year stretch at the height of its popularity. But then something happened; something so devastating that it almost makes me feel bad for the drug companies...almost. Prilosec's patent ran out. Malcolm Gladwell's article is about what AstraZeneca did in anticipation of such a massive loss of revenue. They formed the Shark Fin Project.

Picture the shape of a shark fin. That is what the profit graph looks like for a successful drug. The steep upslope is the drug catching on and then dominating the market. The even steeper down slope is the shape of the massive drop in profit once a successful drug goes generic. The Shark Fin Project, composed of lawyers, marketers and scientists was charged with the task of brainstorming ideas to compensate for the loss of patent by fooling with the Prilosec molecule to create another saleable drug. Here, according to Gladwell, is what they did.

> The Shark Fin Team drew up a list of fifty options. One idea was to devise a Prilosec 2.0—-a version that worked faster or longer, or was more effective. Another idea was to combine it with a different heartburn remedy, or to change the formulation so that

> it came in a liquid gel or in an extended-release form. In the end, AstraZeneca decided on a subtle piece of reengineering. Priolsec, like many drugs, is composed of two 'isomers'—- a left-hand and a right-hand version of the molecule. In some cases, removing one of the isomers can reduce side effects or make a drug work a little bit better, and in all cases the Patent Office recognizes something with one isomer as a separate invention from something with two. So AstraZeneca cut Prilosec in half
>
> (Gladwell 2004, p.29).

And thus was born Nexium. But there was still some work left to be done. The researchers at AstraZeneca cleverly seized upon a complication of heartburn, erosion of the lower end of the esophagus, and compared Nexium vs. Prilosec in healing the erosion. By a hair, Nexium prevailed so the FDA approval was granted. The rest was easy. Really, I mean that. One half billion dollars was targeted to launch Nexium and convince consumers and doctors alike that this was the right pill to be taking for heartburn. It's the *new and improved* purple pill. Of course the ads do have to deal with that cumbersome phrase "esophageal erosions", a term most consumers would not comprehend and most doctors never gave much thought to. But you know what…who gives a damn? That's like worrying about whether saying something like Bipolar One disorder in an ad would make somebody wonder why the "One" label; are there other bipolar disorders? Don't worry, it doesn't. America makes great movies. And we are way, way, way ahead of the curve when it comes to advertising. Give some pros a half-billion dollar budget and they could sell ANYTHING. It's all in the budget.

So that's the Nexium story. I don't have sales figures here but I'm certain it's worked out just fine for AstraZeneca. I am aware of one interesting little paradox that has emerged in the proton pump inhibitor wars. Its worth mentioning because it speaks to the complexity of paying for medicines and medical care. Prilosec was released as an over the counter drug, no prescription required. A thirty day supply costs about $30. It is, as you now know, basically identical to Nexium. Yet I've heard from some doctors I've queried that patients prefer a prescription for Nexium because with their insurance the out-of-pocket co-pay is only $10 on Nexium; so why pay $30 for OTC Prilosec? The retail price of a 30 day supply of Nexium?… about $120.

Okay, back to the Shark Fin pros. Among their proposed patent extending strategies were some that I've already seen employed in the psychiatric drug industry. Let me list them for you:

The Isomer Split:
Celexa split in half=Lexapro

The Metabolite Move:
Effexor Metabolite=Prestiq

Combine with another drug:
Prozac plus Zyprexa=Symbyax

Find new indication and rename and repackage drug:
Prozac to Serafem

Produce extended release version:

- **Paxil CR (controlled release)**
- **Once weekly Prozac**
- **Effexor XR (extended release)**
- **Wellbutrin SR (sustained release)**
- **Wellbutrin XL (extended release)**
- **Ambien CR (controlled release)**

Are these modifications that extend patents also improvements that will benefit patients? In my opinion, generally no. Time release drugs can be an advantage sometimes in terms of tolerability and compliance. For example, Wellbutrin XL is a one dose per day drug while regular Wellbutrin and Wellbutrin SR require two doses a day. Compliance with one pill a day is much higher than two a day. So that helped. But with other drugs like Paxil CR and Ambien CR it is, once again in my opinion, much more difficult to see an advantage in the research or clinically. But let me tell you how these patent extending sustained released drugs are marketed.

Physicians are visited regularly by drug reps. They supply us with information/sales pitches, coffee mugs, pens, clocks and free samples (or at least they used to). The free samples can be very helpful to outpatient clinicians because it allows us to provide our patients with small supplies of a medication to try before they decide whether or not to fill a full month's prescription. Free samples also allow us to sometimes supply patients with full prescriptions of medicines that they could otherwise not afford. Drug companies who are going to lose their patents on a blockbuster drug are aware of this impending deadline years in advance. So they develop, for example, the sustained release form and promote its often dubious "advantages" years in advance as well. They obviously desire both the doctor and patient to switch over to the extended patent drug well before the current drug expires. To promote this early transition they typically (in my experience) do two things. They stop giving us free samples of the expiring drug even if there is a year or more left on the patent. We only get samples of the new sustained release drug to try out on our patients. In addition (and believe me, I feel for drug reps), the reps are no longer given "credit" for sales of the expiring drug, only for the new time-released version. Since a good part of their income is directly tied to these "credits" they are under a lot of pressure to get us to prescribe the new form of the drug. Amazingly, even if we continue to prescribe or even increase our prescribing of the expiring form of the drug, which still results in profits for the drug company, the reps are apparently chastised for not getting us to switch. (If you are wondering how the drug companies and drug reps know what a doctor is prescribing, this will surprise you; it did me. There are companies out there who pay pharmacies for their records on what a particular doctor is prescribing and then sell that information to drug companies. Thus the reps know *exactly* who to target for the hard sell. I used to drive the Paxil people crazy because, for my own reasons, I didn't like Paxil and never prescribed it. They were all over me. I think the Cymbalta people also got the same message. To me, and many other doctors, the fact that drug companies can buy a record of our prescribing practices seems wrong, at some sort of deep personal constitutional rights to privacy level, but the official bodies like the AMA and APA have not risen up against this. I wonder why…Hmmm).

I promised to tell you the Prozac/Sarafem story, so here it is. This patent extension move was so outlandish, even cynical little old me could barely believe it. I'll spare you all of the technical machinations that Eli Lilly performed to make this happen and just get to the crux of the story. Prozac (brand name) is the chemical compound fluoxetine packaged in green and white capsules. Sarafem is ***exactly the same drug***, fluoxetine, only packaged in lilac capsules.

Uh…that's it?

That's the crux of the Sarafem story. The rest of the story is that this maneuver by Eli Lilly was backed by a powerful marketing campaign based on a recently acquired phase four FDA indication for PMDD (Premenstrual Dysphoric Disorder) a (scare words) "clinically significantly" emotional and behavioral reaction to menstruation. Where did Lilly find that diagnosis? In the back of DSM IV where there is an appendix "Criteria Sets and Axes Provided for Further Study". How did Lilly get FDA approval for a diagnosis that isn't even established as official by the American Psychiatric Association?

Uh.

Well, how did they get a patent extension (and further profit) just by changing the color of the capsule?

And how did they convince Ob Gyn's to go along with this and prescribe expensive brand name Sarafem when Prozac became available as a much less expensive generic?

Uh.

Hey, I'm as dumbfounded by all of this as you are. What is that global explanation that seems to justify all actions nowadays? Oh yeah, I remember: "IT'S ONLY BUSINESS." When you add in the phase four studies where existing psychiatric drugs keep trolling for new "indications" (when is DSM V coming out?) and the business side of biopsychiatry is no longer the least bit disguised or hidden. That massive advertising campaigns are incredibly effective is also an undisguised 21st Century reality. But what about other money? What about the "research" grants, the "unrestricted" grants to medical schools, universities, institutions and mental illness "support" groups? What about government lobbying and influence on legislation? And what happens when the drug company is backed up against the wall? Can they and do they play hardball? Apparently there is a lot of money to go around. But this gets a little hairy to document in a publication. I'm not privy to proof of corporate funny business and don't just want to throw around accusations because, in a large sense, it is irrelevant to the theme of this book. It is also so repetitive, the theme of corporate corruption, influence and greed; does anyone really need to hear it again? All I can say for certain is that in my life as a clinical psychiatrist I have seen plenty of evidence that drug companies contribute a lot of money to everything from massive scientific meetings to teleconferences to tons of "mopping up" normal research studies done in universities and medical schools. But there is one story that I would like to share with you to close this chapter. It's because it is about someone kind of like me. His name is David Healy. Well not all that similar in that he has written and published four books about what's gone wrong in psychiatry and this is my first. I met David at a conference about four years ago and he was a pleasant and warm person. His lecture was excellent. The story I want to share is one that I recently read in I book I ordered during the course of writing this book. I liked the title and plan to use material from the book in the next two chapters. The book is called *Prozac as a Way of Life* edited by Carl Elliott and Tod Chambers. It was published by The University of North Carolina Press in

2004. It's an academic, philosophically oriented book but in the introduction Carl Elliott tells the story of something that happened to David Healy that is both shocking and illuminating.

As Carl Elliott reports, in November 2000 "David Healy gave a presentation on the history of psychopharmacology at the Center for Addiction and Mental Health (CAMH), an affiliate hospital of the University of Toronto." In this talk "Healy briefly mentioned his worries that in rare cases, Prozac could result in a higher risk of suicide or violence." This was not a new story. Concerns about Prozac's association with suicidal or violent acts had been raised at least a decade before Dr. Healy's 2000 lecture. It seems, however that Eli Lilly, the makers of Prozac didn't take too kindly to his remarks.

I have to piece a little of this together but I gather that Dr. Healy had just been given a prestigious job at CAMH after, Elliott says, "he had been assiduously courted for more than a year." Shortly after the above lecture the appointment was *rescinded* by CAMH, with no specific reason given. "As it happens" Elliott points out, "CAMH is the recipient of a $1.5 million gift from Eli Lilly. The Mood Disorders Program, which Healy was to direct, receives 52 percent of its funding from corporate sources." The story is that Eli Lilly threatened to withdraw its gift if Healy was hired. Bummer. Does something like this surprise you? Anybody who watches television crime shows knows that the pursuit of money motivates all kinds of deceptive and destructive behaviors. The psychiatric medications annually earn multi-billions!! Sharfstein gave these figures in 2005: Worldwide sales of antidepressants, $13.4 billion. Antipsychotics: $6.5 billion. Nuff' said?

To end this chapter I'd like to return to Dr. Sharfstein's August 2005 column in the Psychiatric Times to wrap up my argument that it is *you*, the *consumer* of modern mental healthcare that needs to get smart because even when psychiatry acknowledges its obvious failings the words are hollow and without substance.

PSYCHIATRY AND PSYCHIATRISTS ARE NOT GOING TO FIX THE PROBLEM FOR YOU. INDICATIONS ARE THAT THE DEHUMANISTIC, REDUCTIONISTIC MEDICAL MODEL WILL ONLY GET MORE POWERFUL AND THAT THE OVERDIAGNOSIS AND OVERMEDICATING OF COMMON HUMAN EMOTIONAL PROBLEMS WILL GET EVEN MORE WIDESPREAD. THE NEXT GENERATION IS GOING TO GROW UP IN A WORLD WHERE BEING LABELLED MENTALLY ILL BECOMES SO COMMON THAT IT WILL SIMPLY BECOME A BARELY NOTICED PART OF EVERYDAY LIFE.

Do you honestly think the pharmaceutical industry will simply settle for their current profits? You do live in America right? The land where basketball and baseball players get angry about "low-ball" offers of merely $50 or $60 million? (See Shaq and the Orlando Magic and LA Lakers for example). Psychiatry's identity and very existence as a medical specialty is now inextricably linked to the pharmaceutical industry. There is no way out. Nevertheless, Dr. Sharfstein, the then newly elected president of the American Psychiatric Association commented that "we must examine the fact that as a profession, we have allowed the biopsychosocial model to become the bio-bio-bio model. In a time of economic constraint, a 'pill and an appointment' has dominated treatment. We must work hard to end this situation and get involved in advocacy to reform our health system from the bottom up."

AND DO WHAT DR. SHARFSTEIN??
DO WHAT??

How exactly do we reform our healthcare system from the ground up? Socialized medicine? That will demand even more cost containment and pressure for PRIME MD-like efficiency. And do you think biopsychiatry and Big Pharma are going to go along with advocating psychotherapy or social intervention in lieu of expensive and profitable psychotropic medications? Good Lord, what if it worked? How would the drug companies react? The CATIE study showed that an old antipsychotic, perphenazine, performed equally good (bad) in terms of compliance in chronic schizophrenia as all of the new ultra-expensive second generation antipsychotics. Do you think psychiatry's collective conscience just perked right up and started to prescribe this affordable drug? What I've seen is article after article after article by our "thought leaders" working to soften the blow and justify current prescribing practices. Did the abysmal results in the STAR*D study launch a clamor for a reform of psychiatry's conceptualization of depression and the role of medication in its treatment? NO way. Because the reform Sharfstein alludes to, the stand he implies psychiatrists need to take, is more than a stand against over-diagnosing and overmedicating emotionally distraught people in 15 minute med checks; it is a stand against the entire corporate and economic structure of 21st Century America, a stand against technology and the quick-fix mentality. Seriously, it is. And that is just not going to happen. There is no revolution on the horizon. But I've told you all along there is hope…hope for you. You can rise above all of this nonsense if you are willing to do just one small thing…***rewrite the story***. What story?

Your story

Chapter Nine:
SO, WHAT'S THE STORY?

> "I didn't anticipate that people would bombard me with hate mail, offer me blood transfusions, advise me to get a bodyguard, threaten to rip me apart, or warn me of assassination unless I recanted."
>
> **Elaine Showalter, 1997**

Wow, what in the heck did Elaine Showalter do? How did she manage to get people so angry at her? What she did was write a book; a book about stories.

At the time of writing her book Elaine Showalter was the Avalon Foundation Professor of the Humanities and Professor of English at Princeton University. The book she wrote that elicited the hate mail and threats against her life is titled *Hystories* (Showalter 1997). That's history with a "y" instead of an "i" and is spelled that way because of what the book is about—hysteria. With that word she is referring to what is defined in the dictionary as a "functional disturbance of the nervous system, of psychoneurotic origin". In plain English that means that the "hysteric" is a person with a wide range of physical and psychological symptoms that are thought to be caused solely by psychological conflicts, fears, repressions and defenses. It is interesting to note that the language used in this modern dictionary definition is more Freudian than biological, revealing the long history of psychiatric concern about this condition. In fact, concerns about hysteria go back much further, to the origins of medicine itself, when hysteria was diagnosed exclusively in women and blamed on the uterus "wandering" around the body. (Boy, speculative medical thinking not requiring physical evidence can get pretty wild, huh?

A wandering uterus; those ancient Greeks! Bipolar spectrum disorder; those 21st Century biopsychiatrists!)

I think most of us hear the word hysteria and start thinking about "hysterical." But in the psychological concept the term hysteria does not necessarily refer to people who get hysterical (although they often do). It refers to people who believe that there is just plain "something wrong" with them and WILL NOT TAKE NO for an answer. They just KNOW that SOMETHING IS WRONG! When modern medicine cannot provide a diagnosis or cure they turn to alternative types of explanations; explanations that are derived from fringe belief systems of their particular culture at their particular time in history. It is in pointing out this historical fact and bringing it into the present day that Showalter got herself into major hot water. Let's look at what else is on the book cover and you will see what I mean. The subtitle of the book is *Hysterical Epidemics and Modern Media* but it is in the list that follows the subtitle where we get our first clue about the disproportionate homicidal response generated by the book. Here is that list:

- **Alien Abduction**
- **Chronic Fatigue Syndrome**
- **Satanic Ritual Abuse**
- **Recovered Memory**
- **Gulf War Syndrome**
- **Multiple Personality Disorder.**

Dr. Showalter is suggesting that we consider that the above named conditions, that people come to fervently believe to be the actual cause of their diffuse and varied physical and psychological problems, are simply today's manifestations of an historically common phenomenon where some pretty outlandish beliefs are invoked to explain the hysteric's "condition". (Demonic possession and being bewitched are examples of past manifestations). She goes out of her way NOT to attack or make fun of people who believe they were abducted by aliens or have "recovered" memories of sexual abuse thirty or forty years ago. Apparently, that was not enough to appease those readers who elected to send the death threats (and other remarks that I decided were too vile to print in this book). They obviously felt attacked even though they were not!

So what, *in essence,* did Dr. Showalter do to these people? She questioned the way they had chosen to understand their lives and their problems; she questioned the legitimacy and coherency of their life "stories." Let's look a little more closely at the concept of a life story.

We all know what stories are; they are so familiar to us that most of us give little thought to what makes something a good story. So I'd like to offer the Carrie Fisher definition. First, though, another:

Roderickism:

I know all these snooty intellectuals that brag about never watching TV. That might be a source of pride to them but I have no idea how you can be a legitimate philosophical critic of the American way of life without it!

I'm proud to say that Rick would be proud of me. I watch lots of TV. That is where I got the Carrie Fisher definition of a good story. (You remember her, Princess Leia from "Star Wars"). She was a judge on one of the new reality TV shows modeled after *American Idol.* It was called *On the Lot* and was a contest between young aspiring film directors to land a one million dollar contract with Dreamwork Pictures and Steven Spielberg. I liked the show; it's interesting to see what goes into making even short, one or two minute films. Here was what Carrie advised and commented about on every film. "A good film tells a story, it has a clearly defined beginning, middle and an end." It is painfully clear when a film does not live up to these minimal criteria…it's a jumbled mess. Stories need to be coherent and make sense. The technical term used to describe a story's credibility and coherency is called its narrative structure. How this is germane to our topic here is that a group of psychologists have embraced the narrative concept in their work as psychotherapists and developed an approach called narrative therapy. The concepts of life-story and narrative underlie and tie together all of the material in this book so we now need to examine the philosophical foundations of narrative therapy.

To do this I want to turn to a book that I haven't mentioned before. It is called, appropriately enough, *Narrative Therapy* and was written by two psychotherapists, Jill Freedman and Gene Combs. It was published by W. W. Norton and Company in 1996. Freedman and Combs identify themselves as postmodernists, just as I do. So you know they are going to be grounded in a theoretical stance that does not believe in a single final truth or fully knowable objective reality. They spell out their position very clearly in chapter two when they say:

1. Realities are socially constructed
2. Realities are constituted through language
3. Realities are organized and maintained through narrative

There are a ton of people out there who would strongly disagree with these three declarations, including those who sent the death threats to Dr.

Showalter. No essential truths? Nothing holding it all together? What about physical reality? What about atoms...I mean quarks...I mean sub-atomic particles...I mean muons...I mean flavors...I mean "strings"?? (And now I need to add...the "God" particle). Whoops; even in the seemingly purely objective and detached world of physics, the deeper the explanation the weirder and more outlandish it starts to sound. I sometimes think about the widely accepted big bang theory of the origin of the universe, you know, the theory that proposes that all matter and energy was condensed into a single point before exploding in a universe birthing event, the big bang. Oh yeah, I can easily picture that in my mind's eye. C'mon.

Okay, back to the concept of narrative (we will get to the idea of the social construction of reality shortly). Since this is a psychological theory derived from postmodern philosophy then narrative is related to the concept of discourse we've previously discussed. In my mind, however, the word narrative has less of an implication of exerting power and control and more of a sense of "storying" (narratives therefore exist *within* and are *strongly influenced* by the dominant discourses we've previously talked about, the "regimes of truth" that guide our thinking). Narratives are also clearly historical. Dreyfus (Dreyfus 1993) gives the example that in 20th Century America you could not truly live the narrative of a Shogun warrior. The conditions for the possibility of that life story no longer exist. Narratives also have degrees of coherency and structural integrity. We are always reading about narrative structure in critical reviews of new movies and books. Even if we don't think in that precise terminology, all of us have a well developed sense of good versus bad narrative structure. A novel or movie with a good narrative structure "holds together", "makes sense", "wraps up the loose ends" and satisfies us to watch or read.

Narrative therapists use this concept of narrative as a metaphor for a slightly different kind of story, the kind they deal with in therapy. They are:

<u>THE STORIES WE TELL OURSELVES ABOUT OURSELVES.</u>

(I've capitalized and italicized this because this is the core central concept of this book. If you are getting a sense of how our lives are essentially all about the stories we tell ourselves about ourselves, then, as an author, I'm doing my job). All of us are storytellers and make sense of our lives a lot like novelists and screenwriters make sense with their books and movies. There is a big difference, however; our lives are infinitely more complex than any novel or movie. And sometimes we lose track of our stories or *don't even know that we are telling one.* We lose track of (another metaphor here) our *authorship* of our life stories. Often the reason this happens is because we have such a limited sense of authorship in the first place. Most people simply feel bandied about by forces completely out of their control. The job of the narrative therapist is to restore the sense of authorship to the client. This can be a very difficult therapeutic process, however, because power driven (and heavily marketed) dominant cultural discourses are often threatened by the personal empowerment that accompanies insights into authorship of our own life stories. Okay, that's a little bit too abstract. How about this: The drug company that makes Abilify (and spends millions putting ads in magazines and newspapers) wants the ***story you tell yourself*** about your moodiness, irritability and general dissatisfaction with life to be the bipolar disorder story so carefully crafted and promoted by the biopsychiatry/pharmaceutical industry. In other words, buy their pills. We talked about the dehumanizing reductionism of the medical model in psychiatry before. Now we are expanding our language with which to describe and understand it. Hey, this is all starting to make some sense:

I'm dissatisfied with my life. I feel lost and lonely. My job is stressful, repetitive and boring. I never go on vacation; I can't afford it. My kids are becoming a burden more often than a pleasure. I don't have enough money saved for retirement. My dad is gone and my mother is sick. The 11PM news is full of scary stories. I'm nervous all the time and can't eat and haven't had a good night's sleep in months. I'm starting to have episodes of crying for no reason.

WHAT IS THE STORY HERE?

If you ask your family doctor *the first seven sentences of your story will be ignored*, only the last two will count. Anxiety, tearfulness, loss of appetite, insomnia; that's the "story" of an illness called depression. It is caused by a chemical imbalance in your brain. It is not your fault and requires medical treatment to get better. End of "story"!

So, you get it? The struggling patient is GIVEN a narrative by his doctor. It gives his story a beginning, middle and end. And it's a very popular and compelling story because the endpoint is allegedly so easily achieved. The point I want to make clear, however, is that this medical narrative is just ONE story, not the ONLY STORY. Let me name two other possible storylines for this man.

1. Alienation
2. Spiritual Hunger

These stories also have a beginning, middle, an end and a satisfactory narrative structure. But here the endpoint of conquering feelings of alienation and spiritual hunger will not be as easily achieved as the promised restoration of the chemical balance of the brain. Thank God. How boring and "Brave New Worldish" history would be if the chemical balance storyline were actually the case.

In a New Yorker cartoon the psychiatric patient is lying on the couch complaining to the doctor: "Can we raise the dose? I'm still having feelings."

Re-storying the problems as alienation and spiritual hunger will not require the dehumanizing reduction of dropping the first seven sentences; in fact the first seven sentences will be the main plot line of the story. But before we go into greater detail about these alternate narratives (which will occupy us for the rest of the book) I want to more deeply examine the issue of how the power of the ruling discourse shapes our narratives and how and why we resist alternate storylines because this is critical. Let's go back to some of my former patients.

My poor beleaguered office staff had learned not to get alarmed when one of my patients departed abruptly from my office with very dramatic door slamming nearly drowning out the "F___ YOU'S" being launched in my direction. I'll give you a composite "case history":

I recall looking over the paperwork on a new patient that I was about to see and saying "uh oh" to myself. The first hint that I was in trouble comes from the fact that the patient was self pay. My charge for an intake exam was $175.00 and for many of the people who lived where I practiced, that was a lot of money. Since I had gotten burned so often by people making self-pay appointments and not showing up, we instituted a policy of needing to be paid one week in advance or automatically canceling the appointment. The next concern was raised by the age of the new patient. Anywhere from 18 to 40 was not good (why are these people in prime working years not covered by insurance?). Then my fear was completed when I looked at the source of the money used to pay for the appointment.

OH NO! THE MOTHER PAID!!
OR WORSE, THE GRANDMOTHER!!

The reason for the appointment my secretaries wrote down on the intake might have been depression or anxiety or bipolar disorder or ADD but that was irrelevant. I knew why they were really coming. I knew. (Remember, this is a composite, not true for every case). They were coming to see me because they were drug addicts or alcoholics. The reason the grandmother or mother was paying for the appointment was that their "child" was in crisis and/or had recently *moved back home and looked and acted very depressed and anxious and angry. Meanwhile Mom or Grandma had read or heard about psychiatry's ability to diagnose and treat the mental illnesses that cause people to "self medicate" with alcohol or drugs. So the stage was set for THE appointment, the one visit that would turn this all around and even though $175 is a lot of money to pay (often it was paid by credit card), it would be worth it to save the child.*

Put into the language we are discussing, mom or grandma and the patient have already applied a story-line to the tragedy of the patient's life. It goes like this. As a child or teen the patient suffered from an unrecognized mental disorder (Hey! How about ADD or Bipolar Spectrum Disorder?). The experimentation with and eventual addiction to drugs or alcohol was a destructive and desperate attempt by the patient to self medicate the symptoms of that disorder and was an understandable response to their suffering. The key to recovery therefore lies in the diagnosis of the underlying, previously unrecognized mental disorder and its treatment by the expert…(that would be me). This is the very popular "dual-diagnosis" narrative. Unfortunately, in my practice, this is where the trouble started. As you already know, I rarely bought the dual diagnosis story.

Unlike most psychiatrists and primary care physicians I *actually treated* drug addiction and alcoholism for years in the days *prior to* the domination of the dual diagnosis narrative. (Hey, I'm not ancient. I'm 58 years old. I treated addiction in the mid to late 1980's and, honest to God, we rarely used any psychiatric medications in our program). We were a traditional 12 Step program that prioritized the addiction and viewed all of the emotional and psychological "symptoms" displayed by addicts as the consequence, not the cause, of the years of substance abuse. We put the responsibility for recovery and emotional healing exactly where we thought it belonged, squarely on the shoulders of the addicts, not on the "clinical psychopharmacologist." We refused to promote a perspective that absolved the addict of personal responsibility. "Victim" was not our storyline because the one we had worked just fine, thank you very much.

Unfortunately my storyline about addiction is as radically different from today's dual diagnosis storyline as Dr. Showalter's storyline about hysteria is different from the hysteric's cherished storylines about chronic fatigue syndrome or multiple personality disorder. Like her perspective, mine actually angers people. (I have not received death threats but I dealt with a small but constant degree of trepidation that maybe this time I enraged the wrong person and someone would be waiting for me outside the office). I once saw a guy in my office that looked like he was going to go into acute alcohol withdrawal right then and there. A week prior his girlfriend had kicked him out because of his drinking, which he told me was about a twelve pack a day.

(Rule of thumb, take the amount the alcoholic or addict tells you they were doing and multiply by two, so I was thinking along the lines of a case a day). He had moved back with his mother and reportedly would just lie in bed and cry. (He secretly admitted to me that he did sneak out to buy "one or two" beers a day). Reacting to his behavior, the mother set up his appointment with me to evaluate and treat his depression. She was understandably very concerned and willing to pay the $175 she could barely afford. When she heard that I *did not* start her son on medication and gave him only one choice, to present to the local public rehab facility for a medical detox and treatment, she called and gave my secretary hell on the phone. (God bless my secretaries). Feeling she got no service for her money, she threatened to call the credit card company and void the payment (I don't know if she did or not). In this case the patient didn't get mad. He was disappointed but I think feeling too sick to argue. In other cases I have had the door slamming and cursing exit when I didn't automatically go along with the dual diagnosis narrative and instead recommended a singular option only, rehab. That would then be followed by the angry phone call from mom or grandma.

In a way narratives are consumable commodities, just like the products we buy. They need to have customer appeal. I think both Dr. Showalter and I know very well what general kind of narrative has the highest level of customer appeal in early 21st Century America—-the "*victim*" narrative. I think we all know and at some level accept this even though we are often repulsed by how more and more people play the "victim card" to escape taking personal responsibility for their actions. This has recently hit a new high (low?) when celebrities who make fools of themselves or pedophilic congressmen or racial hate spewing actors and comedians trundle off to "rehab" because, in this case, it is the drug or alcohol (or uncontrollable sexual desire) that did the victimizing. This trend shows no sign of abating. If you think about it, the victim narrative fits comfortably with the medical psychiatry narrative as well, especially when behaviors such as getting out of the car and beating the stuffing out of a driver who cut you off has recently been "blamed on the brain." It's called Intermittent Explosive Disorder, DSM IV code 312.14. And guess what? It's not your fault.

Before we explore this concept of narrative further and begin to look at how it can free you to re-story your life I want to share with you how the addiction-to-dual-diagnosis narrative change was rooted in and stimulated by that *you-know-what* called money. It's time for me to tell you the story about the birth of the dual-diagnosis concept in alcohol and drug dependence. I feel that I have a right to tell *my version* of this story because I was an eyewitness, standing right there in the delivery room, when this particular narrative was born.

Once upon a time there were two men called Bill W. and Dr. Bob. They were not bad men but they had a bad problem—drinking. They just didn't know what to do about it. So they decided to help each other. Maybe the two of them together could be stronger than either one alone. Thus they started a fellowship that would one day become Alcoholics Anonymous. This movement was founded back in the mid 1930's and has since grown by leaps and bounds despite its spiritual language, lack of scientific validation and, most remarkable to me, it's lack of willingness to participate in or benefit from free market capitalism (See the Twelve Principles of AA). No one is getting rich from Twelve Step meetings, a "commodity" utilized by millions of "consumers" everyday. I find that totally mind blowing. Anyhow, back to the dual diagnosis story…and to the comfort zone of modern capitalism.

To stop drinking or drugging or even gambling it is a heck of a lot easier and safer if you can start your quest for sobriety in a secure environment, immersed in Twelve Step treatment and with no ready access to your drug of choice. That is what a rehabilitation program (rehab) is. It provides for medical detoxification because coming off of alcohol and some drugs is actually physically dangerous, sometimes fatal. Other drug withdrawals are not life threatening but so incredibly difficult (e.g. heroin) that a medical detox and lack of access to the drug of choice is mandatory. So, in the terminology of capitalism there was:

1. ***A demand:***
   Detox and recovery for skyrocketing numbers of addicts and alcoholics.

2. ***A source of profit:***
   Medical insurance, self pay or government funding.

3. ***A product:***
   The rehabilitation hospital.

Rehab facilities began to spring up like weeds in most cities in the country. The model that generally guided treatment in these facilities was "The Minnesota Model", an amalgam based primarily on the Twelve Step philosophy but also incorporating principles developed in programs devoted to heroin addiction such as Synanon as well as psychological theories of motivation, behavior and maintaining a therapeutic community. When there were no cost restrictions, such as in the rehabilitation hospital where I worked, the treatment team would typically be composed of an MD psychiatrist, a PhD psychologist, a certified addiction professional, an MSW social worker/family therapist and a specialized nursing staff. The average length of stay evolved into a traditional "twenty eight days." I liked the job as the team director and was very good at it. Don't get me *wrong, housing thirty heroin and cocaine addicts, male and female, in a locked hospital unit and maintaining a therapeutic environment supportive of Twelve Step Treatment was no cakewalk. It was difficult and exhausting work. I still remember how, as the chief honcho, I came to fear hearing these words when I walked in the door "Oh, thank God you're here", because that meant big trouble. I can't tell you how much those words made me just want to turn around and go home. That is when I would say to myself, "Glad I'm not in this alone" and call an emergency staff meeting. It was a good job, the focus and goals of the program were clear, and I made good money (little did I know at the time that it would be more than I would ever make again as a psychiatrist). The hospital owners and directors could afford to pay me and my staff well because the place was always full, there was a waiting list for beds, and the cost to the patients was around $1500 a day. I enjoyed the job as a rehab doctor and believed we gave high quality, state of the art care. The capitalists involved in building and running rehabs rightfully saw the places as gold mines. Looking back, I realize now that there was just too much money to be made, too damn much.*

That's the trouble with free market capitalism, one that every television viewer is aware of. When something makes good money, everyone wants in on the action. So when a new concept such as the reality show "Survivor" is an unexpected hit, we can expect to be swamped with "Survivor" clones shortly after. Similarly, the rehab business went nuts, overbuilding and finding more and more ways to attract customers. One company made a deal with the Canadian government to treat heroin addiction. I personally know someone who told me she used to drive around Canadian cities in a van looking for junkies and entice them with promises of a free trip to Florida with its warm sandy beaches and daytrips to Disneyworld if they would agree to sign up for rehab. Of course, someone, namely the government and medical insurance companies, had to pay for all of this and at some point it just got to be too much. And who could really blame them; pay out $45,000 for a twenty eight day stay at a rehab for cocaine abuse with absolutely no guarantee for success? So right in the middle of the game, they changed the rules. There would no longer be automatic approval and payment for inpatient rehab (this started at about the same time as the managed care concept was catching on in all of medicine). The insurance companies told the rehabs they would no longer pay for inpatient rehab for heroin, for cocaine, for alcohol or any other substance abuse UNLESS THERE WAS ALSO ANOTHER AXIS I PSYCHIATRIC DISORDER!! Wait...listen do you hear it...the faint cry of a newborn baby? Yes, congratulations. You are a witness to the birth of a brand new storyline...the dual diagnosis narrative.

I know that I am sounding cynical here and maybe even a little paranoid. But I'm telling you the truth. I was an eyewitness to this nearly overnight change in the "understanding" of addiction and the treatment of the drug addict. Fortunately, for the people on the business side of the equation we were dealing with the incredibly flexible pseudo science of psychiatry, not real pathophysiology based medicine. Because, for example, if the hospital was allowed to only admit people with accompanying physical *complications of addiction like hepatitis, AIDS or heart disease, then lab tests or X-Rays or biopsies could be used to determine whether or not the addict met admission criteria. But when the admission requirement was for an accompanying diagnosis of a psychiatric disorder…you do know where I'm going with this don't you? Can't prove a diagnosis of depression or an anxiety disorder but can't disprove it either.*

But you don't have to take my word for it. Here it is directly from the horse's mouth: In a 2004 medical psychiatry textbook on Dual Diagnosis Nunes et al. are discussing the problems of making an objective diagnosis of an underlying primary psychiatric disorder versus diagnosing the mood or anxiety problems arising as a result *of the substance abuse. The latter does have a (rarely used) diagnostic category called Substance Induced Mood Disorder, diagnostic code 293.83. The difference between the two (both present with the same "symptoms") is whether or not the mood symptoms were "substantially in excess" of the expected "mood altering effect" from the substance alone. The authors noted that this differentiation hinges solely on the clinician's subjective judgment:*

> *However, the system continues to present challenges for diagnostic precision and the development of structured instruments. Particularly in those commonly encountered patients with chronic substance use dating to an early age, the differential diagnosis between categories of depression will hinge on interpretation of the terms 'substantially in excess' and 'in excess' of the 'expected' effects of substance use. These are not further defined and thus left to clinical judgment (Nunes 2004).*

Remember our discussion of the GAF scores in chapter three where I mentioned how the Medicaid requirements of a GAF below 40 to justify admission presented no challenge to the psychiatric diagnostic system or to the hospital? Just adjust the scores, who is going to argue? This same plasticity and vagueness of crucial diagnostic terms in the DSM system allowed for a smooth and easy transition to keeping "heads on beds" in rehabs when the rules changed in substance abuse insurance coverage. In MY VIEW the growth and development of the currently dominant "regime of truth" that characterizes the dual diagnosis model (and its destructive concept of "self medication") occurred in direct response to these insurance company requirements.

So the door stayed wide open for a while in the rehabs. Only now the "co-morbid" psychiatric condition had to be validated by something concrete, i.e.

medical treatment. No big deal really. Just put the alcoholic on Prozac. Diagnose the volatile cocaine addict as bipolar and start her on some Depakote. Then, in the Disney tradition of renaming their underpaid employees as "cast members", drug and alcohol treatment hospitals were renamed dual diagnosis treatment facilities. Now all that was left to do was medicate the addicts and teach them and their families a new concept…self medication. Done! (Money still pouring in).

But alas, even the best laid plans…There was to be a lot more insurance company pressure applied for cost containment, including requiring documented medical justification for every single day *in the hospital. The automatic approval for a twenty eight day program was over, even for "dual diagnosis" patients. Denials exploded, paperwork exploded, it just all got to be too much. The rehab hospital industry was extinguished. You are hard pressed to find a single private rehab facility in a large city now. When I moved to Orlando in 1992 there were six private rehabs and a new one being built. Today there are zero. But the dual diagnosis concept lived on. Why? Is there any* other *industry that might benefit by expanding its customer base to include addicts and alcoholics? Could it be the same industry that is now reaching into our nursery schools and kindergartens? Hmmmmmm…could it be?*

End of story, a textbook example of the social construction of truth. Yes, I have been somewhat cynical here and many would disagree with some or all that I have just said. But if they didn't live my professional life and did not happen to live through this birth (or at least explosive growth) of the dual diagnosis concept, directly experiencing the after effects, then they can't just blow off my arguments. After all, what are they going to do, use lab tests and MRI's to prove that addicts and alcoholics have psychiatric disorders and that I'm wrong? Sorry. But they *can* use every resource at their disposal to control the discourse about addiction and that they have done quite successfully. So here I sit, a holdout against the automatic assumption of a dual diagnosis in my patients with drug and alcohol problems, just waiting to get pounced on by angry addicts and their families. I have to tell you, I am not all alone and do not feel all alone in my overall critique of psychiatry but this dual diagnosis business…In my practice I sometimes truly felt totally alone and had to instruct my staff to consult me before accepting any new patients with addiction problems seeking psychiatric medications. I just didn't want to put myself through that anymore.

I hope you are getting a good sense of this concept of narrative and the role it plays in shaping our self understanding and expectations in life. You will see that therapists working from a narrative therapy perspective can exercise a lot of freedom and creativity in helping people "re-story" their lives. There is only one pre-requisite for a successful course of narrative therapy and that is open mindedness (on both sides). Unfortunately, that tends to be a relatively rare commodity nowadays because of the near insurmountable barrier of our continued faith in the illusion called *truth*. Yes, you are right; it is time to return to philosophy to explore what Freedman and Combs mean when they say that "realities are socially constructed" and that "there are no essential truths". Let's tackle the second statement first.

There was a time in history called the enlightenment. Among the many things that has come to mean, the most important remains the compelling notion that we humans are capable of detached and objective rational thinking that allows us to explore and understand the real world. Thus there is a real world out there that we use our minds (which in this scheme is not a physical part of the real world) to understand. In this Cartesian view of the nature of reality (so named because of Rene Descartes), humans are capable of totally detached reasoning, and are not influenced by any subjective goals or prejudices. Many scholars and even scientists no longer believe in the possibility of this, sometimes described in philosophy as the "view from nowhere" or the "God's eye view." But the "enlightenment project" continues to hold sway over most of us as we truly believe that a final full and comprehensive understanding of the nature of reality is possible and can be achieved. In this belief system there are essential structures that make a thing what it is. There are also essential structures that make us what we are (witness the current explosion of interest in the genetic/neurobiological basis of beliefs and behaviors, from antisocial personalities to religious zealots). So in this view there are essential, timeless truths, the accumulation of which will eventually reveal all.

Contrasting this enlightenment thinking is the postmodern thinking we have been discussing. I previously explained how postmodern "relativism" does not mean that any view of reality is just as valid as any other view of reality. It also does not mean that if you believe that you can step in front of a speeding bus and survive that you are simply expressing a point of view. That would be a very short lived idea. Yes, there is a physical world out there separate from our minds and it does have a sort of brute reality that cannot be denied. And we are in possession of a lot of facts about that brute reality that often rationally and safely guide our thinking and behaviors. Recall that Heidegger calls this element of existence "facticity." I like that term. But facticity is NOT what human life is all about because aside from the brute physical world, there is also the very human world of meaning and significance. This human world is the one chock full of beliefs, ideas, feelings, goals, ambitions, successes, triumphs and losses and failures. It is the world of the *meaning* of our lives told in stories and narratives and discourses. When we combine all of the above we capture the actual lived experience of being human. A term used to describe an individual's integration of facticity and narrative is *worldview* and we all have one.

Think about human development and think about your life from when you were born. How did you acquire a worldview? Did you need to touch a hot stove to learn about facticity, the brute physical reality of the interaction of fire and skin? Maybe you did. But did you need to learn that twice? In contrast, did you have problems with self esteem as a kid because you weren't the brightest or best looking kid in class? What percentage of your inner mental life was taken up by that issue versus remembering not to put your hand in a fire or step in front of a moving car? See the point? I know how you learned about the stove but where did you learn about popularity? Who taught you? Is good looking and popular a timeless truth, part of brute objective reality? Just a glance at a history of art book will answer that question. Standards of beauty are truths, but they are historically situated, *socially constructed* truths. These social truths are more than just personal opinion, however; they are social beliefs that are so widely shared that they are subjectively experienced as *actual truths* and affect us in our daily lives much more powerfully than any brute physical facts about the world. Another illustrative example of a socially constructed truth is a culture's standards of masculinity and femininity. Many of us have witnessed a massive shift in these standards during our own lifetimes. It takes only a fraction of our mental time to learn how to deal with the brute physical facticity of the world but we wrestle for a LIFETIME with the social truths such as self worth, success, gender issues and physical beauty. So when Freeman and Combs say that "realities are socially constructed", this is what they are talking about. They are talking about humanly meaningful reality, the "reality" that *really matters* to us. However, when this dynamic interplay between facticity and socially constructed truths is ignored, things can get very dangerous. How? To understand this we need to add the philosophical concept of the *metanarrative.*

A metanarrative is an attempt to keep the Western enlightenment project alive. By definition a metanarrative is the storyline *behind* all the other storylines, the grand story that explains all the others. How is this dangerous? Theologian and philosopher John Caputo puts it this way: "It is just when people are *convinced* they speak in the name of God (or Reason or History)... that they will stop at nothing and that is what puts us at considerable risk" (Caputo 1993, p.26). I hope I don't need to give you examples of how a "clash of metanarratives" has played itself out in human history (or is playing itself out right now in the Middle East). The relevant point here is that when socially constructed truths (human meaning, values, worth and concepts of wellbeing) are wrongly viewed as objective, timeless truths, then disciplines like psychiatry can become destructive. As part of the tenacious clinging to the enlightenment metanarrative, medical model psychiatry shifts human emotion, cognition, behavior and meaning over to the BRUTE PHYSICAL REALITY side of the equation. And the only way to do this is by being, as mentioned many times before, reductionistic (reducing the description of human emotional pain and suffering to lists of "symptoms") and dehumanizing (ignoring the individual biography and social forces shaping our lives) in evaluating and treating its patients. This then generates its own sub-narrative and, with the powerful backing of big dollars, disseminates this storyline throughout the culture, resulting in a socially constructed "truth" that is on the verge of redefining our entire society and way of life.

In the introduction to the book *Prozac as a Way of Life* Elliott says:

> Maybe the best way to understand the cultural phenomenon that the antidepressants have become is to think about the story the drugs tell: I am the person I am, with the problems that I have, because I have this particular mental disorder. It is a story that provides me with a sympathetic listener (my doctor or therapist), a community of like-minded sufferers (my support group), and a coherent narrative (told on television) both for myself and for those to whom I must explain myself. Increasingly, this is a story of biology and the brain, in which biological psychiatrists, pharmaceutical companies, and patient support groups all agree that disorders that respond to the SSRI's must have biological roots. Eventually this story may even create a new set of criteria for what counts as an acceptable identity, one of which will be a response to treatment. (Elliott 2004, p.10)

Is this what we want to be a predominant storyline in this culture? (It's getting there). This makes me once again think about the ads where pharmaceutical companies talk about historical figures that they say suffered from bipolar disorder: Newton, Beethoven, Van Gogh, Lincoln, Churchill… what precisely is the message these ads are supposed to convey? If modern medical psychiatry existed in their days, what would we have done, treated them? We want to diagnose some of the most powerful, creative and courageous figures in history as suffering from mental disorders? And if we did "treat" their "disorders", who would have benefited? I remember a 60 Minute story on the questionable economic relationship between C.H.A.D.D. (a patient support group for adults and children with ADD) and the pharmaceutical industry. Morley Safer interviewed a middle aged man who told Morley that he definitely meets and exceeds all of the criteria for adult ADD. But he would never agree to take medication to help him slow down and focus because he said he feared losing his creativity, feared losing the benefit of thoughts and ideas just popping into his mind. One of those thoughts was the idea for E-Tickets for airline travelers. This adult ADD "sufferer" was the president and CEO of Jet Blue Airlines.

Previously I quoted psychologist Miriam Greenspan's observation that one of the most powerful socially constructed truths in America is that the normal human mood state is "cheeriness", something that would strike most people in other parts of the world and in the past as rather "naïve or nutty." I totally agree. But what do we do about medical psychiatry? Aside from the radical and polarizing rhetoric of anti-psychiatry groups like Scientology, all *balanced and legitimate critiques* (like Greenspan's) recognizes that you cannot and should not simply dismiss the need for or usefulness of psychiatric medications. These thoughtful critiques call for a more sane and reasonable application of medical model thinking to the needs of each individual patient. But what exactly would that look like? What would be the guidelines for the clinician to follow in deciding whether or not to use medications in a particular patient? I do have an answer for that but it will not be a very satisfactory one because it runs counter to everything that guides a "rationalized" society. My answer is that this decision must reside in the *wisdom* of the clinician. In chapter two I characterized the Wizard of Oz as a man of wisdom who saw that the Scarecrow, the Tinman and the Cowardly Lion could be "treated" with placebos. I suppose if Oz were a litigious society like ours he might have been terrified to stick his neck out and recommend anything other than "standardized treatment." But I see no other long-term solution. The decision to use or not use psychiatric medications simply cannot be reduced to rule-driven equations. That is what has gotten us into the mess we are in today.

So have we come to a dead end? I don't think so. The ultimate "solution" here resides in something that would require a radical shift in psychiatric residency training but is not inconceivable. I believe that psychiatric training programs need to be devoted to and directed by the goal of launching the students onto, for lack of a better term, a path to wisdom. And I am not the only one who sees it this way. Here is an excerpt from the extremely thoughtful critique by Bradley Lewis. Doctor Lewis is both a practicing psychiatrist and a humanities scholar at New York University:

> I believe in psychiatry. I believe that secular cultures need the services psychiatry can provide. At its best, psychiatric care provides holding spaces where people may come for help with their confusions, their suffering, and their anxieties without judgment or blame. Ideally, people in need should meet kind,

> thoughtful, and well-trained clinicians who are happy in their work. These clinicians should have a broad education and be aware of the multiple dimensions of human suffering and human flourishing.
> They should also have the generosity of spirit to help wherever they can and the humility and wisdom to recognize those instances where they can provide only companionship and solace.
>
> To nurture that kind of clinician, psychiatry must reconsider its basic priorities, as that caliber of clinician requires scholarly resources beyond the sciences. Although an advocate for psychiatry, I am deeply worried about its soul and its future. I yearn for a psychiatry that lives up to its potential as a helping profession. Psychiatry's current path is taking it further and further from that potential. It is difficult these days to find well-rounded and intellectually nuanced psychiatrists. The best way to correct this imbalance toward science and rationality is to develop alliances on both sides of campus that will bring the tools and insights of the humanities to bear on the training of psychiatrists
>
> (Lewis 2006, p.xiii).

Can't you just feel the good and caring heart behind this quotation? Perhaps you can contrast it with a personal experience of psychiatric care you've experienced in your doctor's office. I have literally seen people whose "depressions" were "treated" by their family physicians by writing a script for a month's worth of antidepressants WITH ELEVEN REFILLS! "See you in a year!" So, what are the chances that Lewis' vision might someday come to fruition? I'll be optimistic here and say that someday I believe it will. Postmodern and holistic thinking is slowly but steadily making inroads into traditional medicine. But the radical change in curriculum and training that Lewis advocates? Clearly, not anytime soon.

As you are well aware I believe that the only immediate solution to the biopsychiatry problem is consumer education and empowerment (which we are going to get back to shortly). To end this chapter, however, I would like to tell you about what is going on in psychiatry residency training today and discuss something called evidence based medicine (EBM).

I'm always perusing the want ads for jobs in psychiatry because I would like to get more into teaching and cut back on my clinical work. Twenty eight years of dealing directly with patients can be a real burn out. So I see this job in the paper. A nearby medical school is looking for a director of residency education. Perfect! So I compose a letter explaining what I believe I can bring to the table that might really benefit the residency program. I explained that I have all the standard qualifications (board certification, good training, publications, teaching experience) but that I also have a strong working knowledge of the new movement in psychiatry called postpsychiatry (postmodern psychiatry). I told them I felt that this was a unique qualification and that their program could develop a curriculum that could separate them from the pack. Unlike other times when I have sent in applications and never heard anything at all, the residency director application did allow me to get someone on the phone to give me some feedback. She told me that the board reviewed my application and found it very interesting. However, "we will not be granting you an interview at this time."

I've heard from friends and acquaintances of mine that have worked as adjunct professors for psychiatric residents that whenever they tried to teach something other than biological theories the students showed little interest. For example, the psychiatrist Alfred Adler has a fascinating theory of human behavior, motivation and developmental challenges throughout the life cycle. He is a major figure in the history of psychiatry. But when my friend tried to get the residents interested in doing some independent reading on Adler, a full 0% expressed the desire or willingness. My friend no longer chooses to do adjunct professor work.

Here is something that will probably surprise you. What I mean when I refer to a residency are the years of specialty training required AFTER medical school to qualify to be a board certified specialist in a particular medical specialty. (After the residency you are then "board eligible"; you still need to pass a monstrous exam to be board certified). The surprise is that a psychiatric residency is four years long while an internal medicine or family medicine residency is only three years! Three years is deemed sufficient for internists and family practice doctors to learn all about the diagnosis and treatment of diseases affecting every organ system in the body (including psychiatric illness) but it takes FOUR years to learn one book (the DSM IV with its 365 diagnoses) and become proficient in using about twenty medications ?? I just don't get it. The four year residency duration made some sense when we were learning multiple perspectives and treatment techniques. When I was in training we carried some psychotherapy patients for all four years, usually under the tutelage of a psychoanalyst. It was called long term psychotherapy. (You would be hard pressed to find a *psychotherapist* doing long term therapy nowadays). I can't imagine why a psychiatric resident would spend time learning about something he or she would clearly never do. When I was a resident we also had much more lengthy hospital stays where the obligation of the psychiatrist went well beyond mere diagnosis and medication treatment.

So it made sense to learn family therapy, group therapy and other disciplines involved in long-term hospitalizations, but not now. Average hospitalizations run three to five days. So what do psychiatric residents do for four years? To be honest, I don't know and am not planning to look into it because I think the answer would only further demoralize me (notice how I didn't use the word "depress"?) What I've heard is that psychiatric residents see themselves as brain scientists and are busy learning all about neurophysiology and evidence based medicine.

Evidence based medicine (EBM) is among the many scary trends in our culture today as we continue to insist on becoming a rational, rule-driven society. Of course "wisdom" has little place in such a culture where it seems like the most powerful challenge is "Prove it!!" That is, of course, the challenge that EBM is designed to meet. The definition of EBM is self evident. You base your treatment plans on evidence of whether a certain treatment works or not in sound scientific studies. That eliminates what is called anecdotal evidence (treatment ideas derived from a single or a few cases) as well as medical "tradition" from consideration. For example, there is no room for psychodynamic concepts in EBM. So "neurosis", "defenses", "transference" are out! So too are humanistic concerns such as Maslow's "self actualization" or the existential concept of "authenticity." No…EBM requires clearly delineated categories of illness (DSM criteria), measurable outcomes (e.g. depression inventories) and easily distinguished treatments (pills versus placebo). So is EBM skewed to favor biopsychiatry? As asked before: Does a bear poop in the woods?

Fortunately, not all psychiatrists, even biopsychiatrists, are enamored with EBM in psychiatry. In a recent editorial in *Clinical Psychiatry News* Robert Michels, M.D., a professor of medicine and psychiatry at Cornell University says:

> Our current evidence base in psychiatry is not totally irrelevant to the clinical task of treatment planning and selection. But it comes dangerously close.
>
> What has been offered as evidence is only data. Evidence is data that is useful in making decisions. Much, probably most, of the data available about treatment in psychiatry fails that test in the clinician's office.
>
> We need evidence relevant to clinical decision making. We don't have that evidence yet. In the current setting *we don't have much of a chance of getting it* (Michels 2007).

Yet another clinician bemoaning the disconnect between psychiatric "knowledge" and clinical reality. But since this is the basis upon which medical education is resting today, wouldn't logic dictate that a recently schooled graduate (totally up to date on the newest EBM) be a far better choice for a doctor than a twenty year veteran who might still be making decisions based on personal clinical experience and God forbid, other non-objective criteria (like gut feelings)? Now, how does that sit with your own life experience and common sense? Does wisdom count for nothing? And seriously, if it is all heading towards EBM, then perhaps the idea of computers delivering medical care should be resurrected. It was a bust during the heady days of artificial intelligence in the 1980's, but that was in part because they asked the top doctors to help program the computers and found that they relied too much on intuition. (See *Mind Versus Machine* in the list of books in the appendix if you want to learn more about this). But that was then. We wouldn't even need doctors to program the computers now, just data sheets on the latest EBM studies. I recently had a personal experience that really brought this home for me. I'll share that with you to end this chapter.

About twenty minutes from my private practice office was an excellent hospital, the Halifax Medical Center. You might have heard of it as the hospital where NASCAR drivers are treated if they are injured in the Daytona 500. (Unfortunately, it is where Dale Earnhardt died). Halifax has a family practice residency program and I have been invited to give a number of lunchtime lectures there. Generally these have been sponsored by pharmaceutical companies so the topic was specific, e.g. the diagnosis and treatment of panic disorder. But I always managed to inject a little bit of my philosophy and skepticism into those lectures even when the drug rep was sitting there watching. This time, however, I elected to give a lecture without drug company involvement or remuneration. Being in the midst of writing this book you can imagine what that lecture was like. I took along Marcia Angell's expose of the drug companies to lend credibility to my talk. I covered the marketing and deceptive advertising so rampant in biopsychiatry today and offered inarguable concrete examples like I do in this book. What I noticed were two things. The first was that I was not seeing the shock and outrage I expected to see from these student doctors. Although surprised by some of the things I was saying, they didn't seem particularly angered or upset about having been manipulated by drug companies and biopsychiatry. I think they believed me; I just don't think they could incorporate what I was saying into the mental schemata they were developing as family practice residents. Then there was the second thing I noticed. The longer I talked the squirmier and more uncomfortable they looked. Finally the residency director interrupted to explain to me that their program was based on the concept of evidence based medicine and now I was suggesting that the EBM emerging from psychiatry could not be trusted. They had no idea where to go with that. I don't think I'll be invited back to give a lunchtime talk there anytime soon. I got the distinct impression they were angry at me because for the first time no one hung around to talk to me after my lecture. Oh well…sigh. Let's move on to chapter ten.

Chapter Ten:
TO PILL OR NOT TO PILL?
Towards a Rational Psychiatry Part One

Primum non Nocere: First, do no harm!

Ethical maxim generally credited to Hippocrates

I think it is the case that most clinicians today practice anti-Hippocratic psychopharmacology without realizing it.

Nassir Ghaemi, M.D.

I know and respect Dr. Ghaemi. He has managed to co-exist in the two worlds of academic clinical medicine and postmodern philosophy. He was the director of the bipolar disorder research program at Emory University and also serves on the executive committee for the Association for the Advancement of Philosophy and Psychiatry. In 2008 he published an article titled "Hippocratic Psychopharmacology" (Ghaemi 2008). The quote above is from that paper. Let's look at what it means and see how Dr. Ghaemi's philosophy of treatment forms the basis for the recommendations I will be making in this chapter.

In his paper Dr. Ghaemi points out that "do no harm" is not precisely the Hippocratic Oath young doctors take when graduating medical school. Hippocrates's position is more subtle and nuanced than "do no harm" implies. Basically Hippocrates's medical philosophy is based on the idea that in medicine: "Nature is the source of healing, and the job of the physician is to aid nature in the process of healing. In contrast, the anti-Hippocratic approach, which has always been quite prevalent, is that Nature is the source of disease, and the physician (and surgeon) needs to fight Nature to effect a cure" (Ghaemi 2008, p.190). Thus, in the Hippocratic approach Nature is viewed as the source of healing and the physician's "job" is merely to assist Nature in doing her work. The anti-Hippocratic position posits that Nature is the source of disease and it is the physician's responsibility to fight disease with all the tools that are available. Where the Hippocratic physician might recommend a treatment plan involving "diet, exercise and wine – all designed to strengthen natural forces in recovery from illness", the anti-Hippocratic physician would utilize every "potion and pill" available, even if questionably effective and "with limited attention to side-effects." Three guesses which approach characterizes biopsychiatry (the first two don't count).

Of course biopsychiatry is alarmingly anti-Hippocratic. That's what this book is about. But is Ghaemi therefore recommending a full conversion to the Hippocratic approach in psychiatry? No. That would be wrong. We have been dealing with obvious mental illnesses such as schizophrenia and bipolar I disorder long enough to realize that spontaneous healing is not the natural course of these diseases. But Ghaemi makes the point that most psychiatrists today have not caught up with the rest of medicine. (I tend to think of psychiatry as being about 100 years behind). In most of medicine the treatment of the underlying disease state by methods and medicines that have the strongest possible solid scientific evidence of efficacy strikes the appropriate balance between the extremes of Hippocratic and anti-Hippocratic treatment (e.g. cholesterol and blood pressure lowering drugs *along with* weight loss and exercise). Most psychiatrists are still stuck in the anti-Hippocratic philosophy of merely treating symptoms with whatever potions and pills are available. He says: "Scientific medicine is the treatment of diseases, not symptoms. Yet today many psychiatrists practice non-scientific symptom-oriented treatment, giving sedatives for insomnia, stimulants for fatigue, anxiolytics for tension, antidepressants for depressive symptoms, and mood stabilizers for lability – leading to an excessive and ineffective polypharmacy" (Ghaemi 2008, p.193). In the rest of the article Ghaemi goes on to examine the solidity of the scientific evidence for the various medications used to treat bipolar disorder and, like I've previously stated, finds that the oldest treatment, lithium, remains well ahead of the pack.

In this chapter I will go through some of the major diagnostic categories in the DSM IV and offer my opinions on:

#1: The legitimacy of the diagnostic category itself
#2: The medical treatments with the strongest scientific evidence of efficacy.

I realize that this is risky, risky business, advising when and when not to seek a medical solution to emotional, cognitive or mental problems. I want to make it **perfectly clear** that what I will be offering here is my opinion on the matter, not some final truth. I am going to go through the DSM IV to organize my recommendations. I will not be able to cover all of the diagnostic categories of course. I will select those that I think create the most pressing problems in today's mental healthcare.

> *"There are certainly downsides to medications," Malloy said.*
> *"But when medications don't work, we are pretty much screwed.*
> *There are not a lot of options."*

"Malloy" is Kate Malloy, the mother of a ten year old boy being treated for behavioral problems with an atypical antipsychotic. The quote is from an article in the local section of the July 30, 2007 edition of *The Daytona Beach News-Journal.* The article is about the soaring number of prescriptions for atypical antipsychotics for children and teens in Florida. Specifically, the article reports that there has been a 500% increase in prescriptions for atypical antipsychotics in Medicaid children in seven years. That's an increase from $4.7 million to $27.5 million, an average of $1800 a year per child. (I told you these pills are EXPENSIVE). The reason I added this quote is because I love that Mrs. Malloy used the word "screwed." It is the *perfect* word to describe what biopsychiatry and the pharmaceutical industry have done to parents in this country. Because the money that used to support all of the non-drug treatment approaches to behavioral and emotional problems in children is severely curtailed! Where did it go? Reread the above. (Hope you taxpayers have some pharmaceutical company stock so you can get something for your money). I really and truly feel sorry for today's parents with less than perfect kids. They are, what can I say? …screwed.

The first section of DSM IV is **"Disorders Usually First Diagnosed in Infancy, Childhood and Adolescence."** I want to be clear that this not an area of great strength for me because I am not trained for or clinically experienced in child and adolescent psychiatry. But because this is such a crucial topic, I will try to give you some basic suggestions. A number of disorders listed in this section of DSM IV are what are called developmental disorders which are usually very obvious and unmistakable in their presentation. This includes mild to profound mental retardation, pervasive developmental disorders (such as autism and Asperger's syndrome) and specific learning disabilities. For these problems and their management consult an expert. Some behavioral and neurological disorders are also obviously abnormal. Examples include Stuttering, Pica (eating non-food items such as paint chips), and Tourette's disorder. Again, consult the experts. For behavioral problems such as bedwetting (Enuresis), self-soiling (Encopresis) and Separation Anxiety Disorder specific behavioral treatment plans and programs are available. Ask your pediatrician.

So far, no problem. Now let's get to the toughies. The first is the extremely worrisome trend of diagnosing "grown-up" mental problems in kids. This, of course, includes depression and bipolar disorder. These conditions, however, are not listed as separate diagnostic categories in this section of DSM IV. We've talked about the deep problems with these diagnoses over and over in this book and you should by now have a well developed index of suspicion anytime someone suggests these diagnoses and medical treatment in children and teens. Be wary and be careful.

***NEWS FLASH: JULY 2007. THE FDA HAS NOW OFFICIALLY EXTENDED THE SUICIDAL WARNING ON ANTIDEPRESSANTS FROM 18 YEARS OLD TO 24 YEARS OLD. YES, THAT'S RIGHT! NOW THE LEGAL, ETHICAL, MORAL AND LOGICAL DILEMMA CREATED BY THE USE OF MEDICATION AS THE EXCLUSIVE RESPONSE TO HUMANS IN DISTRESS HAS CREATED AN EVEN LARGER BOONDOGGLE FOR EVERYONE INVOLVED.**

So, in assessing whether your pre-teen, teen or (now) young adult child should embark on a trial of medication for emotional distress, try to seek out non medical-model professionals to render alternative diagnostic and management recommendations. Use common sense. Use the internet to educate yourself but watch out for drug company supported websites. It will not be easy for you or your healthcare professional to muster the courage to defy mainstream thinking here since American psychiatric leadership really hypes the potential life threatening consequences of not medicating these "conditions"; so be prepared. If it were my kid I would try EVERYTHING else before I submitted to the lifetime diagnosis and medical treatment of a "bipolar disorder." But that will be up to you. All I am trying to do is introduce some reasonable doubt.

That brings us to the subsection of childhood and adolescent disorders labeled **Attention Deficit and Disruptive Behavior Disorders**. These include ADD, ADHD, Conduct Disorder, Oppositional Defiant Disorder and Disruptive Behavior Disorder NOS. I think that these are the second most worrisome diagnoses in children. Diagnosing childhood depression and bipolar disorder is clearly the most potentially destructive in terms of long term effects on self understanding, quality of life and mandatory lifetime exposure to psychotropic medications. ADD and the conduct disorders do not necessarily carry such dire consequences. But once again it will be up to the parents to make the final decision regarding accepting the diagnosis and the medications that follow. Since you are already well educated about the medical model theory of attentional and conduct problems, I want to present to you an alternative narrative about ADD. It is from a book written by a perceptive and well-qualified author, neuropsychologist Richard DeGranpre PhD. The book is called *Ritalin Nation* and was published in hardcover by W. W. Norton and Company in 1999. My suggestion is that any parent confronted with the ADD issue *read this book* before making any decisions regarding treatment. (A paperback edition is available, published in 2000. Page references here will be from the paperback edition). I am going to offer a brief summary here to give you an idea of what DeGrandpre has to say and how it relates to our theme of the social construction of truth.

The basic premise of DeGrandpre's argument is that we are not, as it appears, witnessing an unexplained explosion in the prevalence of the biological defect underlying ADD nor are we learning more about this disorder and therefore uncovering cases that previously went unrecognized. What we are, in fact, witnessing is the misnaming, misunderstanding and inappropriate treatment of an entirely different epidemic in modern American society, *sensory addiction*. As he describes it:

> Sensory addictions, whether in the child or adult, refer to a disturbance of conscious experience in which the person suffers from an inability to cope with *slowness.* As rapid-fire culture gives rise to rapid-fire consciousness—and, for children, an inability to regulate their own behavior—sensory addictions develop, motivating us to engage in more stimulus-seeking behaviors. At the heart of this developmental problem lies the emergence of a phenomenological experience of unsettledness, characterized by feelings of restlessness, anxiety and impulsivity. Hyperactivity and the inability to attend to mundane activities exemplify the type of 'escape' behavior that the 'sensory addicted' child or adult uses in order to maintain his or her needed stream of stimulation
>
> (DeGrandpre 2000, pp. 31-32).

A Roderickism

The problem today is not a lack of information, it's that we've got too damn much information.

So, according to DeGrandpre the epidemic of ADD is rooted in a continual speeding up of our rapid fire culture. Is that argument hard to accept? C'mon, use your common sense, look around you. The amount of moment to moment ever-changing array of stimuli has gone totally around the bend in America. Its nuts and we are being driven nuts by it. Let me quote one other psychiatrist before I get back to how DeGrandpre analyzes the other half of the "ADD as disease" argument, the so-called paradoxical effect of Ritalin. This quote is from a psychiatrist who works at a university mental health center and has to do with a general trend he is witnessing. The psychiatrist's name is Paul Genova, M.D. Speaking about the rising incidence of depression on college campuses he writes:

> In the bigger picture, one wonders what on earth we are doing. Are we using medication to postpone some day of reckoning with the ultimate limits of our biological equipment?
> ...What might they think then of an early 21st century psychiatry that taught them to think only in narrow mechanical ways about their emotional experience, and that did not help them question and explore its social context? (Genova 2005, p.31)

This might seem a little out of context but it really isn't. Genova is asking a very relevant question: what exactly are the limits of our biological equipment? How many tasks can be included in the multitasking demands of modern society before we literally do exceed our mind's capacity to handle it? Are we already there? I know when I've reached beyond my limit and that is when I walk into a video game parlor at the mall. The noise, confusion of lights and frenetic activity is more than I can process or handle and I make a beeline to the exit. But the kids seem just fine in that environment. They've adapted. They are also very good at using their thumbs and fingers to manipulate multiple buttons at one time, resulting in a smooth progression of the video game character from one dire challenge to the next. Then I think about (for some strange reason it is always the same memory) geometry class in high school. I can vaguely picture a male teacher but vividly remember the clock...a typical high school wall clock...audibly ticking away the endless and unendurable parade of seconds until class was over. I can guarantee you that if inattention, daydreaming and fidgeting are characteristic of a "neurological" disorder, I would have met all of the diagnostic criteria in my geometry class. So what about today's kids whose level of sensory input tolerance is clearly so much higher than mine? How do they fare in the quiet boredom of the school classroom? Apparently okay as long as they've taken their Ritalin.

We've already discussed Ritalin and other stimulants in chapter seven and looked at how similar these drugs are to the illicit drugs cocaine and speed.

Here I want to address a *myth* that sustains and supports the medical model view of the biological basis of ADD; it is the myth of the *paradoxical* response to Ritalin and it goes like this: Some of the most obvious and disruptive symptoms of the ADD disorders are the seeming inability of some of these kids to sit still. They disrupt class and distract everyone by this apparently irresistible need to constantly be moving. They are the hyperactive subgroup of ADD, given the acronym label of ADHD. The "paradoxical" effect is that when you give these kids a pharmacologic stimulant...speed...they calm down and sit still. Shouldn't a stimulant make them even more hyperactive? Let's see what DeGrandpre has to say.

DeGrandpre asks a question that no one ever seems to ask because they assume the answer is self-evident; but it isn't. He asks "why do we assume a stimulant will increase our activity level?" (This is obviously a key point in the paradoxical effect argument). That is a very good question. Many of us have heard here or there that some of these ADD kids could, unmedicated, play video games for hours on end without any distractibility or hyperactivity. The assumption has always been that these games offer sufficient real world stimulation to maintain the ADD child's focus. DeGrandpre's argument is that we should look at Ritalin the same way, as an artificial, externally derived source of internal stimulation: "That is to say, by providing an artificial source of stimulation, the drug actually reduces our need to acquire stimulation through our own actions" (DeGrandpre 2000, p.197). Therefore, no need to be "hyperactive" in a quest for "sufficient" stimulation, Ritalin has already taken care of that. I hope this counterargument is clear. It is basically saying that Ritalin would have helped me pay attention in my boring geometry class by chemically enhancing my sense of overall general stimulation, artificially satisfying my otherwise "bored out of my mind" sensory hunger. As DeGrandpre says: "From this standpoint, Ritalin's effects turn out to be far more predictable than paradoxical" (DeGrandpre 2000, p.197).

Sometimes I joke with my patients about what would happen if someone decided that caffeine is bad for us and outlawed it. (They did it with alcohol, so anything is possible). What would happen is that the next DSM could have a new diagnosis...let's see, I'll try to say this in DSM style...

Morning Hypersomnolence Disorder (MHD)

Characterized by three or more of the following symptoms present for at least one week:

1. difficulty feeling fully awake despite adequate sleep
2. feelings of mental dullness and slowing
3. excessive irritability

4. chronic tardiness at work or school
5. late afternoon fatigue
6. loss of a sense of motivation and ambition

Studies have shown a good response to Cafwake, a prescription medication recently released by Pfizer. Okay, point made. Without a morning jolt of caffeine many people would simply not function as well but that hardly means that they have a mental disorder. What if that is also the case for the vast majority of those diagnosed with childhood or adult ADD? They aren't sick; they just do better with pharmaceutical grade amphetamine delivered in measured oral doses. I suspect that if we de-medicalized this ADD issue a very different form of social debate would ensue, perhaps one similar to the steroid controversy in athletes.

Am I saying that there is no such thing as ADD? Actually I am not. I have this general rule of thumb I follow that serves me well but I have no way to validate it. My rule of thumb is that for widely diagnosed disorders whose primary symptoms are numerous, vague, diffuse and ill-defined, about 10 to 20 percent of those diagnosed with the disorder actually have something biologically wrong with them. I'm talking here about "conditions" like fibromyalgia, chronic fatigue, PTSD, ADD, dysthymic disorder etc. My "10 to 20" rule of thumb comes from two sources. One is the fact that about one-fifth as many British and French schoolchildren are diagnosed with ADD versus American schoolchildren. I just generally think the British and French psychiatric systems are somewhat more reasonable, cautious and clearly more philosophically sophisticated than ours. The second has to do with some historical information about a condition that, unlike psychiatric disorders, relied directly on laboratory abnormalities to validate the diagnosis. The condition is called reactive hypoglycemia (RH) and was widely diagnosed in the 70's and 80's. Here's the story:

The "symptoms" suggesting a possible diagnosis of RH included complaints of tiredness, anxiety, difficulty concentrating, irritability, depression etc.... you get the picture. Bring your problems to the medical world, get a medical diagnosis. The theory was that RH was a defect in the processing of glucose that led to a drop in blood sugar to a level that was so low that the cells in the body were not receiving sufficient fuel, thus the wide range of physical, emotional and cognitive symptoms. The diagnosis of RH was *confirmed* by a laboratory test called the Glucose Tolerance Test (GTT). In the GTT the patient was asked to drink a concentrated dose of glucose (called glucola) and would then have their blood sugar level measured at various time intervals. If the blood sugar dropped below 50 then the diagnosis was confirmed. Millions of people were diagnosed with RH based on their complaints and the results of these tests. There was no specific treatment for RH except the suggestion to eat six small meals a day and to avoid ingesting high sugar foods. But at least these millions of people had a laboratory validated diagnosis and many were relieved to know exactly what was wrong. But… did they?

Along the way somebody got the idea to ask the question of whether the laboratory finding of low blood sugar on the GTT was *actually directly correlated* with the symptoms that the diagnosis was meant to explain. Two things were done. First GTT's were run on people without complaints of RH symptoms. It turns out that under the conditions of receiving an abnormally high glucose load (the glucola) a lot of people have their blood sugars drop to below 50 yet *have no symptoms*. The second thing done was to take patients *already diagnosed* with RH and measure blood sugars only when the patient complained of symptoms. Under those conditions only about 10% of the patients ***already diagnosed*** with RH actually had low blood sugars when symptomatic. So, for what its worth, that and the British and French ADD data (and my clinical experience and intuition) is where my 10 to 20 percent rule of thumb comes from.

I don't see kids or teens in my practice, so have I ever newly diagnosed and treated an adult for ADD? Rarely. But then there was Larry…

If there is one thing I feared in my private practice it was someone presenting for an evaluation that might be so disturbed that I would need to call the police to take the patient directly to the hospital on an emergency commitment. I feared this because the one and only time I had to do it was on a Sunday morning when I agreed to see one of my depressed patients who had apparently flipped into a dangerous state of mania. He had no insight, was euphoric and giddy but easily agitated. Throughout the weekend he had been making threats to various family members, particularly his wife. The family had called the police but when they arrived at the house the patient would pull it together just enough to not get hauled off to the psychiatric hospital. (The police, rightfully, hate to do this). After a brief evaluation I decided that he definitely needed involuntary commitment and called the police myself. I explained that I was a doctor, had already filled out the necessary commitment papers, and needed someone to come ***right away*** *because the patient was escalating and I feared might become dangerous. The police arrived ONE HOUR after the initial (and three additional) phone calls. I suppose if we were all dead when they arrived there might have been a review of procedures but that experience really scared me. So I didn't relish the idea of an out of control psychotic showing up at the office. At first glance, I thought that Larry just might be one.*

Larry was a middle-aged man who presented to me because he had experienced a failed abdominal surgery two years prior and had not been able to return to work. Not working was driving him up the wall and he had been feeling increasingly agitated and depressed. This was his stated reason for the consult. What I observed was a muscular man with uncontrollable hyperactivity, loud rapid talking and an inability to maintain his focus on one topic for more than one or two sentences. Fortunately, his incredibly agitated state was not accompanied by a psychosis. I was not dealing with a psychotic manic needing hospitalization. So what was I dealing with? I took a careful history. A long time concern with ADD (since childhood) was mentioned. But how had this guy made it so far in life, (married, kids and gainfully employed in construction), until medical problems kept him from working? Had he ever tried any medication? Once he tried his wife's Wellbutrin but said it agitated him and he couldn't sleep for three days. Another time a friend had given him an Adderall (an amphetamine used to treat ADD) and said that it made him feel "grounded". I decided to give the ADD treatment a try. It took a while to find the right dose and I would hardly describe Larry as totally normalized but he was able to concentrate and focus much better and landed a new job. Reports from his family confirmed his impressive improvement. So Larry was one of my 10 to 20 percent. I have seen a number of adult patients that other doctors had diagnosed with ADD that are nothing like Larry, have not had a clear-cut response to meds (although most like the amphetamine effect), that comprise my 80 to 90 percent overdiagnosis category.

Moving on. The next major category of disorders in DSM are what used to be called organic brain syndromes to distinguish them from the other psychiatric disorders that used to be called "functional". This distinction was meant to convey the fact that in organic brain syndromes there is demonstrable tissue pathology where in functional syndromes there is not. Since the new message in psychiatry is that, in essence, all disorders are organic (we just haven't as yet found the biological cause of the vast majority of disorders) the organic label was dropped. The DSM III-R published in 1987 still had the organic category; only DSM IV doesn't. So the category is now **Delerium, Dementia and Amnestic and Other Cognitive Disorders.** These disorders are actually dealt with by neurologists more than psychiatrists and I won't spend much time on them here. I just want to briefly touch on the subject of Alzheimer's disease because my psychiatric journals and newspapers are loaded with ads for drugs to treat this condition.

It is generally agreed that Alzheimer's dementia is a true organic illness because at autopsy there are definitive physical abnormalities in the brain. But these do not show up on X-Rays or MRI's of living brains, so Alzheimer's is one of those diseases diagnosed on the basis of clinical findings alone. Therefore, there is some wiggle room in making the diagnosis. Why am I telling you this? Did I mention that my journals and newspapers are loaded with ads for drugs to treat Alzheimer's? Might the manufacturers of those drugs want to exert some influence on the frequency of the diagnosis of this disorder? That's all I really want to say here. Just be wary. Alzheimer's dementia is a terrible disease...it is incredibly tough on the families. I generally recommend that an evaluation at a specialized memory clinic should be done to distinguish age-related memory loss from Alzheimer's. (Please don't rely on just the opinion of your PCP or family doctor in uncertain cases; this is where drug companies exert their influence. A lot of older people have memory problems but are not demented). If the diagnosis of Alzheimer's is clear, I urge the families to get a book called *The 36-hour Day* by Mace and Robins to begin to educate themselves about dementia and its impact on the family. One last thing to mention; as I told you in Chapter seven the FDA recently issued a warning that the second generation antipsychotics are associated with a higher all-cause mortality rate when used to control psychotic or behavioral symptoms in elderly patients with dementia. Just another wrench in the works you should be aware of.

The next section in DSM covers **Substance-Related Disorders.** This is the first of many diagnostic categories we will encounter in which the role of medical model psychiatry is not clear. As thoroughly discussed in chapter eight, the way medical model psychiatrists and their pals in the pharmaceutical industry have bullied their way into substance abuse treatment is through the unproven (and, of course, un-disprovable) concept of dual diagnosis. Whenever I pine for the good old days of running a substance abuse treatment program again I quickly learn that the role of the psychiatrist in rehabilitation programs is now the clearly delineated and extremely limited task of assigning the psychiatric diagnosis and providing the medication. I mentioned earlier that Dreyfus pointed out that you could no longer be a Shogun Warrior even if you wanted to be because the conditions for the possibility of living that narrative are gone. In fact, they have been gone for centuries. It has been disheartening for me to learn that social conditions for the possibility of narratives can change a lot more rapidly than over the course of hundreds of years. As far as I can tell there aren't any jobs left like I had less than thirty years ago at any rehabilitation hospital in the country, including the granddaddy of them all, Hazelden. When I visited Hazelden recently I found that nearly every client I talked to was indeed on some sort of psychiatric medication. At my old job, with precisely the same patient population, I would guesstimate that about two out of thirty clients were on psychiatric meds; today I would bet it is just the opposite. So what is my message to you? The system is broken and can't help you? No, that's not the message. Actually it is the same singular message I am trying to communicate to you throughout this book, the same message that consumer advocates have been promoting since Ralph Nader: Caveat Emptor, Consumer Beware. An example:

In June 2007 I first saw a patient in whom I believe that the dual diagnosis concept, invoked way too early in her "treatment", created such a muddled mess that I am not sure there is any way out. Here is the story: We'll call this patient Lynn.

On one of her follow-up visits to me (after I had hesitantly restarted her on Xanax) Lynn was a nervous wreck. Her AA sponsor had actually suggested that she talk to me about her possibly being bipolar because the sponsor "had observed a pattern of ups and downs in my moods." Okay, no surprise there, right? Of course that advice coming from her spiritual guide, her AA sponsor, is just more evidence of the invasion of speculative mental illness diagnosing into our daily lives and interaction with others. I dismissed this, but still had to deal with how to address her obvious pain and desperation. I felt especially bad when I glanced at her psychotherapist's note, a well-intentioned and skillful helper, who said: "Apparently, she is back on Xanax??? This strongly compromises our work." This therapist and I generally saw eye to eye. And he was right. Putting her back on Xanax was a bad idea. (Fortunately, I put her on the sustained release form and she didn't like it and didn't abuse it. In the past she had used up a thirty day supply of regular Xanax, 120 pills, in one week). So how did this case get to the point where I found myself prescribing Xanax? It started well before I saw her for the first time.

In her teenage years Lynn was what we call a garbage-head. If it altered consciousness, she took it. As is often the case, in her twenties she gave up the insanity of polysubstance abuse and settled on the legal and freely available intoxicant, alcohol. For many years she was a full blown alcoholic. The idea that she was mentally ill, however, came from her family doctor. At the time Lynn was what I would call "toying" with sobriety. She was in and out of AA and had frequent relapses. Her family doctor had tried her on five different antidepressants but none had helped with the overwhelming feelings of anxiety and depression she complained about. Of course, as discussed previously, alcohol dependence could easily be understood as the true source of her distress and that commitment to total abstinence and immersion in AA the necessary AND sufficient treatment. But, as I explained, those days are over. Doctors can barely contain themselves in their enthusiasm to run multiple medication trials on their unhappy and nervous patients, whether they are addicts or not.

Finally Lynn's family doctor found something that really helped her: Xanax. For a patient like Lynn, Xanax is basically a drink in pill form. And she didn't disappoint. One of the many pithy sayings in AA is that for the alcoholic "One drink is too many and a thousand is not enough." Lynn lived up to that prediction with the Xanax as well. The referral to me was prompted by Lynn "abusing Xanax."

In retrospect I think I got a little bit suckered by Lynn who really didn't give me the whole truth about the extent and duration of her addiction. She came across as pretty together and I opted to try sustained release Xanax to help quell her constant anxiety. (This is one way to cut back on the abusability of Xanax). I started Effexor and Ambien as well. I truly realized from the beginning that due to her previous indoctrination as biologically impaired I would simply not be able to convince her to go back to the beginning and prioritize recovery treatment. The dual diagnosis concept and psychiatric medication started four years before the above mentioned follow-up visit. In those four years she had multiple relapses and had been on and off psychiatric medications; the mess that this case had become really hit home on her most recent visit. As I mentioned I had reintroduced Xanax XR to her on the previous visit. Her father had been diagnosed with lung cancer and she was spending 17 hours a day in the hospital with him. I felt sorry for her. But Xanax XR didn't help. She was still on Effexor and it wasn't helping. She couldn't sleep even with Trazadone and Ambien. I knew what she needed… alcohol; because for her entire adult life, she could only truly function "normally" with alcohol. Now she had an AA sponsor suggesting she get treated for "bipolar" disorder. What a mess. When I brought up the possibility of totally prioritizing the alcoholism as THE problem, getting off all psychiatric meds and finding herself a traditional orthodox 12 Step counselor, she was terrified. The dual diagnosis concept did real harm to this woman.

So how do you know if you or a loved one has a drug or alcohol problem? When does "use" become "abuse"? There are guidelines in DSM and elsewhere, some diagnostic, some legalistic. I'm sure you know that I'm not going to have some formulaic answer for you. If I was compelled to put it into one sentence I would say that you know you are having a problem if you keep repeating the behavior (drinking, drugging, gambling, binge eating etc.) despite obvious, frequent and significant consequences. That hardly covers the topic. I told you before that we cannot avoid complexity simply because it's "too complicated." A society cannot deal with the complexity of life at the level of general rules and guidelines. Neither can any profession. There will always be distortion and oversimplification. There is only one person who can even begin to handle the complex question of whether an individual is merely using or abusing a drug. That person is the user!! The drinker, the drug user, the gambler… they know when it's spun out of control. They might exercise some BIG TIME DENIAL…but they know. The sheer genius of the 12 Step program of recovery is that they have recognized this from the very beginning. They made meetings available to anyone who wanted to come but they never went out and dragged people in. Because they knew that unless the alcoholic or addict was personally ready to ask for help, had truly hit their personal bottom and realized that they were powerless over their drug of choice, then everyone trying to help was wasting their time and breath.

I strongly suggest that anyone dealing with a family member or loved one with an addiction watch a show called *Intervention* on A&E network because that show is the real deal and it is not the least bit pretty nor all that encouraging...true reality television. There is a lot more to say about addiction treatment but I am going to reserve that for chapter thirteen. That entire chapter will be devoted to the 12 Step programs and recovery. I will just deal with one last issue here that may be on some readers' minds. If I worked at a rehab where patients were brought by their families, employers and/or court orders to treatment how can I say that the only way to get an addict sober is when they themselves hit bottom and truly want help? I am saying that because it is true. Many if not most of the clients at the rehab I ran were not fully motivated for recovery; they had not yet hit the proverbial bottom. Our job at the rehab was to "raise the bottom" for them so that whatever brought them in would be sufficient motivation to commit to sobriety. Getting fired from a job or a second DUI or losing a home or the threat of divorce can be enough if a skilled staff knows how to enlist other addicts to prove that you don't have to reach your lowest personal bottom because if you keep using, it will find you. This could only be accomplished in a structured residential or inpatient program because the only people the addict trusts are other addicts. So the veterans reach out to and help the rookies work on their level of commitment to sobriety. It often works; sometimes, not. Sadly, the bottom for some addicts is the graveyard...and no one can stop them.

Time to move on. The next section of DSM IV is titled **Schizophrenia and Other Psychotic Disorders.** As I've mentioned before, this group of disorders is generally not as controversial in terms of a biologic origin as the mood, anxiety and other disorders. Unfortunately, the biologic basis and underlying cause of psychotic disorders is not known. The biochemical theories of psychosis arose from a backward logic similar to what led to the catecholamine hypothesis of depression; an effective medication was accidentally discovered and then analyzed. The chemical effect of the medication was then hypothesized to reveal the cause of the illness. In this case the accidentally discovered medication, chlorpromazine, brand name Thorazine, (being used to stop nausea and vomiting), was found to block dopamine activity. Thus the theory was born that psychosis is caused by excessive activity in the dopamine tracts in the brain. As I said, I am not going to go into this set of disorders in detail but do need to mention a few key issues.

The term schizophrenia is probably the most historically rooted label left in biopsychiatry. As mentioned before, other historically rooted terms such as neurosis have been discarded in the DSM manuals. I am really not sure why "schizophrenia" survived and there is rightfully a lot of discussion and controversy about whether its diagnostic criteria describe a single diagnostic entity or a wide range of only tangentially related disorders. Based on the course of the illness in people diagnosed with schizophrenia it has become pretty clear that the diagnosis describes a very heterogeneous group of conditions. What that means is that the diagnosis itself is insufficient to dictate course of treatment or prognosis. At its worst, at one time the schizophrenia label was immediately attached to anyone that displayed psychotic symptoms. That was very common when the only medicines available in psychiatry were for schizophrenia. And since Thorazine was such a powerfully sedating compound, nearly all agitated people were calmed (to put it mildly) by this drug. It is obvious now that many people with psychotic symptoms reflecting an underlying Bipolar I disorder were previously misdiagnosed as schizophrenic. But we need to return to the "cutting nature at its joints" issue, or, in other words, ask if our diagnostic criteria reflect what we see in the real world? I think most everyone in psychiatry would answer no but there are clearly a range of conditions where psychosis (delusions and hallucinations) are the hallmark symptoms. Some conditions are so severe that they simply do not respond to treatment. These unfortunate souls used to end up in state hospitals, or jails, or on the streets or dead. I think the general feeling is that state hospitals were snake-pits and that their closing is a good thing but I don't agree. My disagreement is based, by the way, on first-hand experience.

I did my psychiatric residency at Maricopa Medical Center in Phoenix, Arizona. The Arizona State hospital was directly behind our psychiatry building and we all rotated through there. It was a clean, uncrowded and well-staffed hospital Many of the patients were pitifully ill and would not last a week outside of the hospital, medicated or not. The state hospital in Arizona at the time of my residency represented the most humane and *realistic* societal response to the nightmare of severe chronic psychotic illness. AND IT STILL DOES. I don't know if that hospital still exists but I know that Florida and, I believe, the rest of the country, has been systematically shutting down all state hospitals except those for the criminally insane.

But let's switch gears and talk about a larger group of patients with chronic psychotic illness, that for the lack of a better term, I'll call ambulatory schizophrenics. Because for them I believe that antipsychotic drugs are truly helpful. I'll tell you about some of my private practice patients.

I had about eight or nine patients in my practice that came to me with pre-existing diagnoses of schizophrenia. They were all on antipsychotic medications and stable. Because I was in private practice I was only seeing those patients that were not severely ill and had family based support systems. Some were on the new antipsychotic drugs, some on the older ones. A few had movement disorders (muscular tics of the facial or trunk muscles) but, as a whole, they seemed relatively well. So well in fact that I, as you might have guessed, questioned the validity of their diagnoses. But I don't anymore. Because I personally witnessed five of these patients go off their meds (not, by the way, at my request but of their own choosing) and experience a psychotic breakdown. Despite being a psychiatrist for twenty eight years and having had jobs where I worked with extremely ill patients, I still find psychosis shocking. It truly is like demonic possession, the degree to which the delusions and hallucinations take over. And it usually responds to antipsychotic medication, often in just a few days. I am not saying that appropriately medicated people with what I am calling "ambulatory schizophrenia" are 100% well. All of my patients led limited lifestyles, were mildly to extremely socially uncomfortable, and had blunted emotions. But I am saying that the discovery of antipsychotic medications has liberated a large number of people from the previous fate of ending up on back wards of state hospitals: As long as they take the meds. And, as they say, there lies the problem.

In chapter seven I mentioned the C.A.T.I.E. study where they found that around 75% of chronic schizophrenics DO NOT take their medicine as prescribed. Why don't they take their meds? What can be done about this? The answer to why is very complicated but let me offer this one thought. How long would you comply with medications that cause side effects like tiredness, muscle cramps and weight gain if you didn't believe you were sick? I said that the delusions and hallucinations take over when a schizophrenic is actively psychotic. With the medication they don't necessarily go away, they just lose their hold on the person. That doesn't mean however that the person with schizophrenia will truly understand (and buy the fact) that their false beliefs and sensory experiences were merely symptoms of a brain illness. Many still secretly (but quietly) believe that the delusions were not delusions and that the hallucinations were real. To get a schizophrenic patient to comply with medication usually takes some outside support. This is a recognized fact. Now let's add a few more facts to the equation. The first is the above reported increase in cost of antipsychotic *medications* prescribed for Medicaid children in Florida; from $4.7 million in 2000 to $27.5 million in 2006. The second fact is that facilities like Act Corporation (the public sector provider of mental healthcare services in Volusia County, Florida), the "community mental health centers" created to take over the job of state hospitals, are going bankrupt. To save the agency Act laid off a number of employees, including 50 out of their 52 caseworkers. There are extremely limited funds for mental healthcare in these state supported agencies. When the medication costs eat up all the resources then something has to give...like Act firing their caseworkers. The only problem is that the caseworkers' job was to visit schizophrenic patients at their homes or residences to help insure medication compliance! Drop them out of the picture (especially for patients that don't have families), and there goes your compliance.

This is admittedly a gross oversimplification of a huge and controversial problem. I just want to make the point here (in support of my contention that I am not anti-medication), that I have seen medical progress in the treatment of chronic psychotic illnesses and I pray it keeps going but, like everything else, it's complicated! To wrap up this section on schizophrenia I want to briefly acquaint you with another side to the schizophrenia argument. There are some brilliant thinkers, both providers and recipients, who strongly question the use of medication in what we call schizophrenia. I want to focus here on the work of one man who died recently. His name was Loren Mosher.

A Stanford and Harvard trained psychiatrist Dr. Mosher was the Chief of the National Institute of Mental Health (NIMH) Center for the Studies of Schizophrenia (1968-1980). That is about as mainstream as you can get. Yet in a 2003 newspaper article (DeWyze 2003) the then sixty nine year old Dr. Mosher is quoted as saying: "I am completely marginalized in American psychiatry. I am never invited to give grand rounds. I am never invited to give presentations. I am never invited to meetings as a keynote speaker in the United States." What had Dr. Mosher done to go from a big shot at NIMH to a totally marginalized member of the American psychiatric community? He dared to openly question the medical model. (Remember Foucault's concept of dominant discourses, "regimes of truth" and marginalization of opposing perspectives?). But more than that, he attempted to demonstrate that antipsychotic drugs could actually do more harm than good. He recommended an empathetic therapeutic milieu as treatment for the people we call schizophrenics and actually demonstrated success in programs he set up in California, the best known being Soteria House. Not only was his philosophy about minimal to no use of medication a threat to mainstream psychiatry and the burgeoning psychiatric drug industry, his use of non-professional staff to treat schizophrenics was a threat to the whole mental healthcare power structure and regime of experts supporting it. Oh yes, he was marginalized alright. But he had a voice! And he was respected, admired and remembered fondly by many. For more detail about Dr. Mosher and his philosophy of treatment I recommend the above quoted newspaper article. It can be found on the web at http//www.moshersoteria.com/crazy.htm.

As my tribute to this man I want to wrap up this chapter with a reprint of Dr. Mosher's resignation letter from the American Psychiatric Association. He submitted it to Rodrigo Munoz, the then president of the APA on December 4, 1998.

Loren R. Mosher M. D.
2616 Angell Ave
San Diego, CA 92122

December 4 1998

Rodrigo Munoz, M.D., President
American Psychiatric Association
1400 94 Street N. W.
Washington, D.C. 20005

Dear Rod;

After nearly three decades as a member it is with a mixture of pleasure and disappointment that I submit this letter of resignation from the American Psychiatric Association. The major reason for this action is my belief that I am actually resigning from the American Psychopharmacological Association. Luckily, the organization's true identity requires no change in the acronym.

Unfortunately, APA reflects, and reinforces, in word and deed, our drug dependent society. Yet, it helps wage war on drugs. Dual Diagnosis clients are a major problem for the field but not because of the good drugs we prescribe. Bad ones are those that are obtained mostly without a prescription. A Marxist would observe that being a good capitalist organization, APA likes only those drugs from which it can derive a profit - directly or indirectly.

This is not a group for me. At this point in history, in my view, psychiatry has been almost completely bought out by the drug companies. The APA could not continue without the pharmaceutical company support of meetings, symposia, workshops, journal advertising, grand rounds luncheons, unrestricted educational grants etc. etc. Psychiatrists have become the minions of drug company promotions. APA, of course, maintains that its independence and autonomy are not compromised in this enmeshed situation.

Anyone with the least bit of common sense attending the annual meeting would observe how the drug company exhibits and industry sponsored symposia draw crowds with their various enticements while the serious scientific sessions are barely attended. Psychiatric training reflects their

influence as well; i.e., the most important part of a resident curriculum is the art and quasi-science of dealing drugs, i.e., prescription writing.

These psychopharmacological limitations on our abilities to be complete physicians also limit our intellectual horizons. No longer do we seek to understand whole persons in their social contexts rather we are there to realign our patients' neurotransmitters. The problem is that it is very difficult to have a relationship with a neurotransmitter whatever its configuration.

So, our guild organization provides a rationale, by its neurobiological tunnel vision, for keeping our distance from the molecule conglomerates we have come to define as patients. We condone and promote the widespread overuse and misuse of toxic chemicals that we know have serious long term effects: tardive dyskinesia, tardive dementia and serious withdrawal syndromes. So, do I want to be a drug company patsy who treats molecules with their formulary? No, thank you very much. It saddens me that after 35 years as a psychiatrist I look forward to being dissociated from such an organization. In no way does it represent my interests. It is not within my capacities to buy into the current biomedical-reductionistic model heralded by the psychiatric leadership as once again marrying us to somatic medicine. This is a matter of fashion, politics and, like the pharmaceutical house connection, money.

In addition, APA has entered into an unholy alliance with NAMI (I don't remember the members being asked if they supported such an organization) such that the two organizations have adopted similar public belief systems about the nature of madness. While professing itself the champion of their clients the APA is supporting non-clients, the parents, in their wishes to be in control, via legally enforced dependency, of their mad/bad offspring. NAMI, with tacit APA approval, has set out a pro-neuroleptic drug and easy commitment-institutionalization agenda that violates the civil rights of their offspring. For the most part we stand by and allow this fascistic agenda to move forward. Their psychiatric god, Dr. E. Fuller Torrey, is allowed to diagnose and recommend treatment to those in the NAMI organization with whom he disagrees. Clearly, a violation of medical ethics. Does APA protest? Of course not, because he is speaking what APA agrees with but can't explicitly espouse. He is allowed to be a foil; after all he is no longer a member of APA. (Slick work APA!)

The shortsightedness of this marriage of convenience between APA,

NAMI and the drug companies (who gleefully support both groups because of their shared pro-drug stance) is an abomination. I want no part of a psychiatry of oppression and social control.

Biologically based brain diseases are convenient for families and practitioners alike. It is no fault insurance against personal responsibility. We are just helplessly caught up in a swirl of brain pathology for which no one, except DNA, is responsible. Now, to begin with, anything that has an anatomically defined specific brain pathology becomes the province of neurology (syphilis is an excellent example). So, to be consistent with this "brain disease" view all the major psychiatric disorders would become the territory of our neurologic colleagues. Without having surveyed them

I believe they would eschew responsibility for these problematic individuals. However, consistency would demand our giving over "biologic brain diseases" to them. The fact that there is no evidence confirming the brain disease attribution is, at this point, irrelevant. What we are dealing with here is fashion, politics and money. This level of intellectual/scientific dishonesty is just too egregious for me to continue to support by my membership.

I view with no surprise that psychiatric training is being systemically disavowed by American medical school graduates. This must give us cause for concern about the state of today's psychiatry. It must mean, at least in part, that they view psychiatry as being very limited and unchallenging. To me it seems clear that we are headed toward a situation in which, except for academics, most psychiatric practitioners will have no real relationships, so vital to the healing process, with the disturbed and disturbing persons they treat. Their sole role will be that of prescription writers, ciphers in the guise of being "helpers".

Finally, why must the APA pretend to know more than it does? DSM IV is the fabrication upon which psychiatry seeks acceptance by medicine in general. Insiders know it is more a political than scientific document. To its credit it says so, although its brief apologia is rarely noted. DSM IV has become a bible and a money making best seller - its major failings notwithstanding. It confines and defines practice, some take it seriously, others more realistically. It is the way to get paid. Diagnostic reliability is easy to attain for research projects. The issue is what do the categories tell us? Do they in fact accurately represent the person with a problem? They don't, and can't, because there are no external validating criteria for

psychiatric diagnoses. There is neither a blood test nor specific anatomic lesions for any major psychiatric disorder. So, where are we? APA as an organization has implicitly (sometimes explicitly as well) bought into a theoretical hoax. Is psychiatry a hoax, as practiced today?

What do I recommend to the organization upon leaving after experiencing three decades of its history?

1.. To begin with, let us be ourselves. Stop taking on unholy alliances without the members' permission.

2.. Get real about science, politics and money. Label each for what it is - that is, be honest.

3.. Get out of bed with NAMI and the drug companies. APA should align itself, if one believes its rhetoric, with the true consumer groups, i. e., the ex-patients, psychiatric survivors etc.

4.. Talk to the membership; I can't be alone in my views.

We seem to have forgotten a basic principle: the need to be patient/client/ consumer satisfaction oriented. I always remember Manfred Bleuler's wisdom: "Loren, you must never forget that you are your patient's employee." In the end they will determine whether or not psychiatry survives in the service marketplace.

Sincerely, Loren R. Mosher M. D.

Rest in peace Dr. Mosher.

Chapter Eleven:
TOWARDS A RATIONAL PSYCHIATRY
Part Two
Mood Disorders, Anxiety Disorders & Why Can't I Sleep?

> "To most of us who have experienced it, the horror ofdepression is so overwhelming as to be quite beyond expression...It kills in many instances because itsanguish can no longer be borne."
>
> William Styron
> *Darkness Visible*

We have already talked extensively about depression and bipolar disorder in this book. But we still need to directly address a very pragmatic black and white issue. How do you, as a consumer of mental healthcare, decide whether or not you (or your loved one) should try a mood medicine (antidepressant or mood stabilizer) because, as I'm sure you know by now, your doctor will have an extremely strong bias towards medication and will not help you rationally weigh the options. (Many will nearly force the medication on you). This "certainty" is extremely difficult to resist. William Styron, despite the depth of his despair, emerged from his episode of depression with a negative view of antidepressant medications, feeling as if they actually delayed his recovery. So even in very severe depressions you will not find a 100% agreement that medical treatment is a necessity. Additionally, the vast majority of people diagnosed with depression in today's world are not experiencing such severe symptoms. So somebody has to decide whether or not "to pill." I wrote this book so YOU can weigh the options! You will not be able to fully accomplish this until you finish the book but we will examine the medication issue now by revisiting and expanding the list of the potential hazards of antidepressants:

1. Sexual side effects
2. Drug-drug interactions
3. Birth defects
4. Worsening of emotional state, especially increased anxiety or agitation
5. Precipitation of suicidal ideation
6. Withdrawal syndrome
7. Unknown structural changes in brain: short-term & long-term
8. Unknown functional changes in brain: short-term & long-term

In all honesty this is not a list that is so astoundingly frightening that it alone would lead to banning these drugs in comparison to the risk of other drugs we routinely take for medical problems. I think it should cause *someone*, however, to pause and reflect a bit before just whipping out the prescription pad for anybody expressing unhappiness for any reason. But I'm afraid that is going to have to be *you*, not the doctor. So how do you decide? Are there any criteria? For that matter how do I decide for my patients (and, incidentally, for members of my own family)? The answer is that I weigh a totally different set of risk factors that I call the *spiritual risk factors* in taking antidepressant medications.

The human spirit...amazing. The final two chapters of this book will be devoted to thoughts about healing and nourishing the human spirit so let's take a look at that concept. I'll start with the Oxford dictionary definition because I like it. The definition of spirit in the Oxford dictionary is: "the vital animating essence of a person or animal." Vital animating essence... how much more do you need to say? I think we all have our personal inner definition of the human spirit but as a species all humans share a strong sense of what we have chosen to label spirit. Spiritual practice disciplines abound throughout human history often linked to religious beliefs or other holistic perspectives. Spirituality *defies* the reductionism that seeks to demystify our lives, something that sociologist Max Weber has called the "disenchantment of the world" (Weber 2001). Weber did not live to see the reductionistic, rationalized perspective applied so directly to the human spirit as it is now in biopsychiatry but I'm sure it would not surprise him because, like Heidegger, he saw where this was all heading.

Okay...hold on a second...Weber, Heidegger, the human spirit...what does this all have to do with my deciding whether or not to take Zoloft for my "depression"? Isn't this taking it a little too far? Well, yes and no. We'll start first with the yes; it's taking it too far. Certainly the fate and future of mankind doesn't rest with one person's decision to try antidepressants. So, from that perspective one person trying an antidepressant is no big deal. But let's look at it from a slightly different perspective, one espoused by the famous German philosopher Immanuel Kant. I am going to explain one of Kant's maxims somewhat simplistically and out of context but I really like the basic concept it represents. It's called the Categorical Imperative and has to do with morality and ethics. Kant said that in deciding to perform an act, in making a choice to act one way rather than another, the best ethical guidepost is to imagine that you declare through your action that you endorse this action for everyone else. You have made a categorical decision, not just a personal one. Confusing? Here is a simple example. "Should I cheat on my taxes... perhaps overvalue some junk I gave to the Salvation Army to increase my charitable deduction?" I don't think the U.S. economy will stand or fall on that individual decision. But what if the "decider" (I love that word now... Bush pops into my mind every time I use it), considers that if he or she cheats on taxes that it is a moral endorsement of that act for everyone. It is saying, in essence, that cheating on taxes is morally and ethically okay *for everyone.* Of course if everyone did cheat...that WOULD have an impact on the economy. Do you see the point? Let's look at the decision of whether or not to try antidepressants through the same lens.

Every time that I reread parts of Dr. Bradley Lewis' book on postmodern psychiatry the more I appreciate his brilliant mind. In discussing the broader issues affected by the dominance of biopsychiatry he says:

> The new biopsychiatry, as a way of talking about and organizing human pain, minimizes the psychological aspects of depression—personal longings, desires and unfulfilled dreams—and it thoroughly erases its social aspects—injustice, oppression, lack of opportunity, lack of social resources, neglected infrastructures, and systematic prejudices.
>
> As a deeply conservative discourse, biopsychiatry benefits the currently dominant groups. To state the case polemically anyone unhappy with the status quo and the emerging New World Order, Inc. should shut up and take a pill!

(Lewis 2006, pp.133-34)

Obviously, this is the "no" side to the yes/no question on whether I am making too big a deal about an individual deciding to take an antidepressant. In essence I am saying that it is a very big deal indeed and, to put it polemically, that the act of accepting the biopsychiatry "storyline" about unhappiness and despair and simply taking a pill endorses the idea that all unhappy people should just "take a pill and shut up." I believe that for most people who are unhappy there are identifiable social and spiritual issues at work generating the despair and pain that they are feeling. Whether it is a relationship problem, a physical problem, an economic problem or simply the reflection of living in a shallow, mean-hearted, impersonal and money-grubbing society, one can view the desire for antidepressants as a lack of willingness to address the deeper issues, or, not unrealistically, a sense of powerlessness to do anything about them. The act of surrendering, however, to the seduction of the "antidepressant" concretizes that sense of powerlessness and going along with the crowd that, historically, as we have seen, has not ended well. We saw it in the STAR D* study and you will find it clearly spelled out in the literature on conditions such as post-partum depression—environmental, economic, race, gender, social, vocational variables…they all play a *central role* in the emergence of and response to treatment of this "condition" we are calling depression. These are central human spiritual and social issues. We'll get to them in detail in chapters twelve and thirteen because now we need to get a little bit more pragmatic and realistic since a social revolution isn't likely to happen soon.

The other clear-cut impact of embarking on a trial of antidepressants has to do with the previously discussed "story we tell ourselves about ourselves" because a trial of antidepressants, especially one with the most common outcome, namely, ambiguous results, can and often does *permanently* alter your self-understanding. Yes, as Perot would say…It's that simple. Let's face it, until about twenty years ago very few people's self narratives had a chapter on brain chemicals as an explanation for anything! So this is a very new narrative but apparently very, very appealing. Yes, we still get to blame others for what's gone wrong in our life but the power and appeal of those explanations pale in comparison to the technical brain chemical narrative because brain chemical problems are so easily repaired. Or, as you now know, that is what they want you to believe. AND IT'S WHAT **YOU** WANT TO BELIEVE! (My goodness, just like Disney gets us to believe what they want us to believe… sounds familiar). This probably accounts in large part for the characteristic placebo response rate of 20% to 40% we see in studies (Fink 2006). But that is not the main concern here. For the sake of argument let us assume you have some sort of emotional pain relieving response to an antidepressant. Maybe it's just a response to a surge of serotonin, maybe it's the "what-the-hell" effect or maybe it's something more, a lifting of the doom and gloom in your head. Here are the new questions that then come to the surface:

1. When do I stop the medication?
2. How can I distinguish antidepressant withdrawal from a return of the symptoms?
3. What about my sex drive; will it come back?
4. If I get off antidepressants and then start to feel down or anxious or upset again, should I go back on medication?

All these questions are problematic but it is #4 that represents the biggest problem because if your narrative, your self story, now contains a belief in chemical correction of negative moods HOW WILL YOU EVER ENDURE A NEGATIVE MOOD THAT LASTS EVEN A FEW DAYS AND NOT SEEK BIOCHEMICAL RELIEF?

You probably won't because you've entered the tent;
You are in Psychiatryland!

I don't have the numbers but my observation is that for many, many people that first antidepressant pill presages a lifetime commitment to psychiatric meds. You'll become just like the Tinman, terrified to be even a few feet away from your oil, your prophylactic antidepressants.

OK Dr. Phill, you made your point. So what's the alternative? Suffer? Never try an antidepressant because once I do I am signing on for life? C'mon. That is a bit harsh isn't it? Let's turn for an answer (of all places) to science. There is an interesting movement in the field of psychology (along with the effort to get prescribing privileges) that attempts to even the playing field with biopsychiatry by doing scientific studies and providing empirical "evidence" of the effectiveness of certain psychotherapy techniques, sometimes doing direct head-to-head comparisons with medication. One particular brand of therapy called cognitive or cognitive-behavior therapy has historically shown a consistent pattern of similar or superior effectiveness in study groups of "mild to moderate" depression. So has a routine of regular, vigorous aerobic exercise (Dunn 2005). I will have a lot to say about cognitive therapy in the next chapter and will have recommendations for further reading in the appendix. For our purposes here I just want to point out some strikingly apparent differences between cognitive therapy for "depression" versus medication treatment. That difference is that in cognitive therapy (or even in embarking on an exercise program) you will:

1. Learn Something
2. Actively participate in your treatment
3. Develop new skill sets and coping mechanisms to deal with (and maybe even prevent) future episodes of emotional pain.

Let's face it. Taking a pill prescribed by your doctor is a completely passive and non-participatory act. You play almost no role, learn nothing new about yourself and the world, and develop no new skills to cope with or prevent future problems other than calling the doctor. Cognitive therapy, on the other hand, involves a therapist (or program), a guided examination of your patterns of thinking, an identification of your excessively harsh and irrational beliefs and *practice* putting more reasonable and rational beliefs in their place. It's work. Cognitive therapy has homework assignments and if you don't do them you don't progress. Good cognitive therapists do not coddle or sympathize with the patient; they actually should (and sometimes do) refuse to see the client if he or she isn't doing the work. Again, for what it's worth, cognitive therapy is empirically proven to be as effective as medication in mild to moderate depression. Common sense tells you that it would clearly have a lasting effect by teaching a new skill set to prevent future depressions. Hey... what about a *combination* of medicine and cognitive therapy; would that work better than either alone? Funny you should ask that...

There used to be an antidepressant called Serzone manufactured by Bristol Meyer Squibb. They don't make it anymore because some cases of total liver failure seemed to be caused by the drug...a very, very small number but obviously a terrible side-effect. (This compound is still available as a generic drug called nefazadone, so the FDA did not insist it be pulled from the shelves). Anyhow, the makers of Serzone once sponsored a large scale study assessing the effectiveness of Serzone alone versus cognitive therapy alone versus combined therapy in subjects with chronic major depression. The study was published in the New England Journal of Medicine in May 2000 (Keller 2000). The bottom line (and remember that there are serious inherent flaws in any psychiatric study) is that in terms of response, not total remission, 55% of the subjects responded to medication alone, 52% responded to therapy alone but **85%** responded to combined medicine and therapy. Regardless of the questionable diagnostic and assessment procedures in psychiatric studies, nothing has ever come close to an 85% response rate to anything. You'd think that this study, published in such a prestigious medical journal, would have launched a new standard in care in the treatment of chronic depression. But you know what: You'd be wrong! Because, as it was provided in this study cognitive therapy is expensive (and the wrong people, *the therapists*, are getting the money).

In this study the subjects receiving cognitive therapy (either alone or with medication) were given twice a week hourly sessions for 8 to 10 weeks. The therapy was highly structured and doing the homework was mandatory. This, unfortunately, created a completely artificial scenario because few insurance companies would allow (i.e. pay for) this many therapy sessions and few "consumers" would commit to it outside of a controlled study environment. Then there is one more thing. To my eye (and this should not necessarily be seen as true for all parts of the country), there are fewer and fewer therapists actually doing cognitive therapy. As we discussed before, making demands on clients isn't good for business. I can tell if someone is actually getting cognitive therapy because it will be reflected in their vocabulary. They will start using words and phrases like "automatic thoughts", "irrational beliefs", "catastrophizing" and "shoulding myself to death" during our visits (kind of like how patients in AA start using recovery language, something that I *do* see). So even when one of my patients tells me that their therapist is giving them cognitive therapy, I know they aren't because the expected vocabulary change simply isn't there. That is except for good old George...an unlikely candidate for improvement from cognitive therapy...except it actually happened.

George's felt like another hopelessly muddled case. He came to me after moving to Florida about two and a half years before our appointment. His story was that he was injured on the job when a steel girder hit him on the head. He had a headache for a solid year. After exhausting standard medical options George was referred to a psychiatrist. This was probably because George was one of the most neurotic (driven by worry) persons you will ever meet. Of course his psychiatrist addressed this problem exactly as expected, he medicated him. The particular drug he chose was Paxil. This was to become the beginning of one of the most neurotic and obsessive relationships between a patient and antidepressant that I had ever seen.

George would measure the effectiveness of Paxil and the dose based on the presence or absence of head and neck pain. He was CONSTANTLY self adjusting the dose and imbuing these minor changes with incredible power. He would obsess and obsess about the precise dose, his head, his mental clarity and his drug-induced sexual dysfunction to the exclusion of all else. Yes, George had sexual dysfunction from Paxil and was very upset about it, but not so upset that he would consider giving up his precious magic pill. When I first met George there was no evidence of any capacity for self reflection or any other therapeutic thinking. But he was very good at complaining. He would present with lists of complaints and then just sit back and wait for me to come up with a plan. Here are some excerpts from my notes:

"Says he got down to 5mg. of Paxil and all hell broke loose. Back up to 30mg. Then he felt fine. Went to Vegas last week and felt great. Came back on Friday

and feels like a train wreck since then. He says 'I wish I could come off Paxil. It is crushing my sex life.' Slept all day today; couldn't even get out of bed."

He agreed to try a switch to Prozac, a much longer acting drug than Paxil. The goal would be to use Prozac to prevent Paxil withdrawal and then take him off Prozac, which doesn't have withdrawal symptoms. But even with the Prozac on board:"Seems like he has been a train wreck. Again, trying to come off Paxil and having an incredibly dramatic reaction. He is clearly psychologically/physically dependent on Paxil and trying to get him off is only exacerbating this incomprehensible case."

Next visit: "He is back on the Paxil. He says he couldn't sleep, felt nauseated and was belching on the Prozac." And so it went. I eventually got him to a headache specialist I know who tried a number of interventions but without lasting success. He even tried switching him over to Cymbalta...that was a disaster. I wrote: "Now this highly neurotic patient with self-defeating negative projections is given another opportunity to worry and worry, the primary problem that is never addressed. His only hope is the Midwest Center program or this will just keep on going on and on."

The Midwest Center Program for Stress and Anxiety... sound familiar? Perhaps you've heard radio or TV ads by its founder Lucinda Bassett. (I have no business ties to this program. Honest.) The Midwest Center program is something that I looked into because of the above mentioned problem with finding any therapists who actually do traditional cognitive therapy. The Midwest program advertised itself as a self directed program based on the principles of cognitive therapy. It has CD's, DVD's, printed materials and a workbook. So I ordered one for myself. It was around $400 and, much to my chagrin, no professional discount. It turns out that the program is exactly as advertised. There are 16 "sessions" on audio CD's with titles such as "Self Talk: The Key to Healthy Self Esteem", "Expectations: How to Expect Less and Get More" and "Put an End to 'What If' Thinking." Excellent. The package also includes a workbook and some DVD's. I have recommended this program to at least 50 of my patients. I know it would really help them, especially the neurotic worriers and chronic depressives who characteristically get little to no relief from medications. Thus far, of all people, George was one of only a few patients who not only ordered the program but worked it. It is hard to describe how much better he did. He spoke cognitive therapy language and had insight. He "owned" his neurotic worrying and saw a light at the end of the tunnel. He got off Paxil!! All he took was an "as needed" tranquilizer, Ativan.

So let's get back to the point of this before we stray too far off course. It is an examination of the factors that go into the decision of whether or not to try antidepressants in the first place. The primary issue George's case exemplifies is the natural (and very American) tendency to not only go the technical route and take pills, but to then put all of the eggs in that basket. In part this is because it requires the least effort but it is clearly also because it's what the doctor recommends. In my mind it was a mistake to put George on antidepressants in the first place. His tendency to neurotic worry was so visibly profound, cognitive therapy alone would have been the perfect treatment plan from the beginning. Six years were wasted with med trials and minute dosage adjustments. I think cognitive therapy alone would be best for many of my patients or, as demonstrated in the Serzone study, as a complementary addition to medication. But, as we've said throughout this book, this recommendation IS NOT going to come from the medical community and less and less from the mental health professional community, including from the psychotherapists. I told you in the introduction that alternative non-medical paths to emotional and mental wellbeing are ALREADY IN PLACE. But you are going to have to go get them.

There is just one last topic I'd like to touch upon before leaving the antidepressants and that is the surprisingly necessary question of how to judge whether or not your antidepressant is "working." Let me give you an example of what I would call a clear response to medication.

Kyle was a bright and thoughtful man. He came to me because he was having very dark thoughts. He said that he could barely resist the impulse to drive his car into a tree. There were plenty of precipitants, most related to economic stressors and job dissatisfaction. He was already on an SSRI antidepressant when he came to see me. It was, naturally, prescribed by his PCP. He thought "maybe" the SSRI was helping but was still having suicidal thoughts. Digging a little deeper I found that Kyle, like me, was really struggling with the changes in his chosen profession. It seemed that the winners in his business were the ones who could manipulate the best and get their customers to purchase the greatest number of unnecessary products and services. Aha I thought. We will try to work this through therapeutically and philosophically. In the meantime I also changed him to a different medication, one of the SNRI's (Effexor XR). Okay, long story short: The philosophical approach really didn't hit home with Kyle but apparently the medication did. Within a month he was feeling better, no longer having dark thoughts or considering suicide. For me though, this was not enough to convince me that he was truly responding to the medication. I've seen hundreds of people report an initial positive response to antidepressants only to have the effect "wear off" shortly afterwards and then jump onto the medication merry-go-round of frequent medication adjustments and changes for years and never truly get better; but not Kyle. He maintained a positive response to the SNRI at the initial dosage for six years. We tried to get him off of the medication a couple of times but unfortunately Kyle's medicine has a rather severe withdrawal syndrome that we were never been able to get around. He did have sexual side effects but Viagra helped.

So what are the characteristics of what I personally consider indicators of a genuine response to antidepressants? Here is my list:

1. *Undeniability of positive response*: The positive response to the medication should be both clear-cut and consistent. It should be more than just numbing your emotions or decreasing your reaction to stress (more than just the "what-the-hell" effect). This inarguably positive "lifting of the cloud and feeling the desire to once again embrace life" response does happen...on occasion. It might take a week; it might take up to three months but you'll know it. I am not saying that the more non-specific effect of numbing pain is by definition a total failure of the drug but it is not the true "anti" depressant response experienced by some and will not sustain or satisfy you in the long run. Thus far there are no factors in either my personal experience or the psychiatric literature that can predict who will have a positive and lasting response to an antidepressant. Certainly it's clear that meeting DSM IV criteria for Major Depression has almost no predictive validity. Sorry.

2. *Trials of no more than three antidepressants:* Even the biopsychiatry literature supports the observation that failure on one antidepressant lessens the likelihood of response to a second. If you keep pushing the medical model too long you arrive at the concept of "treatment resistant depression." Check back to chapter six to see what this implies. (Hint: electricity, scalpels). In my mind if you don't have an unambiguous response after three medications that should stimulate more vigorous efforts to utilize non-medical ways of helping yourself.

3. *Never rely on medications alone:* Even if there is such a thing as a chemical imbalance that "causes" depression you should never try to deal with this life crisis with just medication. This is a huge problem in mental healthcare today. Many psychiatrists and nearly all PCP's rarely if ever recommend anything but medication. In following this treatment plan you will, at the least, lose an opportunity for some pain induced opportunity

for emotional growth and maturation. (It's true you know, no pain—no gain). Worse, you could end up (as so many do) just spinning your wheels, waiting for the medicine to "work."

Granted, these are not the most specific guidelines in the world, but it is the best I could come up with. It's a little easier for me to advise what to do if your PCP or therapist or psychiatrist speculates that you are "bipolar spectrum" and need a mood stabilizer. Then just follow the advice about children given earlier in the book: HIDE! Seriously…be very leery of this diagnostic speculation…no matter how much the idea of mood swings being "stabilized" appeals to you. Go back and review the material on bipolar disorder in this book; remind yourself about the terrifying yet rapidly growing trend to diagnose bipolar spectrum in young kids and everyone else. Look up the advertisements in Newsweek and Time to remind yourself about the drug companies' economic investment in the bipolar diagnosis. If that isn't enough call your pharmacy and ask how much a 30 day supply of Abilify, Seroquel or Lamictal will set you back (and compare that to the cost of leasing a nice car). Finally, review chapter seven to reacquaint yourself with the safety and side effects of mood stabilizers. Yes, Bipolar I disorder clearly needs to be treated. But that diagnosis is real obvious. The worst anti-Hippocratic medicine in psychiatry clearly involves the rest of the so-called "bipolar spectrum." 'Nuff said!

The next section in DSM IV covers all of the anxiety disorders. Let's agree on a conceptualization of anxiety before we go on. I want to start with an historical tidbit to try and help put this into perspective. Recall that I mentioned that a mere fifty years ago Freudian inspired psychodynamic psychotherapy totally dominated the mental health field. There is a concept in psychodynamic therapy called signal anxiety. The idea here is that anxiety is a signal of an unconscious emotional conflict and that the resolution of the conflict is what would ultimately result in emotional growth and progress in therapy. Today anxiety is rarely viewed that way. As Ghaemi pointed out, it is just one among the "symptoms" that biopsychiatry "treats." It would be rare indeed for a psychiatrist, PCP (or even a psychotherapist) to inquire what anxiety was signaling and pursue that conceptualization in therapy. I am not saying that the psychodynamic approach was correct or even better; I just want to remind you that mental health care is driven by the predominant theory and that this can radically change over time. Since the predominant theory is now biological, anxiety is viewed as merely a symptom. There are a number of distinct disorders described in DSM IV where anxiety is the chief symptom.

The anxiety disorders listed in DSM IV include:

1. Panic Disorder Without Agoraphobia
2. Panic Disorder With Agoraphobia
3. Specific Phobia
4. Social Phobia
5. Obsessive-Compulsive Disorder
6. Posttraumatic Stress Disorder
7. Acute Stress Disorder
8. Generalized Anxiety Disorder…and a few others.

Every one of these disorders has FDA approved medications for their treatment. Would it surprise you to know (I hope not by now) that the approved medications are, in fact, our all purpose "X factor" drugs, the serotonin antidepressants? Do they "work?" Good question. For me, it's hard to say but I will share my clinical experience and on the matter. Let's start with panic disorder.

I conceptualize a panic attack as a biological event. It is the well known fight or flight response that all animals manifest and it is built into the nervous system. A panic attack is a misfire, a setting off of the entire constellation of fight or flight responses with only one element missing: There is nothing to fight or flee from. A panic attack is arguably the most painful acute emotional experience humans have. We immediately begin to formulate plans to avoid this ever happening again. If those plans ultimately lead to trying to avoid nearly everything and refusing to even leave the house, then that has become the worst form of panic disorder that we call agoraphobia. God only knows how many housebound people there are in this country. And that is a shame because in my experience medications really help panic disorder. The serotonin antidepressants are often (but not always) effective in preventing panic attacks. The minor tranquilizers (benzodiazepines) are also effective and can actually stop a panic attack once it has started. But there are some important caveats. One is to "start low and go slow" with the antidepressants. Too large a dose at first can actually precipitate an attack. That is bad news. The patient will never take that medicine again. So, for example, with Zoloft (sertraline), here is what I do. With a target dose of 50 mg. in mind I will start the patient on a ¼ dose, 12.5 mg. the first week and then raise the dose by 12.5 mg. per week, arriving at the target dose by week four. I have seen my share of patients who have presented to emergency rooms or PCP's for their panic attacks and the doctors just didn't know this and started too high a dose which made the panic disorder worse. In genuine panic disorder I am also generous with the benzodiazepines, including the "dreaded" Xanax, a benzo that in my clinical experience is particularly effective in relieving panic. Sometimes a patient will get off Xanax once the antidepressant starts working, sometimes not. In a good number of cases the antidepressants simply don't work and the patient ends up just using the tranquilizers. But in either case, the medication only represents half the battle. And here is where biopsychiatry falls short again.

For panic disorder more than just drugs are required. Even if we conceptualize the panic attack itself as purely biological, psychological factors soon come in to play. The sufferer starts to have "anticipatory anxiety," non-panic level anxiety about having a panic attack. People, places and things that might precipitate panic (e.g. crowded stores, movie theaters, driving on the highway) start to get avoided. Medications are not going to fix this. Cognitive behavior therapy is an excellent adjunct. It has even proven effective without any medication at all. Psycho-education is essential. This means that the patient must be taught the nature of the disorder and fully understand what is going on. Sometimes further help is needed such as relaxation training, meditation, Yoga or the like. But as you can see; when it comes to panic disorder I'm pretty much in the biopsychiatry camp but, as always, believe that medication alone is not enough.

Another really nasty anxiety disorder is Obsessive Compulsive Disorder (OCD). Unfortunately this is also a condition that is widely over-diagnosed. Like so many other human traits, our degree of obsessivesness with order, neatness, cleanliness and the like is on a continuum. But where is that magic line between normalcy and pathology? Like for the rest of the psychiatric disorders it no longer seems to be related to severity of symptoms. You will often get a diagnosis of OCD simply by expressing concern to a biologically oriented mental health professional or your PCP. So it's the "make an appointment" phenomena again. Genuine OCD is, in my mind, easily diagnosed and distinguishable from problems of excessive concerns with neatness, cleanliness and order. And let me tell you, real OCD is something you wouldn't wish on your worst enemy. It is an exquisite mental torture. Again, I have no problem conceptualizing this as a biological condition. If you want to see a good cinematic depiction of OCD rent *As Good As It Gets* with Jack Nicholson. It's a pretty accurate description, including his lack of responsiveness to medication. Yes, you guessed it; the backbone of medical treatment is again our good friends, the serotonin antidepressants. Only in this case the advice is higher than usual dosages for longer periods of time.

But wait a second Dr. Phill, isn't there a medication specifically designed for OCD? I think it's called Luvox. Correct! And an interesting story. Here it is:

Luvox is the brand name for fluvoxamine and it is simply an SSRI. In fact it is the oldest SSRI, older even than Prozac. It was manufactured by Solvay pharmaceuticals but, at first, marketed only in Europe. It was first prescribed in 1983 and was at one time the most widely prescribed *antidepressant* in Europe. And yet is has never been marketed as an antidepressant in the United States? Why is that? Well, if you want to market a European drug in the United States you need to submit studies proving efficacy to the FDA. European data doesn't count. For some reason Luvox either never submitted or couldn't come up with the two "better than placebo" studies required, at least for depression. They did manage, however, to submit the necessary studies to get FDA approval for the treatment of OCD. The rest is clearly, now how did Rick Roderick put it? Oh yes: "All about that s—t called money".

The following is a list of all of the FDA approved medications for OCD. I think most will be quite familiar: Prozac, Zoloft, Paxil, Lexapro, Celexa, Luvox and one older antidepressant that is not an SSRI, Anafranil. Let's see. That's seven drugs. So how is it that Luvox has so successfully implanted itself in the minds of both doctors and consumers as *the preferred and best* treatment for OCD? Is it *more* effective? No. All approved psychiatric drugs are of equal efficacy. Is it because it is more tolerable and has fewer side effects? No, it displays the whole range of SSRI side effects. Is it because it was the first SSRI approved for OCD and therefore launched an extensive and expensive advertising campaign to influence both patients and doctors to form the *impression* that Luvox is specifically and uniquely effective in OCD? Bingo. Welcome once again to Psychiatryland! Remember the social construction of truth? These are not just obscure philosophical concepts. They are descriptions of lived reality. I really hope you totally get this by now.

So why wasn't Jack Nicholson cured? Why was he (and everyone around him) so plagued by his OCD symptoms? He had a psychiatrist. He would "drop in" on him every once in a while and in their brief dialogue it was made clear that Jack had been on trials of medication. Was it just cinematic license to keep the love story going? I bet if you think about it, you already know the answer. In my opinion, real OCD is clearly a brain illness. But when it comes to the specifics—like what part of the brain and what precisely is wrong; WE DON'T KNOW THAT FOR ANY PSYCHIATRIC ILLNESS. So throwing a serotonin raising drug at the brain…that's what we do for just about everything. It's not going to specifically *cure* anything! It might attenuate the symptoms. And, as with all complex mental problems…more is needed. In *As Good As It Gets* that "more" was the love of Helen Hunt. For her Jack was able to willfully reduce his own anxiety, even stepped on a crack in the sidewalk once. So love is the answer? All you need is love? Well… What you do need to cope with and recover from something as devastating as real OCD is understanding, concern, caring and education from support groups, specialized therapy programs and good counselors. So maybe all you do need is "love", at least in this broader sense of the word. After all, it cured my OCD…honest.

My father died when I was 9 years old. It sucked. It still does. I have very clear and distinct memories of that event in my life. And I also clearly remember what "symptoms" I developed to cope. I was in the third grade. I would sit in class and periodically violently shake my head from side to side. It was a movement that neurologists call a tic. But in my mind, unbeknownst to any observer, I was counting these head tics, trying desperately to keep track of whether there was an even or odd number of tics. I needed to have an even number. I have no idea why but that is characteristic of OCD, a sense of impending doom (the obsession) tied to completely irrational ritualistic behavior (the compulsion). The reason OCD is included in the anxiety disorders is this ungrounded fear of something terrible happening if the rituals are not carried out. I also remember thinking that somehow my rituals were invisible, that people wouldn't notice. But of course they did. Only back then, in 1960, we were not nearly as "educated" about psychiatric illnesses as we are now and neither the school nor my mother thought to take me to a counselor or doctor. Instead she took me to California. Well actually, my great uncle and aunt, in an act of true compassion, invited the whole family to come stay with them for the summer. And they gave us the full Southern California experience; the beach, Knott's Berry Farm, Disneyland, and daily visits to a Boy's Club. I was kept busy every day. I have very vivid and positive memories of that summer. My tic and counting rituals totally disappeared and never came back. That's why I am so concerned about things today. In today's world I wouldn't be given a chance to work through my brief episode of OCD. I would have been diagnosed and put on medication. For all I know, I would still be on it today. Like most psychiatric disorders, OCD is conceptualized as a chronic illness requiring chronic medical treatment. True story.

There is a specific type of therapy that is showing promise in true OCD. It's called Exposure and Response Prevention (ERP) and involves the totally simplistic yet effective intervention of making someone do a feared activity (e.g. putting their hands in dirt) but preventing the usual response (such as washing the hands) for three hours. Eventually desensitization occurs and less anxiety is produced by the feared activity or intrusive thought (Foa 1991). This is very similar to a technique used in the treatment of Post Traumatic Stress Disorder called Prolonged Exposure (PE) therapy which I will discuss in detail now.

For Post Traumatic Stress Disorder (PTSD) we need to discuss both the diagnosis and the treatment because this diagnosis is one that is particularly spinning out of control in our society. That really shouldn't be surprising since this is, after all, the ultimate "victim" narrative, and we've discussed what an attractive commodity that has become. So first, some technical issues about diagnosis. The specific diagnostic criteria for PTSD are clearly spelled out in DSM IV and then routinely violated (kind of like the routine violation of the four day duration of hypomania criteria in the diagnosis of bipolar II disorder). The first issue is the definition of trauma. What exactly qualifies as a "trauma" in DSM IV? This is an interesting topic because the definition of what constitutes a trauma has actually been changing in each edition of DSM.

In DSM III-R a trauma was defined as "an event that is outside the range of usual human experience and that would be markedly distressing to almost anyone" (DSM III-R p.250). In DSM IV the definition of trauma is "the person experienced, witnessed, or was confronted with an event or events that involved actual or threatened death or serious injury, or a threat to the physical integrity of self or others" (DSM IV p.426). I've read that the upcoming DSM V will require that the person "directly experienced, witnessed, or was confronted an event that involved actual or threatened death or serious injury, or a threat to the physical integrity of self or others."

Why all the nitpicking? Some of it, not all by any means, has to do with, once again, money. A lot of funding, especially in the Veteran's Administration, is tied to PTSD. There is a boatload of litigation every year related to the enduring emotional impact of one "trauma" or another. The big money in civil litigation is usually tied to this emotional issue. In response to this economic concern the definition has been getting more stringent. (After all, money talks). Here is an interesting true story:

I was at a meeting of some of the big names in PTSD where we discussed the following question: In relation to the horrific event of 9/11/2001, could someone watching the events unfold on television develop a DSM IV validated syndrome of PTSD? (There were actually some lawsuits against television networks for traumatizing people by replaying the pictures of the towers collapsing over and over and over again). The consensus of the meeting was that no, watching the towers attacked on television did not meet the standards for trauma set by DSM IV. So what did? In relation to 9/11 the consensus of the panel was that anybody in (of course) or in the vicinity of the towers would qualify. In addition those witnessing the collapse from afar or on television who had loved ones in or near the towers would qualify as well. This was the consensus at the meeting, not a legal finding. But let me tell you more about that meeting because that is where I really learned something about PTSD.

I've mentioned before that I was a paid speaker for Pfizer, the company that makes Zoloft. We've also previously discussed how drug companies use Phase IV (the less stringently regulated) types of studies to get new indications for an existing drug. Pfizer did just that and, in 1999, became the first SSRI antidepressant receiving FDA approval for the treatment of PTSD. (Since then Paxil has also been approved). How incredibly ironic that my "speaker's training" meeting on Zoloft for PTSD was scheduled for November 2001 *in New York City*. (The schedule had been made well in advance of the 9/11 tragedy). So there I was in New York City sitting at a PTSD meeting with researchers and clinicians who were actively involved in dealing with the emotional fallout of the 9/11 attacks. I learned a lot! I want to share what I learned at that meeting with you because it is not necessarily what you would expect.

First, you don't just jump in and "diagnose" PTSD in anyone who has emotional problems following a traumatic event. We've already discussed above how the trauma must meet certain severity criteria to qualify for PTSD. The characteristic symptoms of PTSD (which includes traumatic recall, reliving the event, nightmares, avoidance of reminders of the trauma and uncomfortable feelings of over-arousal) may not be lasting. Over half the people developing these symptoms after a trauma get better in less than 3 months, usually without any formal treatment. In fact, they might do best just being left alone! Huh? Here comes the real interesting stuff I learned at the conference. (I'll put it in a Q&A format):

Q: What about those crisis counselors who descend on mine collapses, school shootings and other tragedies; that's a good thing…right?

A: Not necessarily. That practice is called debriefing, more technically Critical Incident Stress Debriefing (CISD). I think in this culture we always feel we need to be doing *something* and the idea that professional counselors are descending on the site of a tragedy is reassuring. So I was surprised when I heard at the NYC Zoloft meeting that CISD is not all that helpful (in terms of the subsequent development of PTSD) and may, at times, do more harm than good. I remember that this research info was reinforced by counselors at the meeting who were actually *doing* therapy with firefighters and policemen and policewomen who were at Ground Zero. Many of these "clients" did not want to attend but were required to. They just wanted to be left alone to deal with their emotions with their peers and family. Probably, this is a good instinct. There is some neurobiological speculation that the traditional CISD practice of getting people to talk and talk about the traumatic event (usually very soon after its occurrence) might actually keep stress hormones like cortisol at higher levels causing more lasting and stronger connections between the memories of the trauma and the anxiety promoting parts of the brain.

Q: So what type of therapy *is* good for preventing and/or treating PTSD?

A: This was another surprise. I'd always heard, and common sense dictated, that trauma survivors need very gentle supportive treatment. After all someone who has been raped or in a serious automobile accident or survived the twin towers' collapse is rightfully understood to be fragile and vulnerable. Forcing the patient to recount or relive the trauma would seem to be the last thing you would want to do. And yet, strong research has shown that the best treatment for preventing PTSD (or reducing the symptoms if has already developed) is just that, forcing the patient to relive the traumatic event over and over again. (I know I just said that recounting the trauma in CISD can be harmful. But here we are talking about people who are voluntarily seeking help and who usually come forward weeks, months or even years after the traumatic event). The treatment I am talking about here is called Prolonged Exposure (PE) and has been developed by psychologist Dr. Edna Foa (Foa 2007). She was one of the speakers at the NYC Zoloft meeting. In prolonged exposure therapy the patient commits to nine to twelve ninety minute therapy sessions. There is psycho-education about the disorder and relaxation therapy as you might expect, but then the patient is asked to verbally recount a detailed version of the trauma into a tape recorder. If there is time left, the patient does it again. He or she is then instructed to *listen to the tape* over and over again at home prior to the next session. In the next session, the same process is repeated! In addition the patient is often asked to approach the site of the trauma even though this produces anxiety. The bottom line is; PE works. The goal in this therapy is to reduce the ongoing emotional impact of the trauma (the PTSD symptoms) by desensitizing the brain's connection between the memory and anxiety through sheer repetition. How do I know it works? Because the research says it does.

Whoa…hold on Dr. Phill. You can't have it both ways. First you criticize research and then you use it as support for treatment recommendations. What gives?

What gives is that the research on PTSD is, in my mind, more valid because the specific symptoms being tracked are so easily distinguished from everyday emotional problems such as depression and anxiety. Core symptoms of PTSD—reliving the experience, flashbacks, nightmares about the trauma, and avoidance of reminders of the trauma—are unique to PTSD and are simply not part of everyday human life.

Q: Okay, so what about the pills?

A: It is true that Zoloft and Paxil did get FDA approval for the treatment of PTSD. However, from all I've seen and read, these medications, at best, have a modest benefit, usually by reducing general feelings of depression and anxiety often associated with PTSD but not necessarily the core symptoms of the disorder. It is clearly wrong, to "treat" PTSD with *just* medication but, as you know, the medical community typically responds to FDA approval and the subsequent advertising campaigns launched by the drug company and their cadre of "experts", by endorsing the medications as curative and implying that the meds are all that is needed. Believe me, they are not! So remember... as always...be afraid...and think for yourself.

It's time to go on to the next anxiety diagnosis, Generalized Anxiety Disorder (GAD).We'll start our GAD discussion like I do with my patients, by talking about a couple of animals: squirrels and lions. Picture a squirrel in your mind. Can you imagine a more nervous looking creature? Give a squirrel a freshly cooked cashew and the poor thing will still not be able to relax for two seconds to savor it. Now picture a male lion. How many times have we seen wildlife films in which the lion is actually yawning he is so relaxed (and probably a little bored)? You couldn't think of two more polar opposite animals on the nervousness spectrum. But how do they get that way? We all know that squirrels are prey and lions are predators but how do *they* know? Do they learn through life experience? Do they learn it in squirrel or lion school? Of course not; they are born that way. This means that built into the nervous system of these two animals, biologically hard wired, are two very different baseline levels of vigilance, scanning and senses of danger...what we call in humans, anxiety. I use this story when I see patients (and I see quite a few) who are looking for relief from the anxieties and worries that plague their every waking moment.

Generalized Anxiety Disorder is "officially" diagnosed using the following DSM IV criteria:

A. Excessive anxiety and worry (apprehensive expectation), occurring more days than not for at least 6 months, about a number of events or activities (such as work or school performance).
B. The person finds it difficult to control the worry.
C. The anxiety and worry are associated with three (or more) of the following six symptoms (with at least some symptoms present for more days than not for the past 6 months). **Note:** Only one item is required in children.
1. restlessness or feeling keyed up or on edge

2. being easily fatigued
3. difficulty concentrating or mind going blank
4. irritability
5. muscle tension
6. sleep disturbance (difficulty falling or staying asleep, or restless unsatisfying sleep)

Getting back to the first issue illustrated by contrasting squirrels and lions; is it possible that some humans are hardwired at birth for a higher level of baseline anxiety than others? I would say yes but since environment starts to interact with biology at birth, who can really say? From a Darwinian point of view it seems that a certain level of vigilance and apprehension would be an adaptive trait as compared to recklessness and unbridled confidence. But there is no doubt that some people, usually later but sometimes early on in life, find themselves racked with worry and anxiety. As I've said before, anxiety is a noxious emotion but what can (or should) be done about it? I can tell you the first thing…throw out DSM IV and *talk to the patient.* Aside from insurance coverage issues there is absolutely no value to "making" the diagnosis of GAD. When anxiety is the chief complaint the problem can be anything from existential angst (more on this in the next chapter) to not being able to sell a house in the current market downturn. But this chapter is about medication so we need to look at the medication issue, (to pill or not to pill?), in relation to a chief complaint of generalized anxiety.

Are there FDA approved medications for GAD? Once again, does a bear poop in the woods? Are the approved medications serotonin antidepressants? ONCE AGAIN, does a bear poop in the woods? It's almost amusing isn't it, the games drug companies play? That is amusing to everyone except the patients of course, in whom the "trial" of an SSRI might skyrocket their anxiety to new, never before experienced, heights of intensity.

Again, this is my twenty eight years of clinical experience talking. The FDA has approved Paxil, Lexapro and Effexor XR for the treatment of GAD. I have seen my fair share of patients who meet the diagnostic criteria for this disorder. But it is my impression that these antidepressants rarely "work" as the sole intervention. And they sometimes, especially early in treatment, make the person feel worse. And that includes a couple of my patients who experienced such acute levels of unbearable anxiety after the first or second dose that they actually reported considering suicide. You know that there are more and more warnings about antidepressants possibly causing suicidality. If someone asked for my opinion on the topic I would say that when this does occur it is sometimes related to these drugs precipitating an unbearable level of anxiety more than somehow worsening depression.

Alan was a pleasant man in his mid-eighties that I treated. He was clearly a classic case of GAD with a few panic attacks thrown in. He gave a history of anxiety problems for 35 years. The mainstay of his treatment was Valium, which he had been taking for over thirty years. But each time he would change doctors there would be a reassessment of his treatment plan so even after three decades he still had some cognitive discomfort about taking the Valium (but not too much, especially in light of his experiences on serotonin antidepressants). Once someone had tried him on Prozac and after one dose he felt like committing suicide. Just prior to first seeing me his PCP responded to his anxiety complaints (he never stops complaining) by giving him Lexapro. Once again one dose made him feel suicidal. One time when he came in to see me he presented me with a written list of new complaints, all related to current stressors in his life. He also had a sample pack of Effexor XR. This sample pack had fourteen pills. Only one pill was missing; the one he took that made him feel like committing suicide.

Alan has never been in therapy. To be honest I think there is sometimes some truth to the adage that you can't teach an old dog new tricks. All I ever tried to do was be supportive of him taking Valium and alleviate him worrying about being addicted to it. I think it might be a real good idea not to try Alan on any more antidepressants.

So what about the benzodiazepines, Xanax, Ativan, Valium and the like? Are these good treatments for GAD? I can tell you one thing, I have seen boatloads of people taking these drugs for anxiety; some of them have been on these minor tranquilizers for decades! The research literature might not encourage this practice, but the patients swear by it. As discussed in chapter six, these antianxiety drugs, the benzo's, have a well understood mechanism of action and generally will relieve anxiety, but how sedated and muddle-headed they can make you presents problems. I prescribe a lot of benzodiazepines. I don't believe that for the vast majority of patients the chronic use of benzo's represents any kind of addiction in the traditional sense. The "socially constructed truth" on the other hand, is leaning heavily in that direction. It's kind of sad to see a seventy three year old patient forced to anguish about whether or not they are "addicted" to the 1mg twice a day of Ativan they have been taking for thirty years. But this is not really my major concern when confronted with the chronically anxious worrier we label as having GAD. My concern is more the paradoxical issue and moral dilemma I face.

Paradoxical issue: GAD type people worry. They tend to worry about everything. And that includes their bodies and anything they are putting into them, including medications *for* anxiety! So the paradox is that by trying to medically treat anxiety, you are actually giving that person another thing to worry about. Sometimes the medication and its possible side effects become the *primary* thing they worry about. How do I know? Because I get the phone calls!

Marion is an eighty four year old woman who came to see me once every three months for refills on her anxiety medications. She first came to me having been on these medications, Celexa and Ativan, for years. What's amusing is what we'd talk about on every medication-check visit. Marion is a tiny woman married to a tiny man. They are a sweet couple who obviously love each other. They have been married for 60 years. The topic of conversation is invariably about the medication doses. Like many of my anxiety patients, Marion was convinced that the precise dose of medication was crucial and she would frequently self-adjust the dose and timing of her medicines. Also, like many of my anxiety patients, (especially the elderly), she liked to break her pills into little pieces, often taking ¼ or ½ of the recommended dose. The offshoot of this is that in our fifteen minutes together, Marion and her husband and I typically would talk about only one thing—her new dosing strategies and the physical symptoms she and he thought that this might be causing. "I've been burping a lot lately doctor. Is that caused by Celexa?"

Phil was a fifty two year old man, a real worrier who I saw for about two years. "Consumed by worry" clearly described this gentleman. I'm detailing his case because he really *worried about his medication and gave me permission to quote parts of a note he brought on one of his visits. The note was composed by the patient and his girlfriend. It illustrates not only my contention that the use of antidepressants in GAD gives patients something else to anguish about but also shows how in the "information age" we keep getting way more "facts" than we can handle.*

When Phil came to me he was already on Prozac and Xanax prescribed by his PCP. The problem at that time was that under some new stresses he had used up his 30 day supply of Xanax in less than two weeks and when he called his doctor for an early refill he was referred to me. Phil clearly had the worry disease, big time, but was not motivated to do therapy or buy the Midwest Center program. He just wanted his Xanax and I gave it to him. He continued to get his Prozac from his PCP who he would see once a year and get a one month prescription with eleven refills. But then an article in the paper caught his girlfriend's eye. (Keep in mind he had been on Prozac for five years). The article was apparently one of the many written in the last few years about problems with SSRI's but for some reason this one precipitated writing me a two page note full of questions and concerns. Here are some excerpts from that note:

"Report——Prozac could be a stimulant that could over stimulate the central nervous system, worsening depression."

"Phil is wondering if Prozac is over-stimulating him causing anxiety nervousness and butterflies?"

Then she handed me a bulleted list of his many recent symptoms:

- *patients were given sedatives to reduce Prozac's stimulation*
- *drinking water excessively*
- *Loss of appetite, upset stomach, diarrhea with blood.*
- *Weight loss, easily up to five lbs. in one week*
- *Difficulty sleeping/ obsessive thinking (mind racing)*
- *Sleep pattern worsening over last two months*
- *Purchase of new car (impulsive) caused anxiety*
- *Dept. of Revenue letter shows careless disregard for potential problem*
- *After sugary dessert experiences heart palpitations"*

Here are two of the questions asked at the end of the note:

"Could Prozac be over stimulating him and causing some of these issues?"

"Considering the meds he is taking, shouldn't this help him deal with situations like this car ordeal in a healthier manner?"

In case you are ever wondering about my over-hyping the distorted thinking and psychological impact of the domination of the biopsychiatry business in our daily lives, see the above question. I need to remind you that Phil had been on Prozac for five years before sending me this list of questions. Five years!! His relationship with Prozac and psychiatry was not lifelong. Phil had a difficult and dangerous job during most of his adult life and did not experience significant anxiety. It was only after some very stressful life events, a botched surgery with lasting disability and a very nasty divorce that he turned to psychotropics; without, I might add any clear-cut or lasting benefits; which brings me to the moral dilemma:

What am I doing when I go along with Marion's and Phil's focus on medication for anxiety? I do believe that giving a highly anxious person a calming medication is an act of compassion. But am I also directly endorsing what Lewis labeled the "take a pill and shut up" phenomenon? I believe that in many ways I am. Most of my anxious patients have legitimate reasons to be anxious. They have suffered a lot of losses and traumas in life. I even have a pet theory I call "trauma accumulation." I believe that traumatic experiences register in the nervous system and change us. I believe that the longer we live the more traumas we accumulate. And I believe that trauma accumulation manifests itself in every human being as the loss of ability to be what I call "stupid happy." This is similar to the notion of "cheeriness" as a normative expectation that Greenspan mentions in her critique of American psychiatry (more about her in the next chapter). So as we spend more time on this Earth we grow a little sadder (or madder or anxious) but wiser. Only who values wisdom anymore? We just want to be cheery! So, go to good old Dr. Phill and get some pills. After all there is really nowhere else to go.

What I am really morally concerned about is what Lewis notes when he says that biopsychiatry, in dealing with human pain "erases its social aspects—injustice, oppression, lack of opportunity, lack of social resources, neglected infrastructures, and systematic prejudices" (Lewis 2006 p.134). Because I believe that regardless of the level of baseline biological or childhood related anxiety my patients have, the society we live in is truly anxiety producing for everybody. Nearly all the patients I see for anxiety and depression have one complaint in common…stress. They complain bitterly and ceaselessly about stress. It could be family problems, job problems, economic problems, legal problems, most often a combination of stressors that has me silently expressing gratitude that I am not in their shoes. But here is my question. What do they want me, a doctor, to do about it? Why are they here? Big Pharma and biopsychiatry have taught them that they aren't stressed, they are ill. And I have the pills to make them better.

I don't need to list all of the stressors rooted in the social and societal problems elaborated above by Dr. Lewis. We all know all about the stress of modern American life. I just want to talk about one uniquely American stressor here. To start I will recall a scene from one of my favorite comedies called *What About Bob?* I hope you've seen it. In the scene I am referring to Richard Dreyfus, the psychiatrist, writes out a prescription for the incredibly needy Bill Murray, the titular patient Bob. On the prescription is written "Take a vacation…from your troubles." I think of that scene because I often feel the urge to write a similar but shorter prescription for many of my patients. It would simply say "Take a vacation." Or, maybe "For God's sake TAKE A VACATION!" I don't write that prescription. Most could not "fill it" anyhow because in America we don't take vacations.

In the spring of 2007 the Center for Economic and Policy Research published a report titled *No-Vacation Nation* (Ray 2007). That report detailed something that most Americans already know (that we don't take vacations) and something that we didn't know (nearly everyone else in the industrialized world does!) The facts were downright astounding. Most European countries give everyone four to six weeks of paid vacation a year. Americans *might* get two weeks if they have been with an employer long enough, but the majority of workers do not even use all of their vacation days. And those that do stress out about being away from work. I saw a lot of young people in my practice.

As a rule, they were rarely mentally "ill" and didn't truly require medication. They needed VACATIONS; they needed less stress; they needed more hope; they needed more feelings of security and safety; they needed feelings of dignity and worth where they worked. Instead, they get Zoloft or Xanax so that they can keep functioning under the stress. I feel really sad and bad about this. The last line in the note from my patient Phil and his girlfriend reads:

"*Week of vacation—July 7—14 he was fine—no sleep or stomach issue. He was happy and relaxed.*"

Now here is a big surprise. My stressed out, overworked, non-vacationing patients have trouble sleeping. Who would have guessed? Gee Doctor, does that mean they have a DSM IV sleeping disorder? Well let's think about this for a minute. Millions of people are having trouble sleeping in our high stress society. That *must* be a brain illness. What else could possibly account for it? I know what...let's give them some pills!

Yes, there is a multi-billion dollar sleeping pill market out there. I was a speaker for a number of years for the company that makes Ambien. Because of that I got a lot of education about the science of sleep and I must say it is fascinating stuff. Sleep scientists have stronger scientific data than psychiatry... they can actually demonstrate reproducible records of pathological processes on sleep studies (polysomnograms). I have a book called *The International Classification of Sleep Disorders, Second Edition* published by the American Academy of Sleep Medicine in 2005. Unlike the DSM IV which gives short shrift to sleep disorders (there are only 18 coded diagnoses), the sleep disorder manual lists over 80 different disorders; some of them with names you just wouldn't believe. (One of them, I kid you not, is Exploding Head Syndrome. In this disorder the sufferer "complains of a sudden loud noise or sense of explosion in the head either at the wake-sleep transition or upon waking during the night"). The study of sleep and sleep disorders is fascinating and with all of the intricate brain mechanisms involved, it's a wonder that "sleep" works at all. But this chapter is about medication and I'm afraid that when it comes to sleep and sleep medicines the insomnia business is a lot like the depression and anxiety business... many disorders, few treatments.

When I gave my talks for Ambien about the treatment of sleep disorders we would always have a slide or two on non-pharmacological treatments. Similar to the treatment suggestions for depression and anxiety it was always "officially" promoted that combined drug and non-drug treatments were the best. Among the recommended non-drug treatments were some that we've already discussed such as cognitive behavior therapy and relaxation training. These were particularly targeted at those with the most common sleep complaint, difficulty falling asleep. Patients would most often complain that they simply couldn't stop thinking and worrying about everything. (I would always tell them to stop watching the 11PM news. What is with the "news"? They make it sound like the world is constantly dangerous for every adult, child and pet on the planet. Ease up a bit would you?) My recommendation to stop watching the news is part of a larger sleep-disorder-specific set of recommendations called sleep hygiene therapy.

Sleep hygiene is a list of mostly common sense recommendations about getting a good night's sleep. For example, if you exercise, don't do it in the evening if you then have trouble sleeping; don't nap during the day; don't drink caffeinated beverages after 12PM; keep the bedroom dark, quiet, cool and comfortable…things like that. Research however showed that sleep hygiene education alone didn't do much to improve sleep. Stimulus control therapy did.

Stimulus control therapy is based on the principles of classical conditioning, first espoused by Pavlov (the guy with the dogs). The basic principle here is that after a few nights with trouble sleeping we start to experience "sleep performance anxiety" and begin to condition a negative association between our bedroom and sleeping. This begins to manifest itself as the common problem of going to bed feeling tired and then having your eyes pop open as soon as your head hits the pillow. Sleep is fitful throughout the night. Patients will report precise waking times: "I woke up at 1:17, 2:35, 3:56 and 5:12 AM." That means that they are fully awakening and consciously registering the time on the clock. That is a good sign of ongoing negative conditioning. Here is what stimulus control therapy recommends:

1. Go to bed only when sleepy. If unable to fall asleep within ten to fifteen minutes get out of bed and go into another room to read or watch TV until sleepy again. Do this anytime you wake up during the night.
2. Get up at the same time every day, even on weekends.
3. Use the bed only for sleeping and sexual relations. No TV, no reading and certainly no work projects.
4. No napping during the day

These simple steps have proven effective in chronic insomnia if you follow them. Notice how, once again, like in successful cognitive therapy, work and effort and motivation are required on the part of the patient. So, being realistic, let's wrap this up by looking at the "pill or not to pill" question.

There are plenty of chemicals that people take to help themselves sleep. Number one is alcohol but this is a bad idea. Alcohol sedates you and helps you get to sleep but then tends to turn on you, giving you what's called fractured sleep with abnormal sleep stages. The sleep on alcohol is non-restorative as anyone sleeping off a bender can attest.

Over the counter sleeping pills generally contain diphenhydramine. It is an antihistamine sold for allergies under brand names such as Benadryl. When used for allergies the sedation this medicine produces is seen as an unwanted side effect (refer to Claritin commercials). As a sleep aid, the drying of the mucous membranes (the antihistamine effect) is seen as the unwanted side effect. A lot of people use this medication to sleep. The main problem is that its effects are often felt long after sleep. I call it the "waking up with your head in a fishbowl" phenomenon. Also, some people have an opposite response where the diphenhydramine causes feelings of awakeness and restlessness. Judging from the continued prevalence of expensive TV commercials advertising products such as Tylenol PM and Advil PM I would guess a lot of people use these drugs regularly. Now let's talk about the heavy hitters.

Drugs *prescribed* for insomnia fall into three classes:

1. Sedating Antidepressants
2. Benzodiazepine Hypnotics
3. Non-benzodiazepine Hypnotics.

With the sedating antidepressants we are again seeing the phenomena of what used to be a dose limiting side effect, sedation, now being seen as the desired effect. The antidepressant most commonly used for sleep is Trazadone although Elavil and Sinequan also work well. Of interest here are the dosing strategies. For example, with Trazadone it might take up to 300mg. for an antidepressant effect where for sleep as little as 25mg is sometimes effective. Imagine how sedated patients being treated for depression used to feel. Also with Trazadone there is a warning similar to the ones in commercials for Cialis and Viagra—the "erection lasting more than four hours" warning. This is called priapism and really isn't amusing at all because this condition can result in penis disfigurement and lifetime impotency. I rarely prescribe Trazadone to males for that reason (because there are other choices).

The benzodiazepines are the anti-anxiety drugs we have previously discussed. These drugs are all sedating and any of them can be used as sleeping pills. The ones most commonly prescribed are known by the brand names Restoril and Dalmane but have been available for years as generics as well.

Finally there are the non-benzodiazepine hypnotics. How did they come up with that name? If they are not benzo's, why include that terminology in what you call them? That's like calling tea the non-coffee morning hot beverage. Well the reason is actually similar to the relationship of tea to coffee, the active ingredient. Non-benzodiazepine hypnotics work just like benzodiazepine anti-anxiety medicines only they *selectively* stimulate the sedating brain cell receptors more than the anxiety brain cell receptors. These drugs have the trade names Ambien, Sonata and Lunesta (as seen endlessly on TV). When Ambien first came out a lot of us felt like they had invented a perfect drug. It seemed to treat only the desired symptoms, the inability to sleep. It had very few side effects and there seemed to be little if any decrement in effect over time. There also seemed to be no withdrawal symptoms even though it was a Class IV controlled substance. I loved this drug in my clinical practice because it often gave immediate and extremely helpful symptom relief to my depressed and anxious patients. In fact, I remain intrigued by the idea that sometimes insomnia is the cause of depression, not the other way around as commonly believed. This is because the psychological, cognitive and physical impact of sleep deprivation is so clear. As I remind my patients, to get prisoners of war to break down and talk, we deprive them of sleep.

Ah, but, once again, the bloom does come off the rose, doesn't it? If you've been watching the news or reading the papers you know that there have been some major concerns expressed about the possible dangerous side effects of Ambien and Lunesta and Sonata. There have even been reports of people "sleep driving" on these compounds. They certainly induce amnesia and that in and of itself is disconcerting. So the question for both the doctors and patients is what to do if these pills genuinely help you sleep and that your sleep stinks without them. Can and should they be used chronically?

I *am not* going to answer that question. I am not going to answer any more questions grounded in the domination of medical model psychiatry and its singular focus on drugs. I'm sick of it, in my office and in this book. There is a term used in existential philosophy that describes my feeling about this. It's from the philosopher Soren Kierkegaard: "Sickness Unto Death." Levin defines this as "a sickness in which the Self experiences itself as unwhole, split beyond consolation, and threatened with the specters of a deepening and even more hellish disintegration" (Levin 1987 p.23). That's how I am feeling about the extent to which I am forced to "be" a biopsychiatrist. So I am done—that's it. We are going to switch discourses now and for the rest of this book. So take a deep breath because we are now going to embark on a very different narrative about being a human in early twenty first century America. Our story starts with a completely different concept of modernity that emphasizes the *human price* we pay for our technologically advanced world.

Chapter Twelve:
SO...WHAT'S YOUR STORY?
The "Consumer" Narrative

> I believe that in the post-World War II era in the United States, there are indications that the *present* configuration of the bounded masterful self is the ***empty self***. By this I mean that our terrain has shaped a self that experiences a significant absence of community, tradition, and shared meaning. It experiences these social absences and their consequences "interiorly" as a lack of personal conviction and worth, and it embodies the absences as a chronic undifferentiated emotional hunger. The post-World War II self thus yearns to acquire and consume as an unconscious way of compensating for what has been lost: ***It is empty.***
>
> **Phillip Cushman**
> *Why the Self is Empty*

> There is a spiritual hunger in the world today—
> And it can't be satisfied by better cars on longer credit terms.
>
> **Adlai E. Stevenson**

Our goal in this chapter is to develop a new "storyline" for you to use as a framework (narrative structure) to understand your life, your pains and your joys, and to help you, when needed, to heal and grow. The dominant "storyline" that exists in our culture, that you are merely a complex biological "machine", is clearly damaging and has led to the unchallenged domination of medical model psychiatry and its reductionistic and dehumanizing approach to emotional pain. Our new storyline is suggested by Phillip Cushman's concept of the "empty self."

The quotes by Cushman and Stevenson summarize the central paradox of the empty self narrative. The paradox I am alluding to is that modern society and the global economy have mandated the configuration of an "empty self" to serve as the foundation for the constant mindless consumption required to keep capitalistic economies thriving. And yet, this manufactured "emptiness" can never be satisfied by consumption. We have talked about this throughout this book. We have seen the terms alienation, spiritual emptiness, nihilism, the "herd" and "standing reserve" used by our great thinkers to describe the human condition in modern capitalistic western societies. And I have seen, in my practice and in the field of psychiatry, the emergence and dominance of a consumable commodity designed to fill the emptiness, namely psychiatric diagnoses and medications, promising (but not delivering) relief from our sorry state. But I said in the introduction that there is hope, there is always hope. To *gain access* to the resources that offer this hope however, you, the reader, must be able to see, accept and then step back from your condition as an "empty self." To do this, we need to look more closely at what Cushman is talking about.

As I've said previously, when Heidegger used the term "standing reserve' and Nietzsche used the term "the herd" to describe modern western humanity they were not being critical, just painfully honest. The same is true for Cushman. He sees the development of the "empty self" as an inevitable consequence of the post World War II economy:

> I believe that after the war the configuration of the empty self coalesced and finally became predominant as a consequence of the loss of community and in order to match the needs of a new economy. Without this particular self, America's consumer-based economy (and it's charismatically oriented political process) would be inconceivable. New discourses and practices such as the advertising industry and the field of psychology were modified in order to respond to and further develop the new configuration of the self. Practitioners in both fields are placed in the position of being responsible for curing the empty self without being allowed to address the historical causes of the emptiness through structural societal changes
>
> (Cushman 1990, p.603).

You may recognize how the social construction of reality that we discussed in chapter nine is the basic philosophical foundation in Cushman's ideas. So beyond society's "construction" of empty selves there would naturally be a socially constructed response to meet the needs of empty selves. Cushman outlines these in a section of his paper titled "Advertising and the Life-Style Solution." Do I need to say more? This is already familiar territory. Remember my quote from Rick Roderick about how the only thing left resembling the shared human spirit (geist) is advertising?

So where do we go from here? I'm choosing Phillip Cushman's narrative of the empty self to replace the medical model narrative to account the epidemic of the "depression and anxiety disorders" plaguing our society. Yet I am saying (and have said before) that we can never truly rise above and separate from the cultural configuration of reality that we were born into and are bathed in twenty-four hours a day. But we can *modify* it.

Recognizing and modifying the empty self narrative framework opens the door for the pursuit of a more fulfilling and emotionally satisfying life that does not rely exclusively on "things", including medical doctors and psychotropic medications. From that perspective let's begin our examination of the alternatives that I have told you are ***already in place*** in our culture that offer other ways to heal and grow.

Since I cannot exhaustively cover every alternative to mainstream psychiatry I am going to organize my guide into two general categories. The first category is options *within* the field of psychology that, therefore, have a scholarly literature, professional practitioners and some research validation. The second category will be options *outside* of the academic world of psychology and will include what might be called mystical, "new age" or simply spiritual perspectives. Specifically I will be discussing the following options:

Within Psychology:
1. Positive Psychology
2. Cognitive Behavior and Rational Emotive Therapy
3. Philosophical/Existential Psychotherapy
4. Postmodern theories and therapies (constructivism, social constructionism and narrative therapy)

Outside Psychology:
1. Spiritual healing as articulated by Carolyn Myss
2. Spiritual healing as articulated by Miriam Greenspan

This should be enough to get you started. Don't forget, there is still one chapter to go where I will deal in great detail with the widespread and readily available Twelve Step programs of recovery.

We will start with the relatively new discipline called positive psychology.

As my reference I will be using the book *A Primer in Positive Psychology* written by Christopher Peterson, published in 2006 by the Oxford University Press. According to Peterson, positive psychology as a distinct discipline was first named in 1998. The driving force behind this was psychologist Martin Seligman, past president of the American Psychological Association. As defined by Peterson, positive psychology does embrace scientism and, according to him, does not struggle against DSM dominated psychiatry. He says: "Great strides have been made in understanding, treating, and preventing psychological disorders. Widely accepted classification manuals—the *Diagnostic and Statistical Manual of Mental Disorders (DSM)*...and the *International Classification of Diseases (ICD)*...allow disorders to be described and have given rise to a family of reliable assessment strategies. There now exist effective treatments, psychological and pharmacological, for more than a dozen disorders that in the recent past were frighteningly intractable" (Peterson 2006, p.5).

As you might guess, I am not totally "on board" with the philosophical underpinnings of positive psychology and its uncritical acceptance of the medical model of psychopathology. But I've included it in my list of alternatives because they have, at least, turned the "scientistic" gaze to the study of topics like the good life, human flourishing and happiness—and have come up with some interesting findings. Put succinctly by Peterson, positive psychology "is the study of what makes life worth living." Using questionnaires, psychological scales and experiments, positive psychology explores aspects of human existence that are not the focus of a pathology-based psychology and are generally simply taken for granted. Based on the chapter headings in *A Primer in Positive Psychology* topics studied include:

1. Pleasure and Positive Experience
2. Happiness
3. Positive Thinking
4. Character Strengths
5. Values
6. Interests, Abilities and Accomplishments
7. Wellness
8. Positive Interpersonal Relationships

This makes for some very interesting reading and opens up new aspects in clinical care. Rather than just relieving pain and returning the client to the previous level of functioning (the stated goal of medical model psychiatry), positive psychology has set the stage to go beyond that in therapy and focus on learning how to make life better. I see this as an important change in direction in both academic and clinical psychology. (Do some googling to find positive psychology practitioners in your area).

A much more established school of thought in psychology that also maintains a linkage to scientism is Cognitive Behavior Therapy (CBT) and its close cousin, Rational Emotive Therapy (RET). Throughout this book I've mentioned a self help CBT program called the Midwest Center for Stress and Anxiety. What these programs share in common is the basic premise that it matters what we think. You might say, "no duh", but historically CBT arose in response to a very powerful school of thought in psychology called behaviorism that basically postulated that it doesn't matter what we think, that we are merely creatures of habit, conditioned by our biology and our environment. You might have heard of one of the major proponents of behaviorism, B. F. Skinner.

Have you ever played a slot machine, dropping quarter after quarter into the thing and barely looking up when you win a few back; almost always losing in the end but unable to stop? What the heck is that? It is psychology, specifically, an application of the principles of behaviorism. The power of the slot machine to shape our behavior (and take all our money) is based in the way it rewards us for continuing to feed in our quarters. There is a certain type of schedule of rewards built into the slot machine. In technical terms it is called a random schedule of intermittent positive reinforcement. It is the most powerful behavior shaping system of rewards ever devised. The formal psychological theory that emphasizes the role of external rewards (and punishments) affecting and conditioning our behavior includes both classical conditioning (like Pavolv's dogs) and operant conditioning which uses various schedules of rewards and punishments to reinforce or extinguish behaviors. Behaviorism employs a simple formula involving the Stimulus (S) and Response (R); S → R. But what happens in between? What happens is merely a "reflex", conditioned by biology and the environment. Behaviorism held a dominant position in the field of psychology for many years and influenced everything from teaching mentally retarded children to punishing criminals to major marketing plans. But it always seemed like something was missing. Psychologists were wary of treating the mind like a mysterious "black box" and behavior theory and treatment strategies were eventually supplanted by Cognitive Behavior Therapy (notice that the role of "shaping behavior" is still included). Where learning theory was summarized by S → R, CBT was as easy as A→B→C.

In CBT and RET the basic theoretical concept is that a stimulus, now called an Antecedent event (A) results in a Consequence (C) after processing by the mind's Belief system (B). So A leads to C after processing by B. Clearly more descriptive of lived reality, CBT monitored the entire process of how stimuli result in a consequence, be it an action or emotion. The linchpin of cognitive theory is that for those experiencing negative emotions or maladaptive behavior, the thoughts and beliefs underlying them are accessible and can be modified. The general idea is that painful emotions and maladaptive behaviors arise from beliefs and thoughts that are themselves negative and maladaptive. And what characterizes these negative thoughts and beliefs is their *irrationality.*

Yes, our old friend rationality lies at the core of CBT and RET theory and therapy. And you know that rationality is a "worry-word" for me because it brings us back into the enlightenment project and scientism. CBT and RET do, in fact lend themselves nicely to the pseudoscientific research surrounding the pseudoscientific diagnoses in DSM. So, for example, a study can be designed that compares the "efficacy" of CBT versus medication in major depressive disorder. This does not push mental healthcare fully in the right direction but it does, at least, offer an alternative to a purely biochemical approach. I've mentioned CBT versus meds before as well as CBT augmenting medication with the 85% response rate in the Serzone study. I want to acquaint you with some of the content of CBT and RET but first I do have to tell you a bit about how they structured the Serzone study because it is such an excellent example of the distortion of normal human experience that scientism imposes on our mental healthcare "studies."

The belief in science is that all of the treatments being studied in an experiment need to be standardized. In other words, everyone in the study gets *exactly* the same treatment or the results will be invalid. Of course, when it comes to pills that is no big problem; everyone takes X milligrams of this or that chemical. But how do you standardize therapy? Does everyone need to see the same therapist? Obviously that would not be possible in a study with a meaningful number of subjects. The only way to standardize therapy then is to try to "standardize" (dehumanize) the therapists. And in the Serzone study, that is exactly what they did.

For the Serzone study they used a very specific form of CBT called the Cognitive Behavioral-Analysis System of Psychotherapy. The details of the therapy aren't important here; what matters is how they attempted to standardize it. Each therapist in the study was taught how to deliver this particular form of CBT without bringing their "selves" as individual therapists into the session. The sessions were monitored and videotaped. If a therapist was judged to deviate from the standard therapy they were either retrained or dismissed from the study. So was this dehumanizing and reductionistic? Did the effort to use the scientific method distort the results of the study? Does a bear poop in the woods?

I couldn't resist this opportunity to once again acquaint you with the consequences of scientism in psychiatry but let's move on. You know already that I try to get a number of my patients to access CBT and bemoan the fact that it is not readily available from psychotherapists. The reason is that when it comes down to a choice between putting all of your eggs in the medical model basket or expanding your ideas about emotional wellbeing by utilizing a program of therapy that meets the needs of the American mindset (which demands "naming" and "fixing" problems), CBT wins over the exclusive medical model hands down. So let me give you a very brief look at the value of a cognitive therapy program.

Suzy is a young woman who came to me seeking help for obsessive compulsive symptoms. She only saw me sporadically and did, one time, choose to try medication. I didn't feel very strongly that medication would help her but as I explained before, I lay out my beliefs for the patient and let them decide whether or not to go the biological route. I also insisted she get the book "Brain Lock" to do some self-help cognitive type therapy. But things didn't work out so well for her. She struggled to make a living and struggled to maintain a relationship. She complained of feeling "depressed" and hopeless and even had some suicidal thoughts while drunk.

One thing I noticed about Suzy from the beginning was that she had a chip on her shoulder and I clearly felt some entitlement vibes from her. I have a very sensitive radar to picking up on patients who like to present me with a wide range of problems in living and then get angry when I don't present an all-encompassing medical conceptualization and solution that works on the first try. (There really is a LOT of pressure to prescribe psychiatric meds coming at doctors from all sides). But why was Suzy so angry and entitled? Because, in her mind, after years of "abusive and traumatic" experiences, she believed that she was truly damaged goods.

Suzy had what is called a "yes-but" response to all of the recommendations I made. "Yes doctor, I understand your recommendation but..." Suzy was not aware she was doing this. Her self-defeating attitude just came out ***automatically.*** *And that is a very big part of CBT, monitoring our so-called automatic thoughts.*

The basic theory in CBT (and RET) is that our moment to moment thoughts that occur spontaneously in response to activating events are rooted in and reflect our beliefs about ourselves and the world around us. The belief that underlay Suzy's "yes-but" automatic responses could be characterized as something like "I am so damaged that I cannot ever be well." You can imagine how living in a culture full of "victim" narratives could easily lead to that being a core belief. And yes Suzy did have a lot of struggles and traumas early in life. But the *extremity* and *rigidity* of her belief that she was beyond repair is what CBT therapists would identify as a core "irrational" belief. In therapy

Suzy would be taught to monitor and record her automatic thoughts as a part of the homework that I've discussed as necessary in CBT. The therapist would then help her see how many of her automatic self defeating thoughts arise from a core irrational belief about being unfixable. She would then be taught a more rational belief such as: "Yes, it's sad that I've had a number of traumatic experiences in my life, but so have many others and that doesn't mean I can never be fulfilled or happy." She would then be instructed to substitute, through practice, the more rational belief whenever an event triggered her self-defeating attitude (and depressed and anxious feelings).

This is the crux of CBT and RET. The following are examples of some of the core irrational beliefs (and related patterns of thinking) frequently encountered in depressed and anxious clients:

1. I must always be perfect (perfectionism)
2. I've failed in the past so I will never succeed (overgeneralization)
3. He/She doesn't love me, therefore I'm unlovable (magnification)
4. I can just tell my new roommate doesn't like me (mind reading)
5. Big deal, so I got one A this semester (disqualifying the positive)

These are just a few examples. There are literally hundreds of core irrational beliefs identified in CBT. I think there are people for whom CBT or RET are the best treatments for emotional pain. It is a very different approach from simply submitting passively to chemical manipulation by a doctor. Are the two compatible? In a sense the answer is yes but I am concerned that the utilization of medication will both distort and minimize the power of the self healing that CBT alone can teach. Ideally, in many cases

a concerted effort to recover with CBT alone should precede any consideration of a trial of medication. But can I tell you how likely that is to become standard practice? Zero! Can't you just see this in a package insert? "Drug Company X recognizes the inherent risks and likely side effects involved in a trial of antidepressant medication, and therefore recommends a course of CBT for all cases of mild to moderate depression or anxiety prior to medical intervention."

Uh…no.

It's time to move forward now, by taking a giant leap backwards (at least in time). I want to acquaint you with the concept of philosophical therapy (in general) and with existential psychotherapy (as conceptualized by Irving Yalom) in particular.

In my Google search for philosophical psychology I was surprised to see that there is a website for the American Society for Philosophy Counseling and Psychotherapy (ASPCP). I knew that philosophical counseling had begun in Europe in the 1980's but was not aware it had caught on here at all. As always in philosophy there is some bitter controversy. I read a scathing critique of a book designed to popularize philosophical counseling titled *Plato, not Prozac; Applying eternal wisdom to everyday problems* by Lou Marinoff (Harper Collins, 1999). The critic viciously attacked the book as gimmicky, being neither legitimate counseling nor legitimate philosophy. While that controversy is beyond the scope of what we are dealing with in this book, I just wanted to bring to your attention that there is an organization that supports counseling for emotional problems being delivered by people with advanced degrees in philosophy, not psychology. If you tend more towards this approach to your problems, this might be a very interesting option to pursue. Just go to the ASPCP website to get started. I want to turn now to Irving Yalom's book *Existential Psychotherapy* published by Basic Books in 1980.

Dr. Yalom's book and the book *Existence* by Rollo May were the most powerful early influences in my academic life, dictating the direction I tried to take as a professional. (How did I ever end up writing prescriptions for a living?) Yalom's main contribution in his book is not the *form* of the therapy (he wrote this book in the era of the dominance of psychodynamic psychotherapy); it is in the *content* of therapy. Labeling them "ultimate concerns" Yalom brought the following four topics to the forefront of his psychotherapy:

1. ***Death***
2. ***Freedom***
3. ***Isolation***
4. ***Meaninglessness.***

Let's look at these in greater detail one at a time.

DEATH:

Yes, the great equalizer, right up there with taxes, as the unavoidable consequences of existence. Yalom describes his "take" on the psychological impact of the issue of death this way:

> The fear of death plays a major role in our internal experience; it rumbles continuously under the surface; it is a dark, unsettling presence at the rim of consciousness.
>
> To cope with these fears, we erect defenses against death awareness,

> defenses that are based on denial, that shape character structure, and that, if maladaptive, result in clinical syndromes. In other words, psychopathology is the result of ineffective modes of death transcendence (Yalom 1980, p.27).

Wait a second! I thought that psychopathology was the result of chemical imbalances in the brain; no? Perhaps you can see why my heart hurts when I recall the rich traditions of psychology and psychiatry and contrast it with the latest Adderall XR ad blaming everything from divorce to unemployment on adult ADD. Yalom clearly believes that the issue of death, our awareness of its inevitability, and how we emotionally handle it, are central defining features of human psychology. And, of course he is not alone. He cites thinkers, writers, poets and others dating back to the earliest times in recorded history who believe that death and death awareness are critical issues in human life. One of the historical figures Yalom cites is one we've talked about in this book, philosopher Martin Heidegger.

Heidegger made a very big deal about death, in particular, death awareness. And he wasn't talking about awareness of the fact that everyone dies, but awareness of the fact that **I** am going to die, what he called my *"ownmost"* death. A conscious awareness of your personal, inescapable mortality was what Heidegger saw as the key to escaping the scripts and storylines followed by the masses (as merely a part of the "standing reserve") and writing your own emotionally charged, personally meaningful narrative. The latter he labels "authentic" existence.

This notion of "authenticity" has undergone an academic roller coaster ride over the years but the basic point is clear: Life is more charged with personal meaning and the possibility for joy and gratitude when the *fact* of one's own mortality is no longer repressed and put on the back burner but is right up front as a constant conscious awareness. For Yalom the group of people whom he saw as liberated and brought to life by death's inevitability were group psychotherapy patients diagnosed with untreatable, terminal cancer. Of course his hope in developing an existential psychotherapy with death as an important issue in therapy was to make this joy and liberation available to us psychologically without having been told we have a few months left to live.

FREEDOM:

Yalom's second existential theme is freedom. Let me point out right off the bat however that there is a big difference between the existential view of freedom and someone like George Bush's definition. In fact, one of the major figures in existential philosophy, Jean Paul Sartre, called it "terrible freedom." How could freedom be "terrible?"

The fundamental existential position stated by Sartre is "existence precedes essence." Perhaps you have heard this. What it means is that the existence of humans as *meaning-giving* beings comes *before* any notions of what life is all about. Humans have to be in existence for life to have meaning, even if they determine (as has often been the case) that humans do not ultimately create the meaning of life. In more concrete terms, even if in actuality God runs the universe, without humans around to meditate about God and what He wants, then the whole idea makes no sense. Conversely, of course, humans could also decide (as many have) that there is no God and the whole of reality is merely cause and effect interactions of physical objects. Or…anywhere in between… or anywhere else. Can you see what I am driving at as the core concept of existentialism, that humans *give* life its meaning? They are *free* to believe what, at some level, they choose to believe, and that can be a terrible burden.

Yalom titles his first chapter on freedom *Responsibility.* Revisiting this book reminds me of just how powerful and compelling this therapy still is. The basic theme of responsibility, as it relates to existential freedom, is that most of our troubles in life, our complaints, and our depressed and anxious feelings are our fault and our responsibility. Yalom gives the example of how he experiences feelings of guilt whenever he sits back writing in his comfortable home and thoughts about millions of starving people in other parts of the world cross his mind. Like most of us, he feels a momentary twinge of guilt, but then goes about his business. After all, what choice does he have? He can't solve all the problems of the world…or can he? This is what Yalom says:

> There is, as I write, massive starvation in another part of the world. Sartre would say that I bear responsibility for this starvation. I, of course, protest: I know little of what happens there, and I feel I could do little to alter the tragic state of affairs. But Sartre would point out that I choose to keep myself uninformed, and that I decide at this very instant to write these words instead of engaging myself in the tragic situation. I could, after all, organize a rally to raise funds or publicize the situation through my contacts in publishing, but I choose to ignore it. I bear responsibility for what I do and what I choose to ignore. Sartre's point in this regard is not moral: he does not say that I *should* be doing something different, but he says that what I *do* do is my responsibility (Yalom 1980, p.221).

I hope you are beginning to catch on to this existential concept of "terrible" freedom. And it doesn't have to be about something as dramatic as starvation (or genocide or the death of Rebecca Riley). This "terrible" freedom extends down to every aspect of daily life, because we are making choices all the time. I'll give you a much more pedestrian but true example from my life right now: I went to a jazz camp one summer because, although I am a decent trombone player, I cannot play jazz well at all, a problem that has been haunting me since I played in a jazz-rock band in college. I play jazz solos all the time, I just don't play them well (unless by sheer accident). So I went to learn from the pros. And I found out exactly what I already knew. Learning to play jazz requires a tremendous investment of time spent practicing. My combo instructor was kind and caring. He complemented me on my sense of rhythm and then "suggested" that I needed to work on "learning the language of jazz." I can assure you that learning the language of jazz is a formidable, seemingly insurmountable challenge. But he had a suggestion. He told me to listen to jazz trombonists and find a two bar jazz passage (called a "lick") that I liked. Then I should learn the passage and practice it along with the record; just one a day. This might involve 30 to 45 minutes of my time and the results would not be immediately apparent. But in a year, I would be more acquainted with the language of jazz and it would start to show in my playing.

What I have *chosen* to do instead is feel (in my mind, rightfully) totally overwhelmed by the prospect of doing what I have to do to learn jazz and therefore not doing anything beyond continuing to muddle through jazz solos, hoping one will sound good. I'm bringing up this personal example because I want you to understand that I am fully aware of the fact that I am making a *choice* and that the next time I stand up in front of an audience to play a jazz solo (I am already committed to a couple of gigs) I am setting myself up to get an "attack" of low self esteem and its accompanying feelings of depression. And I could be doing something about it: I could even start today. This awareness helps me locate the responsibility for my "depressive" feelings right where they belong, on my own shoulders. An awareness of existential responsibility and its "terrible" freedom doesn't necessarily feel good…but it does feel right. A long time ago in this book I mentioned how in postmodern thinking you need to somehow "negotiate" which interpretation of a phenomenon is the "most right." I don't think that there is much argument that some devoted trombone practice would help alleviate my trombone related low self esteem.

Let's move on to Yalom's last two existential topics, isolation and meaninglessness.

ISOLATION:

Yalom's existential issues are certainly not cheer-me-ups and the existential concept of isolation is no exception. We are not talking here about temporary episodes of isolation and loneliness; we are talking about the "ultimate concern" of true lifetime isolation. As Yalom puts it we are talking about "an isolation that persists despite the most gratifying engagement with other individuals and despite consummate self-knowledge and integration" (Yalom 1980, p.355). So what is this happy topic all about? It's the same as death awareness and terrible freedom; it is another "ultimate concern" hovering at the fringes of consciousness, rarely considered but sometimes experienced. For example, when lying in a hospital bed, frightened about your health, your spouse home sleeping and the nurses busy with other patients: that is a time when existential isolation and the chilling anxiety that accompanies it is sometimes felt. Perhaps your mind then turns to an assessment of the meaning of your life, or maybe the meaning of human life in general. From the existential perspective, that too is cold comfort.

MEANINGLESSNESS:

I want to quote the story Yalom tells at the beginning of his chapter on meaninglessness because it is so profound. It goes like this:

> Imagine a happy group of morons who are engaged in work. They are carrying bricks in an open field. As soon as they have stacked all the bricks at one end of the field, they proceed to transport them to the opposite end. This continues without stop and every day of every year they are busy doing the same thing. One day one of the morons stops long enough to ask himself what he is doing. He wonders what purpose there is in carrying the bricks. And from that instant on he is not quite as content with his occupation as he had been before. I am the moron who wonders why he is carrying the bricks
>
> (Yalom 1980, p.419).

Yalom informs us that these "were the last words written by a despairing soul who killed himself because he saw no meaning in life." Yalom then goes on to articulate the theme of this suicide note by asking:

What is the meaning of life?
What is the meaning of *my* life?
Why do we live?
Why were we put here?

What do we live *for?*
What shall we live *by?*
If we must die, if nothing endures,
then what sense does anything make? (Yalom 1980, p.419)

These are clearly timeless and enduring ultimate questions and Yalom's chapter is chock full of musings on the meaning of life from writers and thinkers throughout history. But do these ultimate questions really plague us average everyday folks on a constant basis? Don't we just ignore or repress these thoughts? What good would it do to just sit around questioning the meaning of life every moment? Good questions. Of course Yalom would not be proposing an existential "psychotherapy" if some emotional good did not come of all this. He isn't in the job of promoting meaninglessness and suicide. So let's look at where he goes with his therapy to understand why he believes working directly with these ultimate concerns in life is a good and fruitful approach. Because Yalom does have some very concrete suggestions.

Altruism: Yalom's first suggestion to give meaning and focus to a life that, by the definition of existentialism, lacks pre-given or clear-cut meaning is through altruism. "Leaving the world a better place to live in, serving others, participation in charity (the greatest virtue of all)—these activities are right and good and have provided life meaning for many humans" (Yalom 1980, p.431). No surprise there; I think we all know that service to others, especially those less fortunate, is somehow inherently meaningful and from all descriptions you hear, often deeply rewarding. This is especially true when you give of your full self (e.g. building homes for Habitat for Humanity, traveling to New Orleans to help rebuild) rather than simply writing a check or phoning in a donation. So that is solution #1 to the existential dilemma. Solution #2 is:

Dedication to a cause: This is similar to altruism and Yalom doesn't spend a lot of time on it. I'll just say that for me, personally, dedication to the cause of educating consumers about what has gone so terribly wrong in psychiatry has breathed life into me and given me hope (even on my very worst days when I can barely stand the thought of one more "patient" coming to me for the magic diagnosis and quick cure). Next for Yalom is:

Creativity: The important point here is that beyond the potential for fulfillment in the arts that I think we are all aware of, creativity can be seen as a potential source of meaning in anyone's life. Thus the accountant, the server at a restaurant or the landscaper can also invest creatively in their work and lives. This creativity potential is, unfortunately, often stifled and discouraged in the worldview described by Heidegger as "Gestell" because here the emphasis on ordering and efficiency *for their own sake* would, by definition, stifle creativity. I got a good look at this process at work when I watched a cable television show on the history of the assembly line. The assembly line was pioneered, as we know, by Henry Ford. What I learned in watching the show about the Ford assembly line was how utterly miserable the assembly line workers were. This was not because of wages or even long work hours; it was because of how working on the assembly line was so stiflingly boring and dull. Despite good wages over 50% of the Ford workers quit every year! They just couldn't take it. So where are today's Ford plants? Not in the automobile industry, most of that has been automated. It is, in my eyes, in the tens of millions of jobs where we sit and stare at computers all day long. Next on Yalom's list…you might like this one…is:

The Hedonistic Solution: We haven't talked about plain old pleasure much in this book. In a related vein, I do like that the underbelly of CNS drugs has been further exposed by some warnings that they are now forced to give on the two drugs marketed to treat Restless Leg Syndrome (RLS). The drugs are brand names Requip and Mirapex. (They are "me too" drugs that belong to a class of drugs also used to treat Parkinson's disease). Here are the official *side effect* warnings: Both Mirapex and Requip may cause increased gambling, compulsive overeating and sexual activity!! (If I'm lying I'm dying…look it up). This just cracks me up. All I can think of is Las Vegas. They probably want to put these drugs in the drinking water. But seriously, can you believe we are now officially prescribing drugs that can *cause* us to gamble, overeat and engage in casual sex? I noticed that these warnings were not included in the drug company's initial package inserts for Requip so I have to assume that these "side effect" concerns emerged post-approval. I would *love* to be a fly on the wall at the conversations that these new warnings could stimulate:

"You fat son-of-a-bitch. Not only do you lose $20,000 playing craps, you hired three hookers to come up to your room? Stop eating for a second and talk to me!"

"But honey…it isn't my fault. It's that medicine I'm taking for those uncomfortable crawly sensations in my legs. I couldn't help myself."

Sometimes I just can't believe this is really happening. But it is. I bring this up here to address a misconception about the concept of hedonism because the underlying concept in choosing hedonism as a way to give meaning to life is not simply "If it feels good, do it!" It's more along the lines of when faced with a choice of two options; choose the one with the most pleasant consequences. This widely opens up the definition of hedonism because we might easily choose a more charitable, kind and altruistic option because the results of that choice might well be the most pleasant. We might also choose to deny ourselves momentary peak experiences of bodily pleasure such as casual sex or fattening foods because the eventual outcome of that choice could well be decidedly unpleasant. Speaking of "peak experiences" the next solution offered by Yalom is:

Self Actualization: This is a concept by Abraham Maslow, considered the father of humanistic psychology. Maslow's psychological philosophy is expressed in his well-known "hierarchy of needs" where, he says that humans must first fulfill more basic survival needs such as food, clothing and shelter before they naturally move on to higher levels of development characterized by knowledge, love, charity etc. The ultimate state of development is the aforementioned self actualization, where human beings realize their full *inborn* potential. This notion of an inherent blueprint towards self actualization (finding the "real" you) is an area of great controversy but often forms the basis for what is sometimes called "pop" psychology and self help programs from people like Dr. Phil and other proponents of positive thinking strategies. Of interest is that Maslow conceptualized society as presenting more of a barrier than a pathway towards self actualization "because it so often forces individuals to abandon their unique personal development and to accept ill-fitting social roles and stifling conventionality." Maslow's psychology was popular in the 1970's. Imagine how he would view the pressures to socially conform now compared to the 1960's and 1970's, the decades of encounter groups, "happenings" and free love. Now we attach the word "free" to the President's Freedom Counsel, advocating mental health screening and its forced conformity to acceptable societal standards of behavior by diagnosing and medicating children.

Engagement: Yalom summarizes the various suggestions on coping with the ultimate existential issues of death, freedom, isolation and meaninglessness as all entailing an engagement in life, living each moment to its fullest, a philosophy of life tragically often evident only in his terminal cancer patients. Contrast this with the nature of the psychiatrist/patient relationship today, involving a controlling technician and a passive, disengaged patient and I think you can see the devolution of mental healthcare clearly displayed. Yalom's perspective shouldn't be a dated way of seeing things, discarded alongside our DOS computers. One of the comments on the back cover of Yalom's book says:

"*This book should be read by every psychiatry resident and every clinical psychology intern. It belongs in the library of every psychotherapist.*"

The sad truth is that I am pretty sure that I could not find a single psychiatric resident who has read this book or has even heard of it unless it was in a lecture on the "psychopathology and neurobiological defects in people who have read *Existential Psychotherapy.*"

We are going to move forward now to some current forms of psychotherapy grounded in the postmodern philosophical perspective that we have discussed throughout this book. I mentioned above that the concepts of authenticity and self actualization are controversial topics in psychology (and philosophy). This is true because the foundational concept upon which they rest is itself controversial. This might surprise you a bit because it does not come up in everyday conversation but the controversy is whether there is such a thing as a self or whether the whole idea of individuals with personalities and choices is an illusion.

For this section I am using a book for reference titled *Constructions of Disorder: Meaning-Making Frameworks for Psychotherapy.* This book was co-edited by Robert A. Neimeyer and Jonathan D. Raskin and published by the American Psychological Association in 2000. I have been fortunate enough to get to know Doctors Neimeyer and Raskin and can assure you that they are kind, caring and wise individuals. (Remember I said in chapter two that I want to emphasize the role of wisdom in psychiatry and de-emphasize the role of experiments and scientistic evidence. I cited the wisdom of the Wizard of Oz as an example). Early in his chapter Dr. Neimeyer mentions the most radical view of the disappearance of the self. Quoting Lather, he describes the "extreme postmodern view of the 'death of the self' as heralding the demise of personal subjectivity and its replacement by the cacophonous echoes of incoherent conversations, anonymous media images, and fragmented communication networks that colonize our mental life" (Neimeyer and Raskin 2000, p.209). Odd language—our mental life is "colonized" by anonymous media images and fragmented communication, but when I look, for example, at my still growing collection of adult ADD ads from the Adderall XR company—somehow "colonizing" doesn't sound too far off.

In one of his taped lectures our old friend Rick Roderick tells a story about Jean Baudrillard, the previously mentioned French philosopher and sociologist best known for promoting the idea of "hypereality", the more real than real media and advertising grounded world in which we live. Roderick's anecdote is about when Jean Baudrillard was asked by a French newspaper to report on the Gulf War. He readily agreed and asked to be set up in a hotel room in Paris. No, they said, we want you to go to Kuwait and report on the war. But Baudrillard objected, saying that the war will not be "fought" in Kuwait, but on CNN: "Who will tell us who won or lost the war?" Baudrillard's point was brilliant. Yes, there would be *something* factual (in the "old" sense of the real) going on in Kuwait and Iraq, but *reality* would be determined by how these facts would be spun, packaged and presented on CNN.

Hearing this Roderick commented that "even at my most cynical, I wasn't prepared to accept that Baudrillard's perspective was correct—until I started to think about it and actually spoke to some people who returned from the Gulf." Most striking to him was a returning soldier who worked in supplies telling him that she had no idea what was going on in the war until she came home and watched what her husband had taped on CNN. He also talked to a pilot who enthusiastically reported that the flying a bomber was "very exciting; the bomb sights were just like at the arcade I grew up in." I don't want to belabor this issue because it's a bit off topic but I did want to mention this most radical view that says, in essence, that humans have "disappeared" and won't come back—it's already too late. As Roderick says "There is no sense in talking about the coming apocalypse, it has already happened." This is obviously not the governing perspective in any of the therapies I want to discuss now because if there were no "humans" there wouldn't be a need for something called "therapy."

The three postmodern approaches to therapy Raskin and Neimeyer explore are constructivism, social constructionism and narrative therapy. I wouldn't exactly call it nitpicking but clearly one of the problems faced in trying to mount an attack against the unchallenged dominance of the medical model and DSM in psychiatry is the infighting about technical details that is seen among the various alternative theories of mental healthcare. My concern is that the alternatives will be so busy canceling each other out that the thought leaders in psychiatry will barely be forced to notice. That is why I think that the DSM big shots who attended the philosophy conference I talked about early in the book were able to be so dismissive and unaffected by the topics of discussion there. There *is* a difference between constructivism, social constructionism and narrative therapy and while I will mention those differences, I want to focus more on what these postmodern therapies have in common as an alternative to a medical model approach to mental healthcare.

As in postmodern philosophy, the role of language is a central concern in constructivist, constructionist and narrative therapy. These theorists are keenly aware of the power of language to constitute reality. Thus Raskin attacks a softer approach to DSM diagnostic labeling proposed by a psychiatrist who "sits down with each client at the start of therapy, and she and the client flip through the DSM IV together. Ultimately, the psychiatrist and the client collectively decide which DSM IV diagnoses seem relevant for conceptualizing the client's problems. Furthermore, if the client is using insurance to cover the cost of therapy sessions, the psychiatrist and the client act jointly in determining which DSM IV diagnoses should be submitted to the insurance company" (Neimeyer 2000, p.31). Raskin attacks this more "democratic" approach to the use of DSM IV on two fronts. (We've discussed both throughout this book). He recognizes and points out the potential real world consequences of a DSM IV label that have nothing to do with the more liberal interpretation and uniquely individual understanding of the label allegedly achieved in this doctor patient negotiation. As he says: "The client and therapist may have reconstrued the meaning of the diagnostic label in a new and empowering way, but those at the insurance company and in society at large, have not" (Neimeyer 2000, p.33). We've discussed cases in this book where there have been significant economic and legal consequences to a diagnosis of, for example, bipolar disorder, no matter how often the words "mild" or "spectrum" were used in the medical notes. That's why it is so hard to believe that people come into my office all the time *soliciting* a bipolar diagnosis for themselves or a loved one. And I am sure this will only get worse as the advertising for bipolar drugs (such as the new Abilify and Seroquel XR TV commercials) escalates.

But Raskin is even more concerned about the intrapsychic and interpersonal impact of diagnostic labels. This is where the constructivist, social constructionist and narrative perspectives all have a voice. So let's look briefly at the similarities and differences in these theories using the "DSM label" concern as a common point of reference.

Constructivism is a theoretical perspective first proposed by psychologist George Kelly in, now get this, 1955! Basically Kelly proposed that our understanding of self and world is in the form of mental constructs that can be both accessed and changed. Thus, Raskin explains: "Constructivists emphasize how each individual creates personal representations of self and world as well as the ability to transcend problematic things in wholly new ways" (Neimeyer 2000, p.6). This "wholly new ways" part is where the social construc<u>tionists</u> have a problem. The hinted at notion that there is, in essence, an unlimited number of possible constructed personal realities runs counter to the belief of social constructionists that the range of possible constructions of reality is set by (and also limited by) the foundational role played by culture and society in producing a finite number of constructions of reality or "scripts" to choose from. (I am, of course, a died-in-the-wool social constructionist as I'm sure you've realized). Finally, according to Raskin: "Narrative theorists combine features of both of these perspectives, positing that people are inveterate storytellers who attempt to organize their experience into coherent accounts" (Neimeyer 2000, p.7). These might not sound like big theoretical differences in these various schools of thought and they aren't. But they are enough to send the practitioners on slightly different courses with differing literatures and loyalties. To me this once again illustrates how terrifying the medical model truly is. By attaching itself to the unchallenged dominance of the scientific and rationalistic storyline, the medical model advocates are a*lready strongly unified* around foundational questions such as "What exactly *is* a mental disorder?" and "Who determines what we call mental health?" and no longer ask about or debate these still completely unsettled critical issues.

In actuality constructivist therapists, social constructionist therapists and narrative therapists do very similar work with clients, work that in many ways is the polar opposite of the way psychiatrists deal with patients. Here is what I mean. The "job" of the psychiatrist is to listen to what the patient says and then "fit" what is said into the diagnostic paradigm defined by medical model psychiatry. We've talked throughout this book about what a disaster this has become. The postmodern therapists on the other hand are there to *learn,* not teach. They want to learn how the client sees the world, not impose their view of the world on the client. Then, ideally, in a mutual and democratic fashion, the therapist and the client search for other ways to see things (construct reality) that might be more fruitful and beneficial. The "power" here is not solely in the hands of the "knowing" therapist. (As I said before, the postmodern therapist tries to take a "knowing not-knowing" position). The "power" is actually placed right where it belongs, in the client-therapist *relationship.* It has been known for a long time that the reason that two hundred fifty six different types of therapies, including medications and placebos, seem to "work" is because of the therapeutic relationship. Can I really say that this is true for meds? There is definitely a "relationship" between a medical doctor and an emotionally struggling patient, a type of relationship that many of us seek our whole lives; a relationship between a helpless child (the patient) and an all-knowing, all-powerful parent (the doctor). Only in this case the illusion that supports the power of the doctor is merely the finely crafted and continually communicated profit driven message of biopsychiatry. (It isn't really "daddy" and he doesn't really "care").

So where do you find a good postmodern therapist and who pays for it? Those are legitimate real world questions. Raskin understands the harsh reality of the healthcare delivery situation in our society: "The tension between the demands of a belt-tightening system of managed care and its apparent resistance by many constructivist, social constructionist, and narrative therapists may lead some readers to question the practicality of a postmodern therapy in light of the economic realities imposed by living in a modern world" (Neimeyer 2000, p.7). So, in truth, the effort to develop a postmodern professional therapy is a noble effort and I hope its practitioners, theorists and believers keep working on it and keep holding meetings and conferences and maintain their websites. But the average consumers out there are not going to easily find therapists of this persuasion, and, if they do, be able to afford the treatment. So it's time to turn our attention to other sources of help that are not constrained by economic factors (by that I mean will not require the presence of a professional). In general I suppose you could class these other forms of help under the heading "spiritual", but they also belong to a larger group of programs and plans called "self-help", a huge (and in some cases very profitable) industry in our country. There are a wide range of spiritually based programs and plans available, including the most widely prevalent, available, affordable (and in my mind most effective)—the 12 Step programs. I will devote the final chapter of this book to them. In the remainder of this chapter I just want to introduce you to two of the many spiritually grounded philosophies I've encountered that I believe can be very helpful. The first is articulated by Carolyn Myss and the second by the previously quoted Miriam Greenspan.

Carolyn Myss is not someone whose credentials would automatically attract me to her work. Trained in journalism and theology, she says that she found herself possessing an uncanny ability to intuitively diagnose medical illnesses. So, she is now known as a medical intuit and spiritual guide. What did attract me to her was when my wife got me to watch one of her videotaped lectures because I was struck by both her wisdom and her ability to communicate difficult spiritual concepts using easily understood metaphors. For example, Carolyn wants to help people understand that she believes that we have a finite and limited amount of spiritual energy to devote to our day to day lives. She metaphorically refers to this reserve of energy as a bank account. So, as she describes it, we have a daily supply of one-hundred dollars a day of spiritual energy. She then asks, how much do you want to spend on fruitless thoughts and endeavors, like holding a grudge? You've been through a nasty divorce. You find yourself consumed with anger and a desire for revenge. So how much does that cost, twenty five dollars? Then you are starting your day off with only seventy-five dollars of spiritual energy, energy that could and should be devoted to your well-being and growth. Another ten bucks tied up with your stressing about your boss and fifteen bucks tied up with worry about money and you are already at half strength. Does this strike home with you, make sense? I find this metaphor very appealing and I speak its language in my own mind daily.

In essence Myss teaches that *the path to spiritual well being and spiritual growth is not* ***around*** *the pain but through it!* ***This is the essential message communicated in all good spiritual (and interestingly PTSD) programs of recovery and growth. FACE THE PAIN, OR YOU WILL NEVER CONQUER IT.*** *Can't you see how this is the polar opposite of what psychiatry and most psychologies are all about?*

Carolyn Myss discusses the spiritual journey of what she calls the "modern mystic" in her taped lecture series *Spiritual Madness* (Available on Amazon.

com). She illustrates the difference between traditional therapists and spiritual guides with the following anecdote. A "patient" presents to the therapist with a whole slew of complaints about all of the terrible things that have happened and all of the pain she is in. The typical therapist responds with sympathy and concern, promising to help the patient find ways to reduce the painful emotions. The spiritual guide, on the other hand, might say: "Perfect, you are just where you need to be on your path to spiritual growth. Be prepared, the pain might get worse before it gets better." (Of course the spiritual guide might find that her client elects not to make a follow-up appointment because someone advocating that she embrace, own and take responsibility for her pain might not be exactly what she was *shopping* for). In a similar vein, Myss' take on the issue of consumerism and the "empty self" is voiced as a concern for something she calls "woundology." I love that term. She explains it this way in her book *Anatomy of the Spirit.* Speaking of modern culture she says:

> ...we have become therapeutically fluent, in the process of creating a new language of intimacy that I call "woundology." We now use the revelation and exchange of our wounds as the substance of conversation, indeed, as the glue that binds a relationship. We have become so good at this that we have converted our wounds in a type of "relationship currency" that we use in order to control situations and people. The countless support groups for helping people work through their histories of abuse, incest, addiction, and battering, to name a few, serve only to enhance woundology as our contemporary language of intimacy (Myss 1996, pp.208-9).

Myss is not being insensitive here. She is merely describing a cultural phenomenon that she is witnessing and in many places she expresses both compassion and caring for those who have suffered trauma and abuse. However, in a sense she is saying, okay, enough is enough! It's time to move on from wounded to healing and that requires getting past wallowing in the language of "woundology." She says: "I have [become] convinced that when we define ourselves by our wounds, we burden and lose our physical and spiritual energy and open ourselves to the risk of illness."

Myss' work also incorporates the Hindu concept of chakras. In the foreword to *Anatomy of the Spirit* C. Norman Shealy, M.D. writes: "*The Anatomy of the Spirit* presents an exciting ecumenical way to understand the seven energy centers of the body. It integrates Judaic, Christian, Hindu and Buddhist concepts of power into seven universal spiritual truths" (Myss 1996, p.xiii). The chakra concept derives from the Hindu tradition that locates energy centers in various parts of the body. But as Shealy points out, Myss' use of chakras is not strictly Hindu but represents a blending of traditions from four world religions. To be honest with you, the idea that there are literally energy channels in our bodies (the basic justification for acupuncture, for example) has always been a little tough for me to swallow. But I have no trouble at all believing that there is great wisdom in every religion and, as you recall, I long ago promoted the idea of turning to wisdom literature to develop a foundation for a more humanistic and holistic mental health theory and practice. Caroline Myss' work is exemplary of the effort to blend a modern understanding of being human with thoughts and ideas gathered from all corners of the world and from ancient to modern times. That this is labeled "New Age" is in a way unfortunate because it lumps a lot of diverse thinkers together so that the current guardians of the ruling regime of truth can so easily dismiss them and maintain their unchallenged discourse control: "Oh, that's just that New Age garbage." (As you will see in the next chapter, however, because they are so visibly successful the ruling elite find it harder to be so dismissive towards the 12 Step programs, despite their spiritual, "new-age" feel).

Carolyn Myss is, in essence, calling us out on our language of woundology. But she also offers a path out, a path to healing and growth, and delivers her message with great skill, wisdom and compassion. I will list some of her materials at the end of this book but it is probably easier to just Google her, she is very popular. My favorites are *Spiritual Madness*, a lecture on audiotape, and *Why People Don't Heal,* a book that is also available as a videotaped lecture. I enjoy the videotape the best because watching this woman truly calms the restless soul.

Carolyn Myss' philosophy is characterized as a blending of Judaic, Christian, Hindu and Buddhist wisdom. The work that I've seen and read leans more toward the Christian and Hindu side so I would like to close this chapter by introducing you to a therapist of similar persuasion but with more of (to my eyes) a Judaic and Buddhist leaning, the previously mentioned Miriam Greenspan. In particular I want to focus on Greenspan's use of a growingly popular topic in spiritually driven psychology, the Buddhist concept of "mindfulness."

The following are some quotes from Greenspan's preface to her book that clearly explain her philosophy of healing through the dark emotions:

> This book will argue that our emotional illiteracy as a species has less to do with our inability to subdue negative emotions than it does with our inability to authentically and mindfully *feel* them. What looks like a problem with emotional control actually has

> its source in widespread ignorance about how to tolerate painful emotional energies and use these energies for emotional, spiritual and social transformation (Greenspan 2003, p xii).
>
> In my thirty years as a psychotherapist, I've come to believe that the inability to bear the core triad of grief, fear, and despair is the source of much of our individual and collective emotional ills. These are the emotions we most avoid and that we most need to attend to in our time (Greenspan 2003, p.xii).
>
> In short, aborted grief, fear, and despair are at the root of the characteristic psychological "disorders" of our time—depression, anxiety, addiction, irrational violence, and psychic numbing (Greenspan 2003, p.xiii)
>
> While generally devalued in our culture, the dark emotions have a wisdom that is essential to the work of healing and transformation on both individual and collective levels (Greenspan 2003, p.xiii).

Notice that Greenspan talks about the need for healing on both an individual *and* societal level. Think about how this differs from biopsychiatry's central tenet that emotional and mental disorders are contained in individual nervous systems and are to be both located and treated there. Greenspan openly acknowledges that her perspective on psychotherapy is rooted in her personal experiences of being the child of holocaust survivors and being a mother whose child died in infancy. From this background she tells us how the dark emotions that engulfed her ultimately became the source of her transformation to a state of acceptance and serenity. Specifically, she articulates how through the "alchemy" of the dark emotions we can progress from:

Grief to Gratitude
Despair to Faith
Fear to Joy

And not an antidepressant or mood stabilizer in sight!

Part four of *healing through the dark emotions* is titled "A Home Course in Emotional Alchemy." In it Greenspan spells out thirty-three emotional exercises for her readers. She touches on chakras but many of her recommendations derive from Buddhist traditions of *acceptance* that suffering is a natural part of human life, calming the mind through *meditation* and the previously mentioned concept of *mindfulness.* So what exactly is mindfulness? Here is a good definition that I found: Mindfulness is a state of consciousness "characterized by a vivid and tangible experience of being in the present, a heightened sense of dwelling inwardly in one's body as a whole and feeling what the body is doing, a sharpened and heightened clarity of the five ordinary senses, and the ability to achieve an unbiased and highly objective perspective of life, grounded in direct experiencing alone" (What is Mindfulness 1996, p.1). A state of mindfulness is generally attained through meditation, an exercise to quiet the chatter in the mind. Greenspan recommends the commonly prescribed practice of focusing on your breathing to attain a meditative state. But, she says, "When you practice mindfulness meditation, you don't try to wipe out anything. This is a gentle, nonjudgmental practice. When you find yourself thinking, or when you are distracted from your breath by an emotion or physical sensation, this is not a problem. Just allow the thoughts, feelings and sensations to move through, without trying to stop them or understand them. See them passing through, like clouds moving through the blue sky of your awareness. And gently return to your breath" (Greenspan 2003, p.280).

Of course this is just one of the thirty three exercises that Greenspan recommends to assist in healing through your dark emotions. But here is the essential question to ask: Will anyone really DO the thirty three exercises? Will anyone really practice what Carolyn Myss teaches? For that matter, after you buy the $400 Midwest Center Program for Stress and Anxiety, will you do your part and get your $400 worth? Aside from a select few, the answer is probably no. It won't hurt; in fact it will definitely help to access these materials at any level. Positive thinking-based and Eastern philosophy based materials abound (e.g. Carlson's *Don't Sweat the Small Stuff,* books by Dr. Wayne Dyer and Andrew Weil, M.D.) but all are *self* help and, because of our over-busy, fast-paced lives, will never, I believe, make a real dent in or challenge the dictatorial domination of the *quick-fix* medical model**. BUT...**

There ***is*** an already existing program for emotional problems that I believe can, in fact, make a real dent in the medical model's domination and offer a realistic alternative to those seeking help with emotional problems...a true and lasting alternative. It's a spiritual program but *not* one that you do alone. The strength and power of this program is not just its philosophy or beliefs; it is the much more powerful healing and sustaining power of ***FELLOWSHIP.***

On to chapter thirteen!!

Chapter Thirteen:
IS FREE CHEAP ENOUGH??
Emotions Anonymous and the Salvation of Mental Healthcare

> Many did try Al-Anon. Soon, their visits to my practice decreased. One woman used to come in every month with something, and after she started going to Al-Anon, she stopped coming except for her annual checkup. People also seemed happier.
>
> Marsha Epstein, M.D.
> *Clinical Psychiatry News:* July, 2005

I am going to make a very bold assertion here and then use the rest of this chapter to back it up. Here it is:

> Dr. Epstein's quote is the single most important observation about healthcare in America today!

You will notice I didn't say *mental* healthcare in my hyperbolic statement, I said *all* healthcare. Dr. Epstein is not a psychiatrist even though her quote was in *Clinical Psychiatry News* (Epstein 2005). She is a general medical physician who at the time of writing the quote was listed as the medical director for the South Bay Area of the Los Angeles County Department of Health Services Division of Public Health. I assume she is a very busy doctor who spends at least part of her time seeing patients in a public health clinic. So I want to take a deeper look at what she said about Al-Anon and examine the profound implications of her statement.

Al-Anon is a program devoted to helping the families and loved ones of addicts and alcoholics learn to cope with addiction in their lives. As an outgrowth of Alcoholics Anonymous (AA) it derives from the same Twelve Step and Twelve Tradition philosophy that has been guiding AA since the 1930's. (We will be carefully and thoroughly evaluating these Twelve Steps shortly, but for our purposes now, just understand that Al-Anon is a free of charge, readily available Twelve Step program for the loved ones of addicts and alcoholics). There are no mental health professionals involved in organizing or running Al-Anon meetings.

Okay, now let's talk about Dr. Epstein's patients. In her quote above Dr. Epstein refers to a woman "who used to come in every month *with something.*" Every medical doctor knows what that "with something" means. It's a complaint, an inexplicable physical symptom, a request for a medication change or more medicine, something along those lines. (In psychiatric patients this is extremely common, resulting in the frequent medication changes and polypharmacy previously discussed). We are not talking about the development of an actual new physical disease; we are talking about new symptoms and complaints in already evaluated and treated patients. What we are *really* talking about is **NEEDINESS** and how so many of us have learned to take our feelings of need (rooted in the previously discussed sociocultural problems of alienation, loneliness, stress and spiritual emptiness) to the medical world. And the medical world responds with its emblem of caring: **PILLS**. So, what is Dr. Epstein saying happened to the woman who came in "with something" every month who, after a referral to Al-Anon, stopped coming monthly, showing up only for an annual checkup? What happened to all of her physical complaints and new symptoms? Apparently they weren't *really* physical problems in the first place. She came to the doctor every month because she needed *something* which, apparently, she *got* at Al-Anon. Beyond that, when Epstein says: "People [who went to Al-Anon] also seemed happier". Is she saying that going to Al-Anon makes people happier? ...Really?

I SAY YES!

That is exactly what she is saying. Of course Dr. Epstein is just one doctor and she is expressing an opinion. But is it true? Are there any studies to back her up? As I told you before, I'm not going to argue my point of view in the language of scientism; besides, for reasons you will see as we go on in this chapter, I couldn't if I wanted to (Twelve Step programs don't keep data). But with the skyrocketing cost and decline in quality of medical care in this country, when Dr. Epstein suggests that there is another way to go that will substantially *reduce demand* for medical care and that makes people feel healthier and happier, then don't we all need to play very close attention? Did I mention that Al-Anon and all the rest of the Twelve Step programs are free? So, to all of the politicians, activists, administrators, doctors, social workers, therapists and support groups who constantly argue that *not enough funding* is the core problem in healthcare I ask: How about it?, IS FREE CHEAP ENOUGH??

THE TWELVE STEP PROGRAMS

My biggest problem here is going to be keeping the content of this chapter under control, there is so very much to say about Twelve Step programs and their role in attaining and maintaining physical, mental and emotional wellbeing. Let me start by briefly explaining how I came to be a believer. I am not myself a recovering addict, alcoholic or gambler and have not personally participated as a member of any Twelve Step program. What I did do, as mentioned before, was take a job after my psychiatric residency at a well known psychiatric and addiction hospital, Fair Oaks Hospital in Summit, New Jersey. I was hired as an outpatient physician with a specialty in eating disorders. However, soon after I arrived one of the psychiatrists on the inpatient addiction treatment unit announced she was leaving and I was asked to take her place. My only previous experience in directly treating addiction had been a three month rotation on an addiction unit in the fourth year of my residency. So I was pretty much flying blind; fortunately I had a mentor, Dr. Bill Annito and I learned it all from him. (The real learning in medicine has always been in the form of apprentice/mentor relationships).

I will spare you the details of my growing pains…OW! Suffice it to say that eventually Dr. Annito left and I became the "man" on our unit, treating around thirty heroin and cocaine addicts at a time. As I also previously mentioned, this job was before the days of the insurance company spurred growth in the dual diagnosis concept. My job was to be the team leader and I typically used medication only for detoxification. We rarely used any psychiatric medications on my unit. We had a multidisciplinary treatment team but the core and foundation of the program was the Twelve Step philosophy. Among the staff there were always two or three recovering addicts or alcoholics who would keep the rest of us on the straight and narrow, following an orthodox Twelve Step plan. I was at Fair Oaks for about six years.

After I moved to Florida I kept my hand in addiction treatment as the medical director of a public addiction treatment program but now I have very little to do with this form of treatment. Although I miss it, I stopped responding to rehab hospital medical director job advertisements because it's clear that the only reason they hire psychiatrists now is to validate dual diagnoses. No thanks! I remain a pretty orthodox believer in the Twelve Steps. Put simply, here is why:

IT WORKS!!

Unless you've been an addict or alcoholic yourself, have had a loved one on drugs or booze or have worked directly with them, it is impossible to appreciate how monumental a challenge it is to get and remain sober. To me it remains a source of amazement that *anyone* can do it, yet millions do, primarily through Twelve Step programs. The other reason that I so strongly support the Twelve Step programs will become obvious to you as you read this chapter. The philosophy and guiding principles that form the foundation for Twelve Step work are exactly the ones that I have been promoting as the *core wisdom principles* in positive psychology, cognitive-behavior therapy, existential psychotherapy, postmodern and spiritual therapies; all right there for the taking in a widely available cost free program grounded in feelings of community, caring and fellowship. So let's get to these magical Twelve Steps and first ask: Where did they come from?

They came from the mind of a man named Bill Wilson, a.k.a. Bill W.

Bill Wilson was born in 1895, so he came of age in the roaring twenties and then the depression. By the age of thirty-nine Bill was near death from alcoholism. Despite an incredibly supportive wife and a natural talent for business and the stock market, if Bill didn't stop drinking he most likely would not have lived another year. It was downright amazing that he had made it as far as he had with the incredible amount of alcohol he had consumed before, during and after prohibition. He was a talented business analyst but by constantly drinking himself into states of oblivion he had burned every bridge on Wall Street. He had been in numerous detoxification and treatment facilities of the day, but, like most of the other drunks he met, sobriety never lasted very long. Then two things happened. An old friend entered Bill's life that had attained and maintained sobriety with the help of a Christian movement called the Oxford Group. The second thing that happened was that while he was in a hospital detoxifying, Bill had a transcendental religious experience where he saw a brilliant white light and felt the presence of God (A.A. 1984).

That was when Bill stopped drinking. He decided to devote his life to helping other alcoholics. He remained active in the Oxford Group and started inviting alcoholics to live in his house where he would preach his philosophy of recovery to them. However, very few of them got sober. He would also preach his message to gatherings of alcoholics but that didn't seem to work very well either. It seemed that despite the wisdom that Bill had gained from the Oxford Group's philosophy and his own sobriety, simply hearing a message of hope from a "preacher on a pulpit" didn't help other alcoholics. Bill W. did not give up, however, and continued to work on refining and improving his message. But he also had to survive economically and a business takeover plan led him from New York to Akron, Ohio where he met the co-founder of A.A., Dr. Bob.

Bill's business venture in Akron was not going well and he found himself, for the first time in a long time, really craving alcohol. All of his friends and supporters were in NYC and without them around, Bill was in trouble. He sensed he needed another alcoholic to talk to, someone who could truly understand his plight. He found Dr. Bob, a local surgeon and raging alcoholic. With Dr. Bob's support, Bill did not relapse.

I closed chapter twelve by asserting that the problem with self help programs is that for most people, no matter how strong and compelling the message in sermons, books, on tapes, CD's and in work manuals, they just aren't enough. Bill W. didn't understand this at first. He thought that if he just worked on and refined his self help philosophy, the listening alcoholics would "get it" and recover. And he had good reason to believe this because what he was preaching was truly revolutionary. In the 1930's alcoholism was viewed worldwide as primarily a moral defect of character. There was very little compassion for alcoholics then and many were simply tossed in jail. Bill's message was that alcoholism is actually more like a disease with physical and psychological causes as well as moral ones. Bill's message restored both hope and the potential for dignity to the alcoholic men and women that society had discarded. Why wasn't that enough? The answer came to Bill in Akron. Nobody knew or understood Bill's message better than Bill himself and he had even directly experienced the presence of God in that hospital room. But when the message was no longer enough, when he felt his resolve and commitment weakening, Bill understood, really understood perhaps for the first time THAT HE COULD NOT DO THIS ALONE. What was needed was a *fellowship* of alcoholics, acting not as "teachers and students" but as *equals,* helping each other conquer their otherwise terminal conditions. Alcoholics Anonymous was born.

I want to say a few more things about AA before looking in detail at Emotions Anonymous (EA) and covering the Twelve Steps from that perspective. I mentioned earlier in the book that I found it astounding that AA has survived and flourished as a non-capitalistic venture in a fully capitalistic society. Lest you think I am presenting Bill W. as some sort of saint I need to tell you that part of his motivation to develop a worldwide network of programs and hospitals devoted to treating the disease of alcoholism was his desire to get both rich and famous. He had plenty of profit making schemes for AA; what stopped him was other people, both inside and outside the fellowship. One was John D. Rockefeller Jr. (yes, Bill knew people who knew people). Mr. Rockefeller turned down Bill's request for funding for his worldwide AA plan. Despite Mr. Rockefeller's deep concern about alcoholism, his philanthropic nature, and his untold millions in wealth, he would give Bill only $5000 along with the admonition: "Please don't ever ask me for anything more." Rockefeller's position was actually a reflection of a good number of the early members of the fledgling AA movement. They knew that any commercialization would run the risk of distorting the mission and the message of AA.

Next for Bill came writing the book. He started writing what would eventually become known as the *Big Book of AA* in 1937. He found a publisher who agreed to publish the book and offered him a $1500 advance on royalties. Some of the AA people were all for it. Others objected, and they prevailed. So AA once again steered clear of the negative influence of money. I am going into this in such detail here because I want you to understand that the profit motive and all that goes along with that was kept out of Twelve Step programs *from the beginning*, and still is! That's one of the reasons that I said above that I could not prove "scientifically" that going to Al-Anon decreases the utilization of medical resources or makes people happier. Twelve Step programs don't keep records. They don't make any claims about success rates. They don't endorse anything or lend their name to other endorsements. They do not participate in research programs and certainly would never be in the position to allow for head to head studies against pharmaceuticals. Twelve Step programs are ANONYMOUS. This is a foundational reason for their success. This fundamental philosophy of nonparticipation in the corrupting worlds of commerce and politics were laid out in the *Big Book* by Bill Wilson. They are called the Twelve Traditions of AA. They are also the twelve foundational traditions of the many programs of recovery derived from AA including Narcotics Anonymous (NA), Overeaters Anonymous (OA), Gamblers Anonymous (GA), Sexaholics Anonymous (SA), Al-Anon, Codependents Anonymous (CoDA) and the program to which we are going to turn now Emotions Anonymous (EA).

THE EMOTIONS ANONYMOUS STORY:

AA and other Twelve Step programs were already well established and widely available when, in July 1971, Emotions Anonymous was founded in St. Paul, Minnesota. The roots of EA were established in 1966 when Marion

F. (remember...anonymous!), who had been attending Al-Anon meetings, decided to start a group based on a concept she had read about in a newspaper article. The name of the group: Neurotics Anonymous. Within a year, members of Neurotics Anonymous had started more groups in Minnesota and neighboring states. One group started in Germany. Unfortunately, politics are everywhere, and eventually a schism developed between the Minnesota groups and the main office of Neurotics Anonymous. The Minnesota Intergroups Association voted to dissociate itself from Neurotics Anonymous, eventually renaming itself Emotions Anonymous. Before we discuss the Twelve Steps of EA, I want to look at some important psychological and philosophical implications of that original name: Neurotics Anonymous.

I have mentioned the term neurotic earlier in this book, pointing out how this commonly used and highly descriptive term was dropped from the official psychiatric nomenclature when DSM III was published in 1980. There are a lot of definitions of neurotic, ranging from its commonsense everyday usage to technical psychoanalytic definitions to ones implying a biologically based mental disorder (e. g. The *Oxford Dictionary* 1996 Edition defines neurosis as "a mental illness, characterized by irrational or depressive thought or behavior, caused by a disorder of the nervous system"). Whatever definition you choose, one thing that they have in common is that they are not complimentary. It has never been said that it is desirable to be neurotic. What I want to look at here is the significance of a self-help group formed by non-professionals actually *choosing* to label themselves with this seemingly derogatory term. What exactly were they saying was the problem that they all shared? My answer to that is simply this: *Being human.* I believe that accepting the label neurotic is, in essence, acknowledging that we, as human beings, are *all* flawed, emotionally unstable, imperfect creatures often driven by fear, anxiety, envy, greed, lust, gluttony, despair and all the rest of deadly sins and negative emotions you can think of. Freud often talked about the "psychopathology of everyday life", in essence saying that that we are all, by our very nature, neurotic. What these EA founders did was have the *courage* and *wisdom* to admit it! That was their *starting point*!

Contrast this with medical model psychiatry's unspoken but clearly implied philosophy of "normality" as a functional and achievement-oriented state of existence consistent with adaptation and success in our competitive, high-stress society. Are you unable to keep up with the demands of multitasking? You've got ADD. Not getting over the loss of a loved one in an acceptable period of time? It's Major Depression. Have you given into temptation and abused drugs, food, gambling and/or sex? Clearly you are "self medicating" a psychiatric disorder. (Unless, of course you are taking medication for restless legs; then it is just drug side effects) See what I mean?

So what can a group of laypeople, acknowledging that they are "neurotic", possibly accomplish by getting together and utilizing a Twelve Step program adapted from AA? It's time to go through these Twelve Steps, one by one, and see. I will use the Twelve Steps as articulated in EA but be aware the only difference from the Twelve Steps of AA is in labeling the nature of the "addiction." (As my reference material in exploring EA I will primarily be using the EA "Big Book": *Emotions Anonymous, Revised Edition*, published by Emotions Anonymous International Services, 1978, and revised 1994. All the following page references from that book will be in the form: EA, p. x).

THE BASIC PHILOSOPHY OF EA:

As you know, my beliefs as a psychiatrist are expressed in what I have called the wisdom principles, those views that encompass and value multiple perspectives in trying to help alleviate human emotional suffering. Here is how the EA Big Book puts it:

> Some of us have tried to avoid getting help for our emotional problems by questioning whether we have a physical illness, a mental illness, or a spiritual illness. Body, mind, and spirit make up our total human self. Each is an integral part and each is influenced by the others. We really cannot divide ourselves as human beings (EA, p.14).
>
> In the Emotions Anonymous program *we do not analyze emotional illness. We do not categorize and label everything* (EA, p.14, italics mine).
>
> We keep ourselves from becoming well; no one else does. It is our responsibility to become well. Only when we choose to act on this responsibility will we gain the ability to recover our emotional health (EA, p.15).

What actions are they talking about? Simple; just follow the twelve steps.

STEP ONE

We admitted we were powerless over our *emotions* that our lives had become unmanageable

There is a countermovement to 12 Step programs called Rational Recovery and the first issue they vigorously attack is the concept of powerlessness. They argue (rightfully I believe) that it is counterproductive to teach someone they are powerless over something because it can lead to blindly following a set of beliefs or practices that have not been thought through individually and rationally. Even my good buddy Rick Roderick has called Twelve Step programs "cult-like". And I would agree if I didn't more deeply understand what the Twelve Step programs really mean when they use the term powerless because in Twelve Step programs this is clearly conceptualized as a temporary, not permanent state. You are not *currently and forever will be* totally powerless over alcohol, drugs, food, sex or depression (choose your poison) but the admission of a current state of powerlessness is a critical and absolutely necessary first step in conquering self destructive behaviors and painful emotions. Think of it this way; admitting powerlessness in Step One is really the same as saying "I need help because I don't know what to do." This common language description of powerlessness puts the concept in the right light. But…it is still much harder to admit that you need help than you might imagine.

As normal humans there is generally only one person we ever truly trust, and that is ourselves. It's the only mind we really know. (William James was said to have observed that the greatest distance in the universe is the one between two minds). Thus to *truly* admit powerlessness over behaviors or emotions is actually saying that I need to be told what to think and do because I can no longer trust myself to figure this out. In acknowledging powerlessness we, in essence, are asked to voluntarily and consciously *surrender* control to an "other" in order to help solve our problem(s). I am making a point out of the fact that this is a conscious and voluntary decision to distinguish between what I will call here voluntary and conscious surrendering versus involuntary and "un"conscious surrendering. Let me illustrate this with a couple of simple examples:

INVOLUNTARY, "UN"CONSCIOUS SURRENDERING:

Susan has been feeling increasingly depressed and despondent recently. Last night she woke up with a panic attack, shaking uncontrollably and having difficulty breathing. First thing in the morning, she called her gynecologist and scheduled an emergency appointment. She *will do whatever* the doctor tells her because she sure as hell doesn't want to ever have another panic attack. To no one's surprise who is reading this book (I hope), her gynecologist gives Susan a free sample of Lexapro, a follow-up prescription and re-schedules her for an appointment in a month. Susan is also given a booklet put out by Pfizer that explains the biological cause and diagnosis and treatment of panic disorder and depression.

On the surface it looks like Susan admitted her powerlessness over the panic attack and surrendered to an "other" (her doctor) in deciding what to do about it. But this type of admission of powerlessness and act of surrendering is involuntary and "un"conscious. She is not choosing between options, nor, (for reasons we've discussed), will her doctor likely give her any. Living in America, she has already been thoroughly brainwashed into conceptualizing emotional pain as an illness requiring medical treatment. Without options (e.g. Yoga, cognitive therapy, marriage counseling, stress reduction etc.) being presented and as a result of years of "Disneyfication" by pharmaceutical companies and biopsychiatry, I think we can comfortably agree that while Susan did admit powerlessness and did "surrender" in seeking help for her panic attack, she did so "un"consciously and involuntarily. And you know what? In our everyday decisions and choices you and I do this a thousand times a day, every day. It forms the fabric of a free-market capitalist culture whose primary method of informing, educating and persuading is its "geist", advertising. But there is another kind of surrendering. It is based on a decision made while fully aware that one is voluntarily admitting powerlessness and consciously deciding to surrender. It's this type of admission Twelve Step programs are interested in.

CONSCIOUS SURRENDERING: A TRIP TO THE BAHAMAS

When I was treating alcoholism and drug addiction the typical length of stay in an inpatient facility was twenty eight days. It wasn't fun and for most patients the time seemed to drag on forever. It was not at all surprising then that most felt physically and emotionally exhausted by the time day twenty eight arrived. Many of the patients felt like they had earned, needed and deserved a break. Often, their family and friends (feeling so grateful that their loved one had finally sought and gotten help) believed so as well. So it wasn't unusual at all for a patient and family to plan for a vacation right after discharge. The truth is, however, that despite twenty eight days of being good and following directions, this vacation issue was the first genuine test of surrendering for many patients. Because our answer to the question of whether or not to take a vacation was always the same: "NO!"

Now you might be thinking that this was merely because vacation spots promote and entice people to party and yes, that was a part of the reason that we always said no. But there was a much deeper and more meaningful reason. It was because despite the patients' and often their families' belief that they have indeed worked hard and deserved a break, our message was that they, as yet, had not accomplished or earned *anything!* Staying sober while locked up in a facility without access to drugs or alcohol proved nothing! That was the powerlessness message we needed to deliver to our patients. And their consciously choosing to follow our advice and not go on vacation, even if they desperately wanted to go and genuinely believed that they would be perfectly safe (most had conspired with their families to come up with some sort of plan to keep them away from the temptations of alcohol and drugs) was the first real act of surrendering they would have to make to stay sober. The first of many!

HOW THIS APPLIES TO EMOTIONS ANONYMOUS

Do you ever say or think, "Why does everything have to happen to me?" If so, you are, we believe, powerless over your emotions"...says the EA Big Book. Sound familiar? How about these?

- *We were not able to change just using our willpower.*
- *We could not get well by ourselves, no matter how hard we tried.*
- *We tried analyzing, but it did not work.*
- *You've tried everything from medications to self-help to self-centeredness and yet your emotions keep running you. It's time to give up; it's time to* ***surrender*** *your will and* ***for now, just for now,*** *turn it over to others to lead the way. Because, after all, your life has become...*(EA, p.41)

UNMANAGEABLE.

What does an unmanageable emotional life look like? Is this the right concept to explain what otherwise might be labeled a depression and/or anxiety disorder (a brain illness)? I certainly think so. Having dealt with thousands of clients and patients over the years, it's hard to argue that a sense of unmanageability underlies many presentations for psychiatric help. But, it could be rightfully argued that in today's complex world and as such complex creatures, there are unmanageable aspects to everyone's life. So let's look specifically at what Emotions Anonymous has to say about this idea of unmanageability as an indicator of the need to surrender and seek help in EA.

In line with the seductive appeal of the victim narrative previously discussed, is the deeply embedded idea that if others would only change, somehow our personal miseries would end. This take on life is so common that a term, co-dependency, has been coined to describe it (generating numerous books, self-help programs and even a dedicated 12 Step program, CoDA). EA says: "We think the people around us make life unmanageable, but the more we try to change others the more unmanageable our lives become. We are powerless over other people and cannot change them" (EA, p. 42).

Unmanageability also takes many other forms. Feeling overly-sensitive, self absorbed, socially isolated or paralyzed, overwhelmed and isolated and alone are some of the manifestations of unmanageability EA lists. They also rightfully point out that physical and psychosomatic illnesses are often also symptoms. This is what I was alluding to in the opening quote of this chapter by Dr. Epstein. These are not radical or outlandish ideas. I believe that most physicians (except, perhaps, hardcore biopsychiatrists) clearly see the connection between emotional and psychological problems (not conceptualized as mental "illnesses" themselves) and physical complaints, even physical pathology. It's been interesting to see how the full force of the Psychiatryland marketing machinery has been profitably turned toward this phenomenon in massive ad and research campaigns to convince doctors to screen their troublesome psychosomatic patients for hidden psychiatric illness. No big deal, a two or three item questionnaire will do! What an "out" for an overly busy doctor. No need to discuss a deteriorating marriage with your patient with worsening hypertension and chest pain; just diagnose depression and simply add another pill to your treatment. Ten minutes and out the door...Next!

The final part of step one is the conscious (as opposed to the "un"-conscious) admission that you don't know what to do and need help. This admission is often accompanied by a mental state defined in all Twelve Step programs as "being sick and tired of being sick and tired." Strongly implied here is an accompanying willingness to take personal responsibility and try whatever it takes, no matter how radically different or challenging. Remember the quote from above:

> We keep ourselves from becoming well: no one else does.
> It is our responsibility to become well. Only when we choose to act on this responsibility will we gain the ability to recover our emotional health.

What, no blame game? No magic pill? Taking personal responsibility... Huh?? Unfortunately, whatever the level of willingness many potential Twelve Step participants find their new found sense of enthusiasm strongly challenged, sometimes defeated, when it becomes time to move on to the next Step:

Step Two
Came to believe that a Power greater than ourselves could restore us to sanity.

You might think that in a society where belief in God or a Higher Power is so seemingly widespread and publicly visible that a step in recovery asking you simply to acknowledge that belief would not be some huge psychological or philosophical barrier to participation, and yet of all the steps, Step Two (and even more so Step Three) seem to be the ones that lead to an early dropout from recovery or, more insidiously, serve as the perfect excuse to not even try a Twelve Step program. I can't tell you how many times I've heard the excuse that "I'm not religious" or "I don't believe in God" leading to an outright dismissal of the option of even trying recovery. And I will use the word ***excuse*** here because that's exactly what it is. Despite the language used in the steps, a belief in God is absolutely and positively ***not required*** for a totally successful utilization of a Twelve Step recovery program. This fact is *clearly articulated* in the careful wording of Step Three:

STEP THREE
Made a decision to turn our will and our lives over to the care of God *as we understood Him*

Those italicized words *as we understood Him* are not merely a throw-in to appease any doubters in potential Twelve Step participants. It is a carefully chosen (if admittedly somewhat sexist) expression of the freedom of Twelve Step participants to choose ***whatever*** concept of a Higher Power works for each individual. In the EA handbook, they put it like this:

> This can be any idea of God, the EA group (the power of many people working together for recovery is greater than one person's power), nature (a force certainly greater than we are), the idea of universal principles, or anything we can accept as being greater than our individual selves (EA, p.46).

The Chinese curse "May you live in interesting times" certainly seems to apply to early 21st Century American life. Terrorism, economic collapse, job insecurity and climate change have certainly met the criteria for "interesting" as meant in this proverb. On top of it is now a new debate sparked by the growing voice of atheism. Is there a God? What perverse and destructive role has religion played and is still playing in modern life? This is a fascinating discourse and the atheism "card" is sometimes, although not all that frequently, played in arguing against Twelve Step philosophy. The more common argument is along the lines of why people say they don't go to church every Sunday; they believe in God or a Supreme Being but don't like or agree with formal religious rituals, beliefs and practices. And on the surface, reading the Twelve Steps can certainly bring these formal religion issues to mind. But I want to assure you, this source of resistance is completely off target because even an avowed atheist can receive the full benefit of Twelve Step work, because although the word God is included in five of the twelve steps, the operative term here is really the one stated in Step Two, "A Power greater than ourselves." That "definition" of God is what allows the group, the program, nature or human spirituality to be invoked as that to which you are surrendering and turning your will and life over to in Step Three. Here is a concrete example:

In a compelling autobiographical account of her Al-Anon recovery, *Letting Go With Love,* Julia H. (H. 1987) devotes an entire chapter to her struggle with the God issue. It's clear in reading her book that Julia is a thoughtful, intelligent and resourceful person yet she just couldn't accept the idea that God exists, let alone watches over and cares for her. So her sponsor asks her: "Are you willing to act *as if* you believed there is a higher power?" Julia responds: "I'm willing to believe that the ocean is a power greater than I am." So her sponsor tells her: "Then go to the ocean and take your defects with you. Close your eyes and feel them drifting off to sea, one at a time." Julia found this acceptable and actually went to the seashore and meditated by the ocean. This helped her get past her resistance to Steps Two and Three and move forward in the program. But what happened at the ocean? Did she really turn her will and life over to the ocean? Did this, as promised in Step Two, restore her to sanity?

In my mind, what probably happened to Julia at the ocean wasn't much, certainly not some magical spiritual transformation. What truly happened was a small but meaningful breakdown in her pattern of resistance to allowing herself to be helped by others. Despite all the lip service we pay to being open-minded, when you think about it, we all tend to be incredibly resistant to other peoples' advice, ideas or beliefs. And this isn't because we've learned to trust ourselves because our thoughts, beliefs and behaviors always turned out to be right. The reason is much deeper than that. It is because we have never navigated ourselves out of the center of the universe. This has nothing to do with self-esteem or individual achievements. This has to do exclusively with the previously discussed primary narcissism, expressing itself in our adult lives as self-centeredness, stubbornness and willful resistance to change. The singular goal of Steps One through Three is to poke holes in this powerful barrier, to open us to the *possibility* of a change in ourselves and our lives that we cannot currently imagine or know how to bring about. In Step Two we are asked to believe that a Power greater than ourselves can restore us to sanity. Is that saying that pre-program we are insane (psychotic)? Not from the Twelve Step perspective. The Twelve Step program's definition of insanity is to "repeat the same actions or behaviors over and over again but expecting different results."

H.O.W.

H.O.W. is a central acronym in early recovery. It stands for **H**onesty, **O**penness, and **W**illingness. These describe the attitude and perspective that grows from a successful navigation of Steps One to Three. And believe me; they are necessary because in Step Four you are going to be asked to do something that takes great courage, something that I guarantee you have never done before in your entire life:

STEP FOUR
Made a searching and fearless moral inventory of ourselves

Go take a look at yourself in the mirror. Don't focus on your outward appearance; you've done that a million times. Look into your own eyes and take a glimpse inside at who you are, who you ***really are.*** What are your strengths? What are your weaknesses? What do you believe and what do you stand for? What have you done in your life that you feel guilty about, ashamed of, have never told anybody? No hedging, no self-delusion…just be painfully and totally honest with yourself. Can you do it?

Okay. Now take out a piece and write it all down, everything!

Now, take that piece of paper and sit down with someone and read aloud everything on that paper.

Does this sound like something you would do? Does this sound like something you ***could do?*** Well get ready, because in the Twelve Step program that is exactly what Steps Four and Five will ask you to do. I said it takes courage because it does. This is how EA describes this challenge and how to meet it:

> Our faith in a Higher Power, along with our decision to allow this power to guide us, provides the courage we need to do a personal inventory (EA, p.53).
>
> A thorough and healthy inventory usually includes a balance of assets and defects (EA, p.53).
>
> We do not knowingly exclude anything (EA, p.54).

> Self-honesty brings self-acceptance and a realistic understanding of where and how we can change. We have no defects which are unique; we are all human. Anything we allow ourselves to become aware of can be changed. It is necessary for us to look within. (EA, p.54).

Earlier I discussed my admiration for the EA program originally naming itself Neurotics Anonymous, openly acknowledging the inherent imperfection of the human condition. Steps Four and Five speak directly to this issue but now the challenge goes well beyond a mere nodding acceptance of this perspective to a detailed analysis of how this applies directly to you. As I am writing now, in December 2009, the news is full of stories about Tiger Woods, a public parade of human imperfection if ever there was one. How easy it is to judge him. Maybe even forgive him for giving into temptation. After all, I've heard it said time and time again, "he's only human." But, what about you? You are only human too. Are you ready to confess (for example) your sexual secrets, fully and honestly? Are you ready to write down your secret sexual desires, to document your own past sexual behaviors? To do this, you will indeed need to be fearless. But I don't want to mislead you. What makes steps Four and Five so difficult is not simply that we have to own and confess to thoughts, beliefs and behaviors of which we might feel ashamed. In fact, EA does not really emphasize confessing past "sins." In the section in which the concept of the moral inventory is explained, embarrassing sexual issues are not excluded but the emphasis is clearly on two other common human frailties:

Resentment & Fear

> Among the important things we deal with in our inventories are resentments. These feelings of ill-will toward other people or institutions destroy peace of mind. When we resent someone or something, we unknowingly allow that person or thing to control us. It hurts us, though it may not hurt the person we resent. They probably are not even aware of it. Harboring deep resentments leads only to a life of frustration and unhappiness (EA, p.55).

Once you identify your resentments you then need to ***restate*** them focusing not on the person or institution you resent but on how it affects you and makes you feel. They give the following example:

I *resent* my boss *because* he never gives positive feedback, is critical,

> promoted someone else instead of me. This *affects my* financial security, self esteem, pride, relationships with co-workers. *I feel* I am a failure at my job; fear of failure (EA, p.55).

We've discussed how we cannot change others, only ourselves. Look at how the wording of this admission of resentment makes that possible. It reframes the problem in a language of how someone else's behavior ***affects you*** (something you could actually work on changing) and how someone else's behavior ***makes you feel*** (again, something you could actually work on changing). Why, though, is there that tagline, "fear of failure" added at the end? It's because EA philosophy believes that "When we look at our resentments, we find they are usually a reaction to being afraid" (EA, p.56).

Frederick Nietzsche has a very interesting (but hardly widely accepted) theory on the origin of Christianity. He believed that the appeal and meteoric growth of early Christianity was rooted in what he called "*ressentiment*", a French term close in meaning to the English word resentment. The point relative to this discussion involves looking at who, according to Nietzsche, the early pre-Christians resented and what emotion underlay it. The resentment was in the peasant class in Biblical times and was directed at the Romans, harsh overlords who had all of the power to do whatever they wanted. It must have been terrifying to have a squad of armored Roman soldiers ride up to your farm or shop demanding more tribute to the Emperor. Your family could be starving and there might not be a single bushel of grain to spare, but what could you do? You were hardly in a position to argue.

Now, imagine that an early Christian believer comes along expressing an entirely different story about human existence, telling you that life on Earth is a mere temporary stop-over before ascending to paradise and living in bliss for all eternity. As for the sadistic Roman soldiers, their end-story would be somewhat different…eternal damnation and suffering. Can you see the appeal that this narrative on the "true" meaning of life could have held for the poor struggling-to-survive peasant? I'm not saying I agree with Nietzsche; I brought this up as a teaching example to clarify the concept of how resentment is often rooted in fear. And really, how different is this from the EA example of resenting the boss? Not much. Acting out aggressively against the boss is usually about as smart as pulling the Roman soldier off his horse and trying to beat him up…doomed to failure. Unable to act then we find ourselves, as quoted above, "harboring deep resentments" leading "to a life of frustration and unhappiness."

Okay, so what is the answer? It's NOT SAFE to go after the boss if you want to keep your job. So how do you conquer your feelings of frustration and unhappiness rooted in resentment which is itself rooted in fear, often realistic fear? I know! How about some Prozac? Seriously, what can you do?

To answer this I am going to jump ahead a bit and give you a brief preview of coming attractions. It's called the Serenity Prayer, a mantra recited at the close of 12 Step meetings.

God grant me the serenity to accept the things I cannot change
The courage to change the things I can
And the wisdom to know the difference

At the end of this chapter I will explain to you how this simple saying incorporates all you learn in Twelve Step programs and all the instructions you need to radically improve your daily emotional life. For our purposes here (which is to explore options to resentment and fear that don't involve surrendering to a lifetime of frustration and unhappiness) let me just say that the answer lays in focusing on a goal of personal serenity rather than the right/wrong, justice/injustice issues that typically under gird our resentments, frustrations and fears. A lot more about that later; let's go back to Steps Four and Five and look at how they contribute to the previously discussed crucial goal of displacing yourself from the center of the universe (your primary narcissism).

We've already looked at how there is important wisdom gained in seeing yourself as an inherently flawed creature among other flawed creatures (normal humans) and not to view yourself as especially worse off than or more impaired than those around you. How come we don't already know this? Why do so many of us feel that our problems are worse than and not understood by others?

We tend to think of narcissism as a falsely inflated reading of our assets that results in an egotistical sense of specialness. But when I use the term "primary" narcissism, I am also referring to the tendency for an inflated reading of our faults and negative life circumstances, resulting in low self-esteem and feelings of worthlessness and victimization. Either way, to move forward in Twelve Step work, this background issue needs to come to the surface. And Steps Four and Five are all about that. Here is how EA describes the importance of the words "of ourselves" in Step Four:

> While writing our inventory we concentrate only on ourselves. This is our inventory, not another person's. We consider only our involvement in situations even when something may have not been entirely our fault. In doing so we become aware of how self-centered we are and how our ego keeps us in this self-centeredness. We see where we have contributed to our own difficulties by being selfish, dishonest, self-seeking and frightened (EA, p.57).

EA is certainly not pulling any punches here. Again, this is a *searching* and *fearless* moral inventory, not merely some exercise in self comforting or justification (that I fear is the case in many so-called "therapy" sessions). The purpose is clear; as stated directly in the handbook when describing Step Five: "All of EA's Twelve Steps ask us to go against our normal inclinations. *They all deflate our egos, and this step is perhaps the greatest ego deflator of all"* (EA, p. 57, italics mine). This leaves little doubt as to what needs to be accomplished before moving on to Steps Six to Twelve. A deflation of the ego (also sometimes referred to as "getting humble"), a goal helped greatly by the Step Five requirement to share your moral inventory with your Higher Power and another human being.

Depending on your personal working definition of your Higher Power, this aspect of sharing will vary. If your Higher Power is based on the traditional concept of God, sharing won't be difficult because God already knows what is in your heart and everything you've done. If your Higher Power is nature or the human spirit, then sharing may be a sort of meditation on your written list. Either way, the real challenge comes in choosing another human being with whom to share your deepest and darkest secrets. Here, EA has some very specific recommendations. "The fifth step is best taken with a person who has a working knowledge of the twelve-step program because it is very important that this person understand what we are trying to accomplish" (EA, p.59). It is suggested that the person you choose be "primarily a listener" and should not offer advice or counseling. And clearly, it needs to be someone who can be trusted not to betray your confidence. Who to share with is an important decision and needs to be thought through carefully. I've heard the example that at the famous Twelve Step program, Hazelden, an ordained minister is made available for Step Five work. This establishes a clergy-client relationship where even confessions of violent crimes (not unheard of in addicts) are privileged.

After an honest and earnest attempt at Steps Four and Five ("Progress not Perfection" a Twelve Step saying goes) there is a very good chance that you will immediately feel a great sense of emotional relief, as if a terrible burden has been lifted from your shoulders. This is just the preparation you will need to begin the healing process in:

Step Six
Were entirely ready to have God remove all these defects of character

To illustrate the difference between recognizing and acknowledging character defects (Steps Four and Five) and doing something about them

(Steps Six and Seven) I want to catch you up on what's been going on with me. As you know I started to write this book in September of 2006. It's now December 2009. The reason this is taking me so long is in large part because I have failed to find an agent or publisher willing to take on the book. If you are reading it now there is a good chance I've elected to self publish, although I haven't totally given up on going the traditional route. As it is for all authors, rejections have been painful and discouraging. So painful, in fact, that the book project sat dormant for about a year (with twelve and a half chapters written) as I decided whether I thought the effort was worth it or not (character flaw #1). But that is not the character flaw I want to focus on here. The flaw I want to look at was one that was clearly revealed during the course of what else I have been doing for the past eighteen months.

Earlier in the book I told you that when I was in private practice I had systematically cut ties with institutions, managed care companies and hospitals. For a myriad of reasons too boring to go into here, that plan became untenable and I was forced to (really I chose to…, rigorous honesty and taking responsibility) just go get a job that paid me a salary, had paid vacations and benefits and removed me from all of the pressures of dealing with insurance companies, landlords and office personnel.

With my critical view of psychiatry and how it's practiced you may have guessed that the last place I'd want to work would be somewhere that required me to do little else but see tons of patients and put them on, adjust or change their medications. But that is exactly what I did. I took a job as a "hospitalist", a doctor who works for the hospital, primarily taking care of inpatients. So I didn't just stick my toe back into the water of orthodox biopsychiatry, I dove in headfirst. Why? Because those were the types of jobs that were easily available, paid well and had the best benefits. Once again I took the easy way out (character flaw #2). Well my dear readers, it didn't work out. As I sit here writing today I have quit two hospitalist jobs in less than two years. I won't bore you with the details but the jobs were simply intolerable to me. I bring this up, however, to illustrate the difference between recognizing and acknowledging a character flaw and the reality of actually doing something about it because these two jobs clearly brought one of my worst character flaws right to the surface.

I would definitely characterize myself as having a core low self-esteem. Despite this I did manage to get my medical degree and gain the prestigious title and responsibilities of a doctor. My character flaw involves my being unable (or is it unwilling?) to recognize that along with the prestige and privileges afforded to a doctor comes some important responsibilities to not just your patients but your fellow health care workers as well. Like it or not, the doctor is viewed as the leader of the health care team, the person other health care workers look to for leadership, especially in times of high stress.

Unfortunately, my primary narcissism and low self-esteem acted as a barrier to my keeping that in mind. In concrete terms, what happened was that I would lose my temper. I would curse and gripe and moan and groan about all that was wrong with the world of psychiatry. And I wasn't mindful of who I was complaining to. It could be a nurse, an orderly or administrator. Most often it was the poor person in admissions, calling me for admitting orders in the middle of the night. I have really let loose on them. But I felt justified! Because I wasn't upset about getting woken up at night (I might not have liked it but had accepted it as part of the job). No, I was griping and yelling about the world, the psychiatric profession, the over diagnosis of mental illness, the profit motives of pharmaceutical companies and hospital owners, the abuse of the system by addicts etc., etc. In other words, I was complaining about all of the issues that have motivated me to write this book. And more often than not the person I was griping to would, in principle at least, fully agree with me! Imagine my surprise then when in both jobs I was called in by my respective bosses because the staff had complained about me. On both jobs I was threatened to be fired if I didn't get my temper under control. About many of the issues bothering me, even the bosses agreed, but they also both said the same thing: "You can't be losing your temper like that. You are the doctor!"

I admit that I was nearly completely unaware of this effect my behavior was having on the other health care workers. I was scaring them! The nurses, orderlies and admission personnel look up to the "doctor" and expect and need a mature, rational, calm and reassuring person in that role. I was scaring them with my temper outbursts. It didn't matter what the "subject matter" was; it had nothing to do with it. These workers were under the same pressure, if not more, than me. They were worried about their jobs and they too had to deal with very difficult working conditions and some really scary and crazy patients. All my outbursts did was make them feel more insecure and frightened. Because, like it or not, I was the doctor. It hurts me to think about this and all that I said and did at those jobs that I wish I could take back (See Steps Eight and Nine).

Okay, let's step back here and examine how my story fits into the topic at hand. I see my character flaw as a narcissistically based blindness to the needs of others rooted in my own fears and core low self-esteem. Fair enough; a fearless and searching moral inventory of one of my worst character flaws. Have I never noticed this before? Did I have to do so much damage to others that I was threatened to be fired twice before it came to the surface? No. I've known all about this "side to my personality" for a long time. What I have managed to do in the past, however, was get away with it. In various and sundry ways, (I believed), I was covering over and compensating for the devastating effect my childlike temper had on others. That's not true, of course, and I've suffered the consequences of my actions, alienating others and feeling alone, misunderstood and depressed. I saw my character defect but wasn't *willing* or *ready* to do anything about it. Next week I start a new job in an outpatient clinic for PTSD patients at a VA hospital. No one there really knows me yet. The job involves much more than simple assembly line patient care and writing prescriptions. I will be part of a treatment team, helping patients through psychotherapy and psychosocial treatment along with medication. And no on-call work! I think I am ready to **DO SOMETHING** about my character defect because I have an opportunity now to start fresh and create an atmosphere at work that will contribute to a sense of wellbeing and serenity in me instead of feelings of frustration, anger and despair.

And that, my friends, is Step Six.

STEP SEVEN
Humbly asked Him to remove our shortcomings

Of all of the Twelve Steps, I am least comfortable with the wording of this one. We are now at the stage of recovery where we are trying to do something concrete about our character defects. What I see Step Seven's language telling us to do is, however, is just sit back and wait...God will do the work. It says:

> We need to be rid of our defects in order to correct our behavior and to live happy, serene and manageable lives. As defects are removed assets replace them. All of this will be done by our Higher Power as we demonstrate our readiness and ask that it be done. The efforts are ours, but the results come from God (EA, p.63).

This sounds a bit too much like the admonition to pray to God for something and your prayers will be answered. I'm sure for many this concept will work just fine, but let's briefly explore an alternative conceptualization of Higher Power that might make this step more universally acceptable.

In his book *On Religion*, philosopher and theologian John Caputo proposes that perhaps the best way to conceptualize a Higher Power in our frenzied and hyper-real postmodern times is as "The Force" from the Star war movies (Caputo 2001). As I'm sure most of you recall the force was presented by Lucas as some sort of energy pervading and organizing the universe. And, of course, the main theme was that the force had both a "good" and "bad" side and that we humans can and must choose a side. Thus we have Darth Vader nearly conquering the universe with the help of the dark side of the force and Luke Skywalker saving the day by allying with the good side, a real Biblical drama. But the theme is intriguing. Unless you truly believe that the universe is simply atoms in random motion, then some sort of organizing principle, a greater or "higher" power has a strong appeal. What I personally like about the idea of the force is that there is also an intrinsic morality attached to it. There is a good side and a bad side to the force and we choose (or, I believe, at least sense) what side we are on. For example, in my personal experiences working in mental healthcare I have come to believe that the doctors and administrators who took advantage of the lack of scientific validity in psychiatry as an opportunity to maximize profits are, whether consciously or not, allied with the dark side of the force. I really do believe that "deep down" we humans do know right from wrong and can distinguish good from bad but that we are cover our choices with many layers of nuance and complexity. "I try to maximize my corporate profits for the benefit of the stockholders who rely on and have put their faith in me", says the CEO. This statement and justification leans to the good side of the force but if the follow-up is: "So therefore today I am announcing 10,000 layoffs, the closing of three factories, a cutback in employee healthcare benefits and my personally selling $3million of stock options", then it's pretty clearly leaning the other way. That is just not hard to see.

I don't want to push this force analogy too far. I am simply using it to demonstrate that there are myriad workable conceptualizations of a "Higher Power" that can minimize discomfort and give you a sense of direction in your Step 7 work. So now let's look at the question of how in this program we can, as quoted above, "rid ourselves of our defects in order to correct our behavior and to live happy, serene and manageable lives."

EA teaches that "humility is the key to working Step Seven." Humility is defined as a realistic and honest self appraisal in relation to other people and your Higher Power. Humility allows you to set realistic goals, feel confident about them and to take your time. You aren't going to correct your character defects overnight. But you must work your program or nothing will change. EA gives the example of procrastination as a character defect. To change that defect (always being late) into an asset (getting things done on time) takes attention to the problem, conscious behavior changes (forcing yourself to be on time for dinner, finishing your work project two days early) and humility. Procrastination is a common problem that many people have; you are no better or worse than them. Just take your own inventory, don't worry about others. For example, don't let it bug you after you've made an effort to change that now you are the only one on time for the dinner. And don't try to take on all of your character defects at once. Just keep working your program every day. Ask for help from your sponsor and other experienced members. Keep an open mind, take advice and try new things. Over time your emotional state and daily life will get much better because…THE FORCE IS WITH YOU…honestly.

It's time now to move forward to Steps Eight and Nine where the focus shifts from repairing yourself to now starting to work on repairing your relationships with others.

STEP EIGHT
Made a list of all persons we had harmed, and became willing to make amends to them all

STEP NINE
Made direct amends to such people whenever possible, except when to do so would injure them or others

Earlier in the book I mentioned that many addicts came into the rehabilitation program wanting to skip right to Step Nine so they could get out of the hot water they created with their employers and loved ones. With the direct damage done to others by the behaviors associated with drug and alcohol addiction, it is pretty obvious why amends need to be made. I also mentioned that we stopped our clients from doing this, insisting that they had to work the steps in sequential order because early in treatment they would be incapable of making true amends; they would simply be apologizing and manipulating again, something they had already done thousands of times in the past. But when it comes to EA we need to ask; exactly how have we harmed others by being depressed, anxious, moody and miserable? Let's look at what EA tells you to do:

> In Step Eight we examine our fourth-step inventory to see where we need to improve relationships with people in our lives. From our inventory we begin to list the people we have harmed (EA, p. 65).

Okay, that's pretty straightforward. Use the Step Four work to launch your Step Eight task. A sponsor can and should help with this. There are tendencies to both under do and overdo this list. You obviously cannot list everyone you've ever known as needing amends. There might also be people that you are not ready to deal with. That's okay, take your time. Again: "Progress not Perfection."

The next part of Step Eight involves developing the willingness to go forward with making amends. Here EA addresses an issue that is central to my concern about biopsychiatry's negative impact on emotional growth and healing. EA says that "we do not rationalize that our past wrongs should be excused because we were sick." Really?, asks the biopsychiatry patient; I have to take responsibility for my past behaviors even though I was suffering from an unrecognized and undiagnosed chemical imbalance causing me to have rapidly cycling moods? I hope that at this point I don't have to critique this in detail. Just recall that biopsychiatry promotes narratives that absolve patients from personal responsibility, rendering them passive participants in brain chemistry balancing experiments, hardly the task EA presents here in Step Eight.

The next thing that needs to be understood about making amends is that: "As our understanding grows, we see how the process of making amends is not so much for their sake as it is for ours." That is because: "If we are to transform our lives and become healthy, we have to be willing to clear away as much wreckage from our past as we can. We want loving, healthy relationships, so we have to start practicing the skills that are likely to foster them" (EA, p. 67).

So with the willingness in place and the long term goal of improving all current and future relationships, it is now time to move onto Step Nine and actually start making amends. What exactly does this entail? Let's start with the question of apologies. Does EA suggest that you apologize?

Half-jokingly, I have proposed a business plan to some of my friends in mental healthcare. Here is an ad for that business:

APOLOGY INCORPORATED

- Have you done something wrong?
- Did You Get Caught?
- Do You Need To Apologize?

Don't just jump in unprepared!!

Here at Apology Inc ™ we have trained mental health professionals who will teach you how to:

1. Look Sincere
2. Choose Just The Right Words
3. Sound Remorseful
4. Cry As Needed

5. Make Promises

OUR GUARANTEE:
Be Forgiven...(or your money back!)

I don't know how it is for you, but it has become very difficult for me to witness the apology phenomenon growing in our culture. Sports stars, politicians, celebrities and just plain folks have taken to making public apologies for offenses ranging from racially insensitive remarks to DUI's to sex crimes. But that's just part one! What really blows my mind is that we, the public, (mostly through the media) have taken to judging the legitimacy of the remorse and guilt the apologizer feels by dissecting the sincerity of the apology. How incredibly childlike we've become. Did he/she cry? Did he/she look remorseful? Did he/she promise never to do it again? And on and on; AS IF someone can't fake sincerity and cry on cue. C'mon, apologies are weak. Maybe they are necessary in polite society, but unless they are followed by genuine changes in behavior, they are simply empty and meaningless. EA says: "Making amends is not simply saying we are sorry, although an apology might be part of an amend. We make amends by changing our behavior" (EA, p. 68). For example, let's look at my temper issue described in the Step Six section above. Should I apologize to the workers at my former job, the ones I used to frighten and upset with my tantrums? I believe I should (in fact, I already have). But there will be no real amends until I do something else, control my temper at my new job! It's complicated. I'm not really directly making amends to those who suffered because of my behaviors in the past (although I think apologizing at least validates their feelings); I am instead kind of "paying it forward" by not putting my current co-workers through what my previous co-workers endured. To me, that represents genuine amends that promises to do what EA promotes as the reason for Steps Eight and Nine, to practice the skills that will foster loving and healthy relationships in the future. Here is an example directly from the EA Big Book:

> We do not apologize for having gossiped about a person if there is a chance he or she is not aware of the gossip. To do so would only cause more hurt. But we can make amends by admitting to the people with whom we have shared the gossip that we were wrong to have done so. We can also strive to stop our tendency to gossip or to listen to gossip. This constitutes making indirect amends to the person we had gossiped about and direct amends to ourselves as we practice honesty and humility. (EA, p. 70)

Making amends is a complicated business. People often need help making the difficult decisions necessary in this step. But the payoff is huge. I like to imagine that when I finally leave my job at the VA everyone I worked with will feel good about me and have positive memories about our time together. But, as I must always remind myself, I am not the center of the universe and even if I haven't behaved well and have lost my temper and scared people, this will have only a minimal impact on their lives. The impact that really matters is the one my making amends through behavior change will have on *my* life! Without my temper my life will be significantly better. And it might be nice to think back on my experiences at the VA with positive feelings, unblemished by memories of behaviors I regret. That is worthwhile goal.

At the end of the Step Nine material in the EA book they reprint the Twelve Promises of Emotions Anonymous. Here are six of them:

> Promise #1: We realize a new freedom and happiness.
> Promise#2: We do not regret the past or wish to shut the door on it.
> Promise #3: We comprehend the word serenity, and we know peace of mind.
> Promise#8: Our whole outlook on life changes.
> Promise #9: Our relationships with other people improve.
> Promise #10: We intuitively know how to handle situations that used to baffle us (EA, pp.70-71).

EA understands that this can easily sound too good to be true. They say that the twelve promises "may seem idealistic, exaggerated, or extravagant at first, but they really are possible. At our meetings we see them coming true in those around us. Some of these promises may be realized quickly, others slowly, but they will all develop naturally as a result of honestly working the EA program" (EA, p.71).

So…too good to be true? You'll never know until you try. Okay, things are looking pretty good. But there are three Steps to go. What could possibly be left to do? Remember the old joke; "How do you get to Carnegie Hall?"…… *practice!*

> Realizing the many benefits of practicing this program, we want to maintain our growth. To do this we go on to Steps Ten, Eleven and Twelve (EA, p.71).

STEP TEN

Continued to take personal inventory and when we were wrong promptly admitted it

STEP ELEVEN
Sought through prayer and meditation to improve our conscious contact with God *as we understood him*, praying only for knowledge of His will for us and the power to carry that out

STEP TWELVE
Having had a spiritual awakening as a result of these steps, we tried to carry this message and to practice these principles in all our affairs

So as you can see, the last three steps are all about the same issue revealed by the choice of the word "recovering" rather than "recovered" used by alcoholics and addicts in Twelve Step programs to describe their sobriety, even when sober for decades: Practice what you have learned! Or you might lose it. Isaac Stern, the world famous violinist, was quoted as saying: "If I don't practice for one day I know it; if I don't practice for two days, the world knows it." The task of recovering is a never-ending one, there is always more to do. Without daily practice of your EA recovery program you will not only miss opportunities for continued emotional and spiritual growth, you will also risk a regression to a level of emotional discomfort that you might have believed was permanently behind you. I can tell you one surprising fact for certain: alcoholics with ten, twenty or even thirty years of sobriety have been known to fall off the wagon, some falling so hard that they never get back up. With alcoholism, of course, it is easier to measure and pinpoint a failure of recovery. In the case of EA I think it is a lot more like the phenomenon described by Isaac Stern. The measurable progress made in EA is much more of a subjectively felt phenomenon than the more visible measure of progress in AA, i.e. sobriety. In an EA regression (or "relapse") on, for example, your tendency to resent others, it might very well be the case that at first there are no outwardly visible manifestations of your no longer attending to that character flaw. However, over time, it will become obvious to others as your irritability, complaining and other signs of resentment increase. Like Isaac Stern, you really don't want things to get to that point. So...practice, everyday!

Step Ten reminds us to take a daily inventory. EA warns: "Now that we are aware of our human imperfections, we realize we can easily fall back into our old ways of thinking and behaving. With this inventory we review our day, correct our errors, accept ourselves and others, and plan ways to do better tomorrow" (EA, p.72). But don't take yourself too seriously all the time. It isn't a daily matter of life and death. EA also reminds us: "If we try and fail, at least we have tried. It is often through our failures that we learn more about ourselves. We learn not to take ourselves too seriously. We benefit by gaining a sense of humor. We find that we can laugh at ourselves" (EA, p.73).

The wording of Step Eleven bothers me a bit because, once again, a very traditional concept of God is implied. But, they didn't forget to add "as we understood Him" to remind us that the traditional concept is not mandatory. In Step Eleven prayer is also defined in the traditional sense as some sort of "conversation" with a Higher Power. This is not a problem for many people. If it is, focus on the Step Eleven suggestion to meditate. The goal of meditation is not to communicate with some sort of Higher Power but to quiet the incessant chattering in our minds. It is about achieving a sense of inner quietude and peace. Wonderful insights often emerge from this state of mind. There are many forms of meditation so I will have resources for those interested in pursuing meditative disciplines in the Appendix.

Finally, let's move on to Step Twelve. To explain the essence of Step Twelve we need to take a step back to chapter twelve where we discussed Existential Psychotherapy as described by Irvin Yalom. As you'll recall, Dr. Yalom outlined the painful and inescapable existential truths of human existence: mortality, meaninglessness, isolation and freedom. But he also offered an achievable solution, altruism, service to others. In Step Twelve you are asked to try to carry the recovery message to others. But how, exactly do you do that and what are your goals in doing so? (It's not what you think).

> A paradox of the program is that to keep what we have learned for ourselves, we must give it away. With some degree of recovery resulting from practicing these steps, we can begin to reach out to others and share what we have learned. We share our stories—what we used to be like, what happened as we worked the steps, and how we have changed. This sharing allows us to see our experiences in a new light, and, consequently, we learn more about ourselves (EA, p.79).

So the paradox here is that carrying this message to others is primarily to strengthen your recovery, not to save someone else. It is essential to clearly grasp this concept because of a character flaw that is quite common in we humans...*feeling responsible* for the success or failure of others we are trying to help. Despite having learned during the long journey down the path to recovery that our wellbeing is solely our responsibility, it is incredibly difficult to not try to fix someone else. It's nearly impossible.

By the time you reach Step Twelve you may be ready to become a sponsor, taking a neophyte under your wing (we call them sponsees) and commit to helping them achieve what you have achieved. But what if your sponsee relapses (AA) or winds up in a psychiatric hospital or commits suicide (EA)? Is it your fault as the sponsor? Was there something that you could have or should have done differently? Maybe there was, but you did not elect to become a sponsor because you knew all the answers for someone else. You became a sponsor to assist in YOUR growth and recovery. You cannot afford to dwell on or obsess about someone else's failure, because what someone else thinks, feels or does *never was and never will be* under your control.

Putting it all together: SERENITY

That now brings us to the final, wrap-it-all-up item in our exploration of EA and the Twelve Steps: the serenity prayer, a simple mantra that can keep you on track and allow you to, as they say in Step Twelve, practice your recovery "principles in all your affairs." EA says that the serenity prayer "very simply sums up the aim of the twelve-step program", and I agree. In fact, I'll go even further in stating that the serenity prayer also, in many ways, sums up in a few words the message I'm trying to get across in this very long book. Once again, here is the prayer:

God grant me the serenity to accept the things I cannot change,
Courage to change the things I can,
And the wisdom to know the difference.

Let's skip the God part…it's a prayer…nuff said. The first question to ask is what, exactly, is the serenity prayer referring to in asking you to accept what you cannot change? To address this I want to turn back to our old friend, philosopher Martin Heidegger, who has a wonderfully descriptive concept that speaks directly to this issue.

Heidegger says that as human beings, each one of us is metaphorically "thrown" into the world. It is not a world of our choosing; it is simply a certain time, place and situation where we "find" ourselves. I often picture this idea of "throwness" in my mind as an image of some poor hapless baby falling to Earth from outer space. Where does he/she land? Nigeria, China, England? Is it in a poor family with eight children struggling to survive or is it as an only child of a multi-millionaire living in a McMansion? Is it 1860, 1960, or 2005? Is the family Jewish, Muslim, Catholic, atheist? Does our helpless baby have any say in the matter? That is precisely Heidegger's point. There is no "choice" involved. You cannot get a start-over and choose a different place to be "thrown."

But after that, don't choices follow? The answer to that question is the proverbial yes and no. Yes, it's inarguable that while we do not choose where, when or to whom to be born, we subsequently make tons of choices that affect our lives. So what is the "no" side? Aside from my "throwness" what else do I need to accept as that which I cannot change? A lot! Because yes, you can make choices within the framework in which you find yourself, but as we've discussed before, there are a limited (not infinite) number of narratives about society, the meaning of life, human freedom, and relationships that constitute the frameworks within which we make our choices. Attempting to deny that reality is where we can get ourselves into some real trouble. Remember the example of "choosing" to be a Samurai warrior at a time and place in history where the conditions for the possibility for being a Samurai no longer exist? That "choice" also no longer exists. I suppose you could choose to walk around in Samurai clothes, brandishing a sword and enforcing some ancient Samurai code of honor, but you would simply be treated as a nut-job. Perhaps I can best illustrate this concept, however, by turning back to that which I know best...myself.

I want to take a look at my throwness and the limitations on choices I've been forced to accept as a medical doctor/psychiatrist who finished his training in 1985 in America. As you recall I earlier defined my goals when choosing to go into psychiatry as hoping to play a role in integrating existential philosophy into an eclectic muti-perspectival mental health discipline. In the late seventies and early eighties this was still a reasonable and realistic goal. Psychiatry and psychology were abuzz with new ideas and efforts to integrate diverse psychological, philosophical and biological theories abounded. How was I to know at the time I chose psychiatry that my throwness was into an historical time when all of this would so abruptly end? By the time I finished my residency and started to seek meaningful work in my chosen profession, the 1980 appearance of DSM III had already launched psychiatry down its path to the pseudo-scientific medicalized discipline it has become. How did that limit my choices? For one, few fellow psychiatrists were interested in what interested me and there were few if any jobs where my day to day work would match up with my beliefs. I was forced into a life of compromise and a certain measure of deception in order to put food on the table (and utilize the eight years of study it took to get there). Besides, I believed strongly that I could still make a difference, could play a meaningful role in a reform of psychiatry. After all, I was not alone. So I wrote papers and books, gave lectures and attended meetings with like-minded psychologists, philosophers and psychiatrists. But all of this came with a heavy emotional price. In my work I found myself in a continual state of frustration, with strong feelings of resentment and anger fueled a constant sense of injustice. It made me an angry person, often perceived by others to be a chronic complainer, a troublemaker, "not a team player", just a pain in the ass. But at least I tried…right?

Wrong!

What I was (and am still) trying to do is, I believe, an important, noble and humane undertaking. What I lacked however, was the wisdom to accept the things I could not change and the courage to try to change the things I could. And without that wisdom my emotional life was a mess. Going to work became harder and harder to face.

I know now that I was focused on the wrong goal. I wanted to triumph; I wanted to win. I wanted to watch the psychiatrists behind the dictatorial domination of the bio-bio-bio model in psychiatry be forced to retreat with their tails between their legs. (Some of them have, by the way, thanks to investigations by Senator Grasseley of Iowa, but I didn't really get much gratification out of it). I was doing the right thing but for the wrong reasons. I didn't have a chance. I really needed the serenity prayer.

The serenity prayer teaches us is how to put things in the right order. Set goals, make choices, do all the things we do to make our lives meaningful. But don't do it for the wrong reasons. Don't do it to be proven right. Don't do it for fame, notoriety or power. These may or may not come. But you must always:

PUT SERENITY FIRST!!

Let's look at that prayer again. It says "grant me the *serenity* to accept the things I cannot change…" Serenity doesn't follow acceptance, it precedes it. The "goal" is to achieve serenity and then, from within that state of emotional quietude and stability, identify what truly can and cannot be changed. But how do you achieve serenity in the first place? Simple. You accept the things you cannot change and courageously change the things you can. Wait a second; that is a totally circular argument! Yes it is. So let's go back and add in the rest of the prayer, the reference to "the wisdom to know the difference." Now there is a familiar word. I've been promoting "wisdom" as a source of guiding principles and decision making throughout this book. Wisdom leads to serenity. And where does the wisdom come from? The answer to that is actually pretty simple. It comes from striving for serenity. Okay that's pretty mind-blowing…and impenetrable. Let's go back to my situation to clarify.

When I was striving to fix psychiatry I carried certain expectations that motivated me. I named a few above. I wanted justice. I wanted things to be made right. I wanted validation. I wanted admiration. I wanted and wanted and wanted. And all the clues telling me that I was on the wrong path were there from the beginning in my goal-oriented, expectation driven emotional states of anger, depression, dissatisfaction and frustration. I was hurting myself and all the people around me. How different it all could have been if I would simply have done one thing, put serenity first. Because when the serenity stopped I would gain the wisdom to understand that I was once again not accepting the things that I could not change.

In truth, I never was in control. I could put my ideas out there but I could not control how others would hear them or how they would react. In fact, in general, I couldn't control much of anything outside of myself. All that I could truly control was my attitude towards all the things out of my control. And if I put my own serenity first, then it would become very obvious (and I would gain the wisdom) to understand all of this and stop hurting myself and the people around me.

So you see it really is a kind of circle. Striving for serenity helps me gain the wisdom that will help me achieve serenity. Not happiness, success, triumph or power; just a nice calm feeling of acceptance and a quiet confidence that whatever comes along...I can handle it.

A favorite joke:

You know how to make God laugh?
Tell him your plans.

I am going to end the book now. It feels like the right time. In the appendix I'll give you information about readings and resources and tell you how to get in touch with EA if you would like to find a group near you or even start one up.

January 2010
Finis

Author Biography

Phillip Sinaikin, M.D., M.A. is a board certified clinical psychiatrist and addictionologist who has been in practice for twenty-five years. He has published and lectured extensively in both psychiatry and philosophy and has had numerous national television appearances on shows such as *Good Morning America, The Today Show, The CBS Evening News, Montel Williams and Geraldo.* He currently lives with his wife in central Florida.

Biblography

Alcoholics Anonymous. (1984). *Pass It On: The story of Bill Wilson and how the AA message reached the world.* New York: Alcoholics Anonymous World Services, Inc.

American Diabetes Association. (2004). Consensus development conference on antipsychotic drugs and obesity and diabetes. *J Clinical Psychiatry,* **65**(2): 267-72.

American Psychiatric Association. (1980). *Diagnostic and statistical manual of mental disorders 3rd edition.* Washington DC: American Psychiatric Association Press.

American Psychiatric Association. (1987). *Diagnostic and statistical manual of mental disorders 3rd edition (revised).* Washington DC: American Psychiatric Association Press.

American Psychiatric Association. (1994). *Diagnostic and statistical manual of mental disorders 4th edition.* Washington DC: American Psychiatric Association Press.

Angell, M. (2004). *The truth about drug companies: How they deceive us and what to do about it.* New York: Random House.

Baron, D.A. and Chrisman, A.K. (2007). Understanding the complexity of adult ADHD: Diagnostic and treatment challenges. *Supplement to Psychiatric Times,* Nov. 2007: 2-5.

Baum, F.L. (1999). *The wizard of oz.* New York: Alladin Paperbacks.

Bennett, W. and Gurin, J. (1982). *The dieters dilemma.* New York: Basic Books.

Bracken, P. and Thomas, P. (2005). *Postpsychiatry: Mental health in a postmodern world.* Oxford: Oxford University Press.

Caputo, J.D. and Yount, M. (1993). *Foucault and the critique of institutions.* University Park PA: The Pennsylvania State University Press.

Caputo, J.D. (1993). *Against ethics.* Bloomington: Indiana University Press.

Caputo, J.D. (1997). *Deconstruction in a nutshell.* New York: Fordham University Press.

Caputo, J.D. (2001). *On religion.* London: Routledge.

Cushman, P. (1990). Why the self is empty. *American Psychologist,* **45**(5): 599-611.

DeGrandpre, R. (2000). *Ritalin nation.* New York: W.W. Norton and Company.

DeWyze, J. (2003). Still crazy after all these years. *San Diego Weekly Reader,* **32**(2): Jan 9, 2003.

Dreyfus, H.L. (1993). Heidegger on the connection between nihilism, art, technology and politics. In *The Cambridge Companion to Heidegger.* Guignon, C.(ed). Cambridge: Cambridge University Press.

Dunn, A.L. et al. (2005). Exercise treatment for depression: Efficacy and dose response. *Am J Prev Med.* **28**(1): 140-1.

Dunner, D. (1998). Bipolar disorder in DSM-IV: Impact of rapid cycling as a course modifier. *Neuropsychopharmacology,* **19:**189-93.

Elliott, C. and Chambers, T. (2004). *Prozac as a way of life.* Chapel Hill: University of North Carolina Press.

Emotions Anonymous. (1995). Emotions Anonymous: Revised edition. Saint Paul MN: Emotions Anonymous International Services.

Epstein, M. (2005). Al-Anon referrals pay off. *Clinical Psychiatry News,* **33**(7): 9.

FDA News. (2005). FDA advisory of risk of birth defects with Paxil. December 8, 2005. *http://www.fed.gov/bbs/topical NEWS/2005/NEW01270.html.*

FDA Public Health Advisory. (2005). Deaths with antipsychotics in elderly patients with behavioral disturbances. April 11, 2005. http://fed.gov/cder/advisory/antipsychotics.html.

Fink, P. (2006). Should the diagnosis of melancholia be revived? *Psychiatric Times,* **23:** 33-4.

Foa, E.B. and Wilson, R. (1991). *Stop Obsessing.* New York: Bantam Books.

Foa, E.B. et al. (2007). *Prolonged exposure therapy for PTSD.* Oxford: Oxford University Press.

Foucault, M. (1970). *The order of things: An archeology of the human sciences.* London: Tavistock Publications.

Fournier, J. et al. (2010). Antidepressant drug effects and depression severity. *JAMA,* **303**(1): 47-53.

Frances, A.J. et al. (1991). An A to Z guide to DSM conundrums. *J Abnormal Psychology,* **100**(3): 407-12.

Genova, P. (2005). Shrink on campus. *Psychiatric Times,* June 2005: 29-31

Ghaemi, SN. (2008). Toward a Hippocratic psychopharmacology. *Can J Psychiatry,* **53**(3): 181-96.

Gladwell, M. (2004). High prices. How to think about prescription drugs. *The New Yorker,* Oct. 25, 2004.

Greenberg, RP. and Fisher, S. (1997). Mood mending medicines: probing drug, psychotherapy and placebo solutions. In Fisher, S. and Greenberg, RP. (eds.) *From placebo to panacea: putting psychiatric drugs to the test.* New York: John Wiley and Sons. 115-173.

Greenspan, M. (2003). *Healing through the dark emotions.* Boston: Shambhala.

Guignon, C. (ed.) (1993). *The Cambridge companion to Heidegger.* Cambridge: Cambridge University Press.

H., Julia. (1987). *Letting go with love.* New York: St. Martin's Press.

Hallowell, EM. and Ratey, JJ. (1994). *Driven to distraction.* New York: Simon and Schuster.

Hasin, D. et al. (2004). Epidemiology. Comorbidity of substance use and psychiatric disorders. In Kinzler, HR. and Tinsley, JA. (eds.). *Dual diagnosis and treatment.* Marcel Dekker, Inc.

Heidegger, M. (1971). *The question concerning technology and other essays.* New York: Harper Textbooks.

Kaiser, D. (1996). Commentary: Against biological psychiatry. *Psychiatric Times,* December, 1996. www.mhsource.com/edu/psytimes/p961242.html

Kaiser, D. (1997). Psychiatric medications as symptoms. *Psychiatric Times,* February, 1997. www.mhsource.com/exclusive/bio0297.html

Kaiser, D. (1997). Psychiatry in the marketplace. *Psychiatric Times,* March, 1997. www.mhsource.com/exclusive/bio0397.html

Keller, MB. et al. (2000). A comparison of Nefazadone, the Cognitive Behavioral-Analysis System of Psychotherapy and their combination for the treatment of chronic depression. *N Engl J Med,* **342**(20): 1462-70.

Kirk, S. and Kutchins, H. (1992). *The selling of DSM: The rhetoric of science in psychiatry.* New York: Aldine DeGruyter.

Klein, D. et al. (1980). *Diagnosis and drug treatment of psychiatric disorders: Adults and children. Second edition.* Baltimore: The Williams and Wilkens Company.

Kramer, P. (1993). *Listening to Prozac.* New York: Penguin Books.

Kuhn, TS. (1962). *The structure of scientific revolutions.* Chicago: The University of Chicago Press.

Lewis, B. (2006). *Moving beyond Prozac, DSM and the new psychiatry. The birth of postpsychiatry.* Ann Arbor, MI: The University of Michigan Press.

Lieber, AL. (2002). Bipolar spectrum disorder. A practitioners overview of the soft bipolar spectrum. www.psychom.net/central.lieber.html.

Maslow, A. (1962). *Toward a psychology of being.* New York: Van Norstrand

Mayes, R. and Horowitz, AV. (2005). DSM III and the revolution of the classification of mental illness. *J Hist Behav Sci,* **41**(3): 249-67.

Medical News Today (2006). Landmark STAR*D depression study offers 'sobering' third round results. www.medicalnewstoday.com/medicalnews.php?newsid=46265.

Michels, R. (2007). Is psychiatry evidence-based medicine? *Clinical Psychiatry News,* **36**(6): 11.

Mich News.com (2004). Compulsory mental health screening is coming for adults and children, preschool and up. www.antidepressantfacts.com/2004-08-25-oppose-screening.html.

Minde, K. et al. (2003). The psychosocial functioning of children and spouses of adults with ADHD. *J Child Psychol Psychiatry,* **44**: 637-46.

Myss, C. (1996). *Anatomy of the spirit.* New York: Three Rivers Press.

Neimeyer, RA. And Raskin, JD. eds. (2000). *Constructions of disorders: Meaning making frameworks for psychotherapy.* Washington DC: American Psychological Association.

NIMH National Institute of Mental Health Press Release. (2006). Initial results help clinicians identify patients with treatment resistant depression. Jan. 1. www.nimh.gov/stard.cfm.

NIMH National Institute of Mental Health Press Release. (2006). Strategies help patients become symptom free. March 23. www.nimh.gov/stard.cfm.

NIMH National Institute of Mental Health Science Update. (2006). Switching to a third antidepressant may prove helpful to some treatment resistant depressions. July 1. www.nimh.gov/stard.cfm.

Pajares, F. The structure of scientific revolutions by Thomas S. Kuhn. A synopsis from the original by Professor Frank Pajares. *Philosopher's Web Magazine.* www.des.emory.edu/mfp/kuhnsyn.html.

Parker, I. (1999). *Deconstructing Psychotherapy.* London: Sage

Peterson, C. (2006). *A primer in positive psychology.* Oxford: Oxford University Press.

Popper, K. (2002). *The logic of scientific discovery.* New York: Routledge.

Schwartz, M. and Wiggins, O. (2002). The hegemony of the DSM's. In Sadler, J. (ed.) *Descriptions and prescriptions.* Baltimore: Johns Hopkins University Press. 199-210.

Sharfstein, SS. (2005). Big Pharma and American psychiatry: The good, the bad and the ugly. *Psychiatric News,* **40**(16): 3.

Showalter, E. (1997). *Hystories.* New York: Columbia University Press.

Spiegel, A. (2005). The dictionary of disorder. How one man revolutionized psychiatry. *The New Yorker.* Jan. 3, 2005: 56-63

Spitzer, RL. (1991). An outsider-insider's views about revising the DSM's. *J Abnl Psychology,* **100**(3): 294-96.

Weber, M. (2001). *The Protestant ethic and the spirit of capitalism.* New York: Routledge.

What is Mindfulness? (1999). Teaching tools for mindfulness training. www.mindfulnessclasses.com/mindfulness.html.

Yalom, ID. (1980). *Existential psychotherapy.* New York: Basic Books

Appendix

Resources and Suggested Readings

The following is a list of suggested readings and resources that might be of interest to you. Some of the books are already referenced in the bibliography but most are not. Along with critiques of biopsychiatry I've also listed some books about the philosophers mentioned in this book. Some of the books are pretty technical, written for philosophers, psychologists and psychiatrists while others are written in everyday language and more targeted to a lay audience. A few titles, listed at the end, are self help and new age books. Finally, I will give you contact information for Emotions Anonymous.

TECHNICAL BOOKS

Being-in-the-World. A Commentary on Heidegger's Being and Time, Division One.
By Hubert Dreyfus.
(A readable analysis of Martin Heidegger's most famous work)

Blaming the Brain.
By Elliott Valenstein
(A neuroscientist's scathing critique of biopsychiatry)

The Cambridge Companion to Heidegger.
Edited by Charles Guignon
(A fascinating collection of essays on both "early" and "late" Heidegger)

Constructions of Disorders.
Edited by Robert Neimeyer and Jonathan Raskin
(A social constructivist/constructionist analysis of mental illness diagnosis and treatment)

Deconstructing Psychopathology.
By Ian Parker et al.
(A postmodernist view of mental "illness", mental "health" and treatment)

Deconstruction in a Nutshell.
By John Caputo
(An understandable explanation of the often opaque philosophy of Jacques Derrida)

Descriptions and Prescriptions.
Edited by John Sadler
(A collection of essays critiquing the social, legal and clinical impact of the DSM's)

Disordered Mother or Disordered Diagnosis.
By David Allison and Mark Roberts
(A case study of the extensive damage that can result from speculative psychiatric diagnoses such as Munchausen by Proxy Syndrome)

From Placebo to Panacea.
Edited by Seymour Fisher and Roger Greenberg
(An in-depth technical analysis of the placebo phenomenon as it applies to psychiatric drugs)

Moving Beyond Prozac, DSM and the New Psychiatry.
By Bradley Lewis
(A compelling, heartfelt and convincing argument for the need for the evolution of current psychiatry to a "postpsychiatry")

The Myth of Neuropsychiatry.
By Donald Mender
(A technical evaluation of the flaws and fallacies of neuropsychiatry)

Pathologies of the Modern Self.
Edited by David Levin
(Fascinating essays on the intersection of modernity and psychiatric "illness")

philosophical perspectives on technology and psychiatry.
Edited by James Phillips
(A recently published collection of essays critiquing biopsychiatry, including a chapter by yours truly, Dr. Phill)

Postpsychiatry.
Patrick Brackin and Philip Thomas
(The groundbreaking book that launched the concept of postpsychiatry)

Philosophical Psychopathology
Edited by G. Graham and G. Stevens
(A look at mental health and illness from a philosopher's perspective)

Rethinking Psychiatric Drugs.
By Grace Jackson
(A detailed and technical analysis of the hidden truths about psychiatric drugs)

values and psychiatric diagnosis.
By John Sadler
(Compelling!!! The best of the best scholarly critiques of the DSM phenomenon)

NON TECHNICAL BOOKS

The ADHD Fraud. How Psychiatry Makes "Patients" of Normal Children.
By Fred Baughman.
(An uncompromising, no-holds barred assault on pediatric biopsychiatry)

America Fooled. The Truth About Antidepressants, Antipsychotics and How We've Been Deceived.
By Timothy Scott
(A very readable critical account of the development, testing and marketing of psychiatric and other drugs)

Coercion as Cure.
By Thomas Szasz
(The latest book by this true pioneer in critical psychiatry)

Commonsense Rebellion : Taking Back Your Life from Drugs, Shrinks, Corporations, and a World Gone Crazy.
By Bruce Levine
(This title is self-explanatory)

Confessions of an Rx Drug Pusher.
By Gwen Olsen
(A first-person "confession" by a former drug rep)

Constructing the Self, Constructing America.
By Philip Cushman
(A practicing therapist's social constructionist perspective on psychotherapy)

The Cult of Pharmacology. How America Became the World's Most Troubled Drug Culture.
By Richard DeGrandpre
(A fascinating look at how social factors influence our relationship with both illicit drugs and legal medications)

Disclosing New Worlds.
By Charles Spinosa, Fernando Flores and Hubert Dreyfus
(A hope-filled account of how real and lasting social changes can occur)

Existential Psychotherapy.
By Irvin Yalom
(An engrossing treatise on the "ultimate concerns" in therapy and in life)

Hystories. Hysterical Epidemics and the Modern Media.
By Elaine Showalter
(A courageous examination of the many presentations of "hysteria" in modern society)

Let Them Eat Prozac. The Unhealthy Relationship Between the Pharmaceutical Industry and Depression
By David Healy
(One of the many excellent books by this highly respected critic of biopsychiatry)

Letting Go With Love.
By Julia H.
(A first-person account of recovery through Al Anon)

Mad in America: Bad Science, Bad Medicine and the Enduring Mistreatment of the Mentally Ill.
By Robert Whitaker
(An investigative journalist's account of the history of the treatment of psychosis and a look at current practices. You won't believe the stuff psychiatrists have believed and did (and still do) to the chronically psychotic).

Making Us Crazy. DSM: The Psychiatric Bible and the Creation of Mental Disorders
By Herb Kutchins and Stuart Kirk
(The second of the two books by these most widely respected social critics of DSM. A must read!!)

Manufacturing Depression. The Secret History of a Modern Disease
By Gary Greenberg
(The latest in a long list of books critical of medicalizing sadness)

Mind Over Machine.
By Hubert Dreyfus and Stuart Dreyfus
(How minds are nothing like machines and why computers will never be minds)

The Myth of Mental Illness.
By Thomas Szasz
(The seminal work that launched the ongoing debate over the very existence of mental "illnesses")

Narrative Therapy.
By Jill Freedman and Gene Combs
(The theory and practice of narrative therapy; a reader friendly account)

On Being Authentic.
By Charles Guignon
(A philosophical examination of the "good" life and being true to yourself)

On Religion.
By John Caputo
(An exploration of the personal and cultural role of religion in modern life)

A Primer in Positive Psychology.
By Christopher Peterson
(A somewhat academic exploration of this new field in psychology)

Prozac as a Way of Life.
Edited by Carl Elliott and Tod Chambers
(An examination of the powerful societal impact of the phenomenon that is Prozac)

Prozac Backlash.
Joseph Glenmullen
(This bestseller by Harvard psychiatrist Glenmullen is a strong warning about the dangers of antidepressants and offers alternative therapies for depression)

Psyched Out. How Psychiatry Sells Mental Illness and Pushes Pills That Kill.
By Kelly Patricia O'Meara
(Another book by a journalist harshly assaulting biopsychiatry. How harsh? The chapter on ADHD and Ritalin is titled "Kiddie Cocaine")

Ritalin Nation.
By Richard DeGrandpre
(Extensively quoted in my book, DeGranpre argues that it is not an attention deficit epidemic but rather a widespread stimulus addiction that is plaguing our society. A must read for any parents with kids diagnosed as ADD)

The Selling of DSM.
By Stuart Kirk and Herb Kutchins
(A careful examination of the political and economic factors that so heavily influenced the allegedly scientific classification of mental disorders in DSM III)

Selling Sickness. How the World's Biggest Pharmaceutical Companies are Turning Us All Into Patients.
By Ray Moynihan and Alan Cassels
(Another journalistic account that looks at not only the manufacturing and promotion of psychiatric "illnesses" but at physical "illnesses" as well)

Surviving America's Depression Epidemic. How to Find Morale, Energy, and Community in a World Gone Crazy.
By Bruce Levine
(Another title by this wise and caring therapist in which he advocates for the development of healthy communities to alleviate the dysphoria and distress in our lives)

They Say You're Crazy. How the World's Most Powerful Psychiatrists Decide Who's Normal
By Paula Caplan
(An insider's view of the exclusionary politics involved in the creation of the DSM's)

Toxic Psychiatry. Why Therapy, Empathy and Love Must Replace the Drugs, Electroshock and Biochemical Theories of the "New Psychiatry".
By Peter Breggins
(The best known and bestselling author in the anti-biopsychiatry movement).

The Truth About Drug Companies. How They Deceive Us and What To Do About It.
By Marsha Angell
(As you know, a major reference and source of validation in this book)

New Age, Spiritual, Buddhist etc. suggested readings:

There are thousands of titles in this category, easily accessed in their respective sections in bookstores and libraries. I strongly suggest you also peruse the booklist at Hazelden Books for many well-written 12 Step based and spiritual titles. And, don't forget, I have recommended Lucinda Bassett's self help cognitive therapy program, the Midwest Center for Stress and Anxiety. The website is www.stresscenter.com.

How To Contact Emotions Anonymous

Here is the information I got when I contacted Emotions Anonymous:

"Any two or three persons gathered together for emotional health may call themselves an EA chapter provided that as a group they have no other affiliation."

"If you cannot find EA in your locality, you may write: Emotions Anonymous International, P.O. Box 4245, St. Paul, Minnesota 55104, and this office will assist you in locating the nearest group. If there is no group in your area, they will assist you in starting a group."

Phone Number: 651-647-9712 Website: www.emotionsanonymous.org

On the website you will find a large array of pamphlets and products, some of which are free. In addition they will send you helpful information about how to get groups started in your area. I truly hope this book has inspired mental health professionals and those seeking help to get involved with, support and help to promote Emotions Anonymous. I feel that I have done my best. Once again, to wrap it all up:

God, grant me the serenity
To accept the things I cannot change
Courage to change the things I can
And the wisdom to know the difference.